Health Sector, State and Decentralised Institutions in India

This book describes the transition in the Indian healthcare system since independence and contributes to the ongoing debate within development and institutional economics on the approaches towards reform in the public health system. The institutional reform perspective focuses on examining the effective utilisation of allotted resources and improvements in delivery through decentralisation in governance by ensuring higher participation of elected governments and local communities in politics, policy making and delivery of health services. It discusses the economic (resource) reforms to explain the relevance and expansion of state interventionism, along with its influence on the health sector, accountability and allocative efficiency. It also explores the connections between neoliberal thought that promote privatisation and insurance-based financing in the health sector, and its implications for health service access and delivery. The book offers ways to address long-standing systemic and structural problems that confront the Indian healthcare system.

Based on large-scale surveys and diverse empirical data on the Indian economy, this book will be of great interest to researchers, students and teachers of health economics, governance and institutional economics, political economy, sociology, public policy, regional studies and development studies. It will also be useful to policy makers, health economists, social scientists, public health experts and professionals, and government and non-governmental institutions.

Shailender Kumar Hooda is Associate Professor at the Institute for Studies in Industrial Development, New Delhi, India. He completed PhD in Economics from Jawaharlal Nehru University, New Delhi. He has more than a decade of teaching and research experience. Previously, he taught at the University of Delhi and Maharshi Dayanand University, Rohtak, and he has worked with the National Council of Applied Economic Research and the National Institute of Public Finance and Policy, New Delhi. He works on the political economy of health and healthcare, health economics, financing and policy, governance and decentralisation in health, medical device and pharmaceutical industry, institutional economics and applied econometrics. He specialises in handling large-scale survey data relating to the Indian economy, and in conducting and designing primary surveys. His writings have appeared in magazines, newspapers and reputed journals. He has delivered several projects funded by national and international agencies.

Health Sector, State and Decentralised Institutions in India

Shailender Kumar Hooda

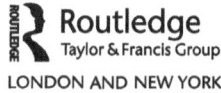

Routledge
Taylor & Francis Group

LONDON AND NEW YORK

First published 2022
by Routledge
2 Park Square, Milton Park, Abingdon, Oxon OX14 4RN

and by Routledge
605 Third Avenue, New York, NY 10158

Routledge is an imprint of the Taylor & Francis Group, an informa business

© 2022 Shailender Kumar Hooda

British Library Cataloguing-in-Publication Data
A catalogue record for this book is available from the British Library

Library of Congress Cataloging-in-Publication Data
A catalog record for this book has been requested

ISBN: 978-0-8153-6101-5 (hbk)
ISBN: 978-1-032-10844-5 (pbk)
ISBN: 978-1-032-10843-8 (ebk)

DOI: 10.4324/9781032108438

Typeset in Sabon
by Apex CoVantage, LLC

Dedicated to my late father (Shri Balraj) and mother
(Smt. Ramrati Devi) for their support and unconditional love

Contents

Figures

Tables

Boxes

Appendices

Preface

This book is an outcome of my research work over the last decade and a half on the development of health sector reforms and policies in India. It contributes to the ongoing debate within development and institutional economics about approaches towards reform in the public health system. It locates the discussion around transition in the healthcare system to understand the changing nature of state interventionism in the health sector.

The book argues in defence of state intervention in provisioning of health services, simply because public intervention in the health sector leads to increase in social welfare through better outcomes, greater equity and more consumer satisfaction. The intervention of the state is significant in areas where other private players fail to provide adequate services; it becomes important in situations of market failure, and it becomes crucial in contexts where the elites and other powerful groups corner greater gains of resources because of uneven distribution of social and economic power.

The extent of state interventionism in terms of resource allocation has always been highly vulnerable to political and economic contexts of a country, and this is so in India. India is a federal country where prime responsibility of the health sector is with the states. States must have ideological differences and prioritise their health sectors differently under different macroeconomic conditions and policies. The book analyses states' allocations and priorities accorded to the health sector under these changing scenarios in Chapter 2.

The size of public investment no doubt has immense importance. Allocated funds, however, may yield little benefit if complementary services are lacking and funds are not well targeted to improve specific targets like preventive care, rural area needs, etc. An inadequate allocation of resource towards medicine, material, supply and equipment limit the ability of health staffs to perform better, rendering the system inefficient. Such inappropriateness and inefficiency is likely to deny treatments and health improvement, and signifies wasted resources in economic terminology. In conditions when tax and non-tax revenue sources are under stress, the effectiveness of every rupee that is spent becomes important. We begin with a premise that elimination of inefficiency from any system acts as a source of finance, as it is equivalent to an increase in the resource availability. The book devotes Chapter 3 to identify sources of functional and allocative inefficiency and discuss ways to improve the resource use efficiency.

Part 2 of the book brings in the idea of institutional reforms. It talks about reforms in decentralised governance that ensure higher participation of elected governments and local communities in politics, policy making and delivery of health services. It argues that elected representatives and governments are more sensitive and responsive towards satisfying the peoples' interests, so as to win the next election. Their greater participation in the electoral process allows political authorities to align their decisions with the interests and priorities of the general public. One can even expect an increase in welfare spending if more excluded groups – including women and minorities – are incorporated into the political process through constitutionally mandated consensual rules. Whether an increase in participation and greater representation of diversified groups in politics leads to concomitant rise in welfare expenditures like health has been analysed in Chapter 4.

The high amount of public spending on health sometimes does not contribute substantially, if the existing facilities or funds are not implemented and managed through proper channels or through effective governance like community participation or decentralisation. This is because the decentralised mechanism improves accountability, effectiveness and efficiency of service delivery by bringing decision makers closer to the people and by enhancing the participation of community in decision making and implementation processes. Their close relation with the local people enables them to know the local problems and needs, and they are therefore in a better position to establish the right priorities than a central or regional government far away. Local governments have more and better information regarding their constituents, and they may be better able to enforce and coordinate policies and programmes at the local level. It promotes intersectoral coordination, increases accountability, reduces duplication and improves implementation of health programmes, which in turn affects the quality and coverage of health services delivery – and thereby, health outcomes. The measurements of decentralisation, however, are context specific. Thus, in order to fully evaluate the gains from decentralisation, the conceptual clarity on what constitutes decentralisation, how it can be empirically captured and what its constituent elements are and how it improve service delivery and health outcomes is empirically examined in Chapter 5.

The gains from decentralisation that involve community, local agents and local governments for effective delivery of services in rural areas depend on how these initiatives have been implemented and enhanced service delivery at ground level. In order to fully understand the benefit from various dimensions of decentralisation, an extensive field survey is conducted at panchayat and health functionaries and household level. From field survey, first the degree of community participation/engagement and extent of decentralisation in the health sector are worked out, and then their impacts are assessed on health service delivery, particularly in improving the access to maternal and child healthcare utilisation and improving the overall health system functioning. Due to the sensitivity of class and caste in a divided society, the Constitution of India provides a clear mandate about the reservation of women and other social categories in Panchayat representation; therefore, these are also incorporated in the analysis presented in Chapter 6.

In addition to the investment (resource) and institutional reforms, in a parallel process, neoliberal thinking heavily tried to justify the rationale of public sector underfunding and privatisation in a liberalisation phase. A need is articulated to promote the private sector and then take advantage of it in service delivery. In addition, the country witnessed economic gradients of inequality in access to healthcare which sharply worsened over time where the rural and poor felt financially squeezed and experienced difficulty in finding services they could afford. This generated a new requirement to find a way to provide financial protection. Devising a financial protection mechanism also emerges as a central policy tool of achieving universal health coverage (UHC) around the world in recent times, including India. The UHC debate focuses more on devising the strategies to finance healthcare, largely through insurance, rather than providing the care. India launched several health insurance schemes for poor funded from public (tax) sources. The financing of an insurance-based system entirely from public sources has led to an important shift in the fundamental nature of healthcare financing in the country. Until recently, public investment on healthcare was almost used for financing public health system for service provisioning; now out of the total health budget, some (tax) funds will be diverted to finance the insurance-based system. The insurance-based financing has now became an integral part of health budget and an instrument to promote privatisation in the healthcare sector. How the private sector took advantage of these initiatives and exploited the Indian healthcare market resulting in unaffordable treatments and inaccessibility towards fulfilling the national health goals, is discussed in Chapter 7, and implications of changing financing nature are then discussed in Chapter 8.

Overall, the book first provides a detailed analysis of state allocations and priorities accorded to the health sector, sources of inefficiency in resource allocation and utilisation. Later, it identifies the public expenditures that best improve health sector outcomes. It then examines the role of institutions in improving the efficacy of allocated resources, as well as access, equity and effectiveness in service delivery. The implications of privatisation in the health sector is dealt with extensively in the last section, which also sheds new light on the politics of health and healthcare financing reform in India.

The arguments of this book have been developed with an extensive use of diverse large-scale data on the Indian economy and a field-based survey conducted in Haryana and Rajasthan and referred at relevant places. I owe a particular debt of gratitude to all informants who shared relevant information to complete this book.

Writing this book has been an intellectually stimulating journey and a humbling experience. This book would have never been realised without the generous assistance and support of many people. The initial idea of this book grew out of my doctoral research on health economics, policy and governance issues. My deepest gratitude and respect must first go to my doctoral thesis supervisor, Professor Atul Sood, for his guidance and encouragement. I have been fortunate to learn several theoretical concepts from him. He shaped my intellectual journey towards locating my research work in the larger interest of society and nation as a whole.

I strengthen my research works on development of health sector reforms and policies further at my parent Institute, where I get enough space and freedom to articulate ideas and develop understanding around politics of health sector reforms. I am grateful to Professor S. K. Goyal and Professor M. R. Murty for extending institutional support and Professor Atul Sarma and Dr Satyaki Roy for academic inputs and motivation from other colleagues at the Institute. I would like to express my gratitude to Shoma Choudhury and Rimina Mohapatra at Routledge for their professional advice and assistance in the publication of the book.

I would like to express my wholehearted thanks and gratitude to my parents (Shri Balraj and Smt. Ramrati Devi), who motivated me to pursue for higher education; unfortunately, we lost them in the initial years of my doctoral study. I am thankful to my younger brother (Sandeep) and sister (Pinki) for being pillars of my strength after my parents. My life partner (Poonam) joined in between and became shelter from the storm, anchor of my soul and pillar of my strength. I thank her for supporting me when I fell and struggled to complete this book, even after missing a few deadlines. She took a lot of pain alone to look after our children (Anshi, Aakarsha and Aviraaj) in the final stages of the book. I thank my children for compromising the quality time I could have spent with them; their cooperation is highly appreciated. I duly acknowledge the immense support received from my mother-in-law (Tarawati) and brother-in-law (Amit) during the completion of the book. This book is a testimony to my entire family unconditional love and support throughout my prolonged pursuit of knowledge.

Finally, I salute the scholars, both past and present, whose work enhanced my knowledge around health and healthcare reforms. I hope the book conveys some enthusiasm among policy makers, health economists, social scientists, public health experts and professionals, government and non-governmental institutions and individuals. This book will be of great interest to researchers, students and teachers of health economics, political economy, sociology and public policy, and development studies.

Abbreviations

ANC	Antenatal Care
ANM	Auxiliary Nurse Midwife
ASHA	Accredited Social Health Activist
AWW	Anganwadi worker
AYUSH	Ayurveda, Yoga and Naturopathy, Unani, Siddha and Homeopathy
AB	Ayushman Bharat
BE	Budget Estimate
BPL	Below Poverty Line
CAG	Controller Auditor General
CBHI	Community Based Health Insurance Schemes
CD	Communicable Disease
CEA	Clinical Establishment Act
CGHS	Central Government Health Scheme
CHC	Community Health Centre
CHIS	Comprehensive Health Insurance Scheme
CHV	Community Health Volunteer
CHW	Community Health Workers
COV	Coefficient of Variation
CPIA	Country Policy and Institutional Assessment index
CPS	Central Plan Scheme
CSS	Centrally Sponsored Schemes
DCPA	Degree of Community Participation and Awareness
DH-District	Hospitals
DIH	Decentralisation in Health
DLHS	District Level Health Survey
DPC	District Planning Committee
DPCO	Drug Price Control Order
DS	Dispensaries
EAG	Empowered Action Group states.
ESIS	Employees' State Insurance Scheme
FDI	Foreign Direct Investment
FE	Fixed Effect Model

FFC	Fifteenth Finance Commission
FPE	For-Profit Enterprises
FRBM	Fiscal Responsibility and Budget Management Act
FRU	First Referral Unit
FYP	Five-Year Plan
GDP	Gross Domestic Product
GFHI	Government-Funded Health Insurance
GMM	Generalised Method of Moments
GOI	Government of India
GS	Gram Sabha
GSDP	Gross State Domestic Product
HDR	Human Development Report
HFA	Health for All
HFS	High-Focused States
HFW	Medical, Public Health and Family Welfare expenditure
HLEG	High-Level Expert Group
HMIS	Health Management Information System
HRH	Human Resources for Health
HWC	Health and Wellness Centres
ICDS	Integrated Child Development Scheme
ICMR	Indian Council of Medical Research
ICSSR	Indian Council of Social Science Research
IHDS	India Human Development Survey
IMR	Infant Mortality Rate
IPFS	Indian Public Finance Statistics
IPHS	Indian Public Health Standards
IRDA	Insurance Development Regulatory Authority
JSY	Janani Suraksha Yojana
LDH	Level of Decentralisation in Health
LHW	Lady Health Worker
LHV	Lady Health Visitor
LPM	Linear Probability Model
LSDV	Least Squares Dummy Variable
MAY	Mukhyamantri Amrutum Yojana
MCH	Maternal and Child Health
MDG	Millennium Development Goals
MGNREGA	Mahatma Gandhi National Rural Employment Guarantee Act
MJPJAY	Mahatma Jyotiba Phule Jan Arogya Yojana
MLM	Multinomial Logit Model
MMR	Maternal Mortality Ratio
MoHFW	Ministry of Health and Family Welfare
MOSPI	Ministry of Statistics and Programme Implementation
MPA	Medical Practitioners Act

MPCE	Monthly Per Capita Consumption Expenditure of households.
MPHW	Multi Purpose Health Worker
NACO	National AIDS Control Organisation
NCD	Non-Communicable Diseases
NCMH	National Commission of Macroeconomic and Health
NCMP	National Common Minimum Programme
NCP	Nature of Community Participation
NDCP	National Disease Control Programmes
NES	North Eastern States
NFHS	National Family Health Survey
NGO	Non-Governmental Organisation
NHA	National Health Account
NHFS	Non–High-Focused States
NHM	National Health Mission
NHP	National Health Policy
NHPI	National Health Profile of India
NHPS	National Health Protection Scheme
NITI	National Institution for Transforming India Aayog
NML	Nested Multinomial Logit Model
NPE	Not-For-Profit Entities
NRHM	National Rural Health Mission
NSS	National Sample Survey
NSSO	National Sample Survey Organisation
NUMH	National Urban Health Mission
OAE	Own Account Enterprises
OECD	Organisation for Economic Cooperation and Development
OLS	Ordinary Least Square Method
OOP	Out-of-Pocket expenditure
PC	Planning Commission
PCA	Principal Component Analysis
PHC	Primary Health Centre
PHN	Public Health Nurse
PMJAY	Pradhan Mantri Jan Arogya Yojana
PNC	Post-Natal Care
PPP	Public-Private Partnership
PPR	Political Participation and Representation
PRI	Panchayati Raj Institutions
QHC	Quality Healthcare
RBI	Reserve Bank of India
RCH	Reproductive and Child Health
RE	Random Effects model
RE	Revised Estimate
RGJAY	Rajiv Gandhi Jeevandayee Arogya Yojana

RHS	Rural Health Statistics
RKS	Rogi Kalyan Samiti
ROHINI	Registry of Hospitals in Network of Insurance
RSBY	Rashtriya Swasthya Bima Yojana
SAP	Structural Adjustment Programmes
SC	Sub-Centres
SDGs	Sustainable Development Goals
SDH	Sub-Divisional Hospitals
SEC	State Election Commission
SECC	Socio-Economic Caste Census
SFC	State Finance Commission
SHI	Social Health Insurance
SHS	State Health Societies
SMS	Sakshar Mahila Samooh
U5MR	Under-5 Mortality Rates
UHC	Universal Health Coverage
UHIS	Universal Health Insurance Scheme
VGF	Viability Gap Funding
VHG	Village Health Guide Scheme
VHI	Voluntary (commercial) health insurance schemes
VHSC	Village Health and Sanitation Committee
WHO	World Health Organisation
WHR	World Health Report

1 Health system dynamics
Evolution of health policies in India

Countries across the world have adopted different approaches to address the health needs of their population and health promotion, and prevention and control of diseases. This is generally guided by their own historical traditions, political and social contexts, cultural value systems and ideologies (Hsiao, 2003). The industrial state and societies have different lifestyles than the developing ones; therefore, prevalence of disease varies considerably. The historical pattern around the world reveals that healthcare system in Western industrial states and societies emphasises largely curative aspects, being limited to health services in the hospitals, medical practice, and pharmacies based on medical technology. Preventive care (prevention of diseases) has relatively little place of value in those economies (Fisk, 2000). Their medicine apparatus in most cases is unaffordable and unfavourable with regards to price and utility for developing countries because of high difference in prevalence of disease pattern (Ourworldindata, n.d.). The majority of the diseases that are prevalent in developing countries are preventable in nature. The primary healthcare system, therefore, is found to be more prevalent in developing nations. In practice, the industrialised/ wealthiest nations have adopted robust healthcare systems, while it is too disorganised in many developing countries; whereas the rich get high medical care/attention, the poor have less access to affordable healthcare, and either they stay sick or die or if they seek care have to pay from their own pockets. Interestingly, however, available research tends to suggest that none of the healthcare systems systematically outperforms the rest; however, some performed really better.

The fundamental questions that thus arise are the following. Why do some health systems work better than others? What features of that system contribute the most to produce favourable outcomes? How can policy makers restructure the existing system to achieve preferable outcome? This depends on how a nation has designed its health system and which type of distinct features and components its health system has (Hsiao, 2003). This study elaborates that health system in general have features of: a) financing, b) organisation of service delivery, c) payment mechanism, d) regulations and e) persuasion.

DOI: 10.4324/9781032108438-1

These features have different characteristics (see Rao, 2017).

Financing has four characteristics, namely: a) financing methods (whether healthcare is financed through government taxes (United Kingdom, Spain, New Zealand, Cuba), employer- and employee-mandated social health insurance (United States, Germany, Belgium, Japan, Switzerland, the Netherlands), government-run/national health insurance (Canada, Taiwan, South Korea) or market-driven healthcare financed through households out-of-pocket (rural India, Africa, South America and, to a degree, China), giving a narrative who control the resources and who bears the financial burden; b) allocation of funds (on different components like medical and nursing education, service delivery, creating physical infrastructure or on staffing, rural and urban setting, primary, secondary and tertiary care), which might impact the access and finally health outcomes); c) rationing (insufficient and unskilled professionals who might impact access, equity and quality); and d) institutional arrangement of financing (like centralised or decentralised, through taxes, user fees or insurance, which helps to understand how equitable and fair the system would be and which types of moral hazards and adverse selection problems it would encounter).

Organisation of service delivery means: a) whether there is monopoly or competition in service delivery; b) how efficient the vertical integration of (primary, secondary and tertiary) service delivery is (like the US focus is more on curative tertiary, while India it is on primary care; each one neglects the other side of care); c) ownership of providers – public, private-for-profit or not-for-profit – as ownership describe the kind of care provided, type of patients seen, nature of disease treated and extent of denial of care happens due to unaffordability); and d) decentralisation of health service delivery, which is often considered a good mechanism to ensure that benefits reach the intended and local government can plan better to the need of local people. Its benefits, however, depend on how this concept is conceived and implemented.

Payment mechanism means incentive system like the mode and amount of payment (fixed-budget, fee-for-services, reimbursement, capitation or salary) which impact the behaviour of different actors like the patients, providers and insurers, which in turn can affect cost, efficiency and quality of care provided.

Regulation is generally enforced by government to impose certain boundaries within which the professions have to function or the manufacture and sale of pharmaceutical products and medical devices have to be organised. These are important to ensure patient safety, equity, efficiency and quality and correct market distortions.

Persuasion – whether by governments or private players – can influence peoples' beliefs, lifestyles, expectations, preferences and behaviours through advertising campaigns and dissemination of information. Persuasion also affects the supply side, justifying governments to regulate and organise medical education as service providers profoundly affect the availability, efficiency and quality of healthcare through the medical ethics and beliefs they uphold (see Rao, 2017).

The health system of any country might consist of a mix/overlapping of these profound features (Hsiao, 2003). The nature of health system evolution, however, is not constant. Its dynamics change over time. It is either guided by growing healthcare needs, changing health profile and burden of diseases (communicable to non-communicable), or influenced by changes in global health policy and advocacy like from a 'health for all' agenda to achieving 'universal health coverage' targets in recent times. There have been tendencies to borrow other countries' best experiences to model their own healthcare system, as well. In addition, the macroeconomic conditions and changes also influence the health system dynamics. The healthcare structure in India has an evolutionary and organic history, where the state over time has tried to reorient its approaches while absorbing the changing dynamics of health profile and policies.

India's state interventionist approach in healthcare

When India became independent over 70 years ago in 1947, the country had several challenges on health as well as on socio-economic fronts. Of the total 36.1 crore population (GoI, 1951), only 18.3% were literate. Female literacy was at 8.86%. Only 1 of every 11 women were able to read and write. While tracking India's progress in health sector after 70 years of independence, Zodpey and Negandhi (2018) reported that overall life expectancy at the time was 32 years. The infant mortality rate (IMR) was 146 per 1000 live births. Maternal mortality ratio (MMR) in the 1940s was 22.2 per 1000 live births. The country was facing a high burden of communicable disease. The number of doctors across the country was only 50,000 and primary healthcare centres only numbered 725 (Zodpey and Negandhi, 2018). The country had no proper healthcare system. The average per capita gross domestic product (GDP) of a citizen was very low at Rs. 1705 ($81.3) in 1960. This means people had low capacity to pay with high prevalence and burden of diseases, largely the communicable ones.

India constituted several committees to suggest measures to address the prevalence of diseases, as well as to invite suggestions on how the Indian health system should be designed. India tried to follow a principle that health is a 'public good'. India's foremost Health Survey and Development Committee encompassed around the principle that 'nobody should be denied access to health services for his inability to pay' (Bhore Committee, 1946: 17). After independence, India constituted more than 25 committees to work for a strong public healthcare system. Several committees on health of independent India (like Sokhey [1948], Mudaliar [1962], Chaddha [1963], Kartar Singh [1974], Srivastava [1975] and Joint Panel of Indian Council of Medical Research-Indian Council of Social Science Research ICMR-ICSSR [1980]; see Table 1.1) considering the diseases burden (like diarrhoea, lung

Table 1.1 Committees, commissions and expert groups on health in India

Year	Committee/Commission/Group	Year	Committee/Commission/Group
1946	Bhore Committee, Health Survey and Development	1977	Sidhu Committee
1947	Sokhey Committee, National Planning Committee	1978	Group on Alma Ata
1948	RN Chopra Committee	1980	Working Group on Population Policy
1958	Udapa KN Committee, Ayurveda Research Evaluation	1982	Krishan Committee
1954	Shetty Committee	1983	Mehta Committee on Medical Education Review
1957	Balwant Rai Mehta Committee	1987	Bajaj Committee on Health Manpower, Planning, Production and Management
1959	Lakshmanswami Mudaliar Committee	1989	High Power Committee on Nursing Profession
1960	Renuka Roy Committee	1992	Review of state of India's Health
1963	Chadha Committee	1996	Bajaj Committee on Public Health System
1966	Mukherjee Committee	1997	Independent Commission of Health
1966	Jain Committee	2000	Task Force on Conservation and Sustainable use of Medical Plants
1967	Jungalwalla Committee, Integration of Health Services	2001	DGHS Committee Report on Spurious Drugs
1968	Mukherjee Committee, Health Services	2003	Mashelkar Committee on examining the Drug Regulatory Issues
1973	Kartar Singh Committee	2004	National Commission on Macroeconomics and Health
1974	NMEP Committee to Determine the Alternative Strategies	2004	Health Sector Reforms Report
1975	Srivastava Committee on Medical Education and Support Manpower	2007	Health Sector Reforms Report
1975	Hathi Committee	2010	High-Level Expert Group Report on Universal Health Coverage

Source: Author's compilation from individual committee, commission and expert group documents, Ministry of Health and Family Welfare, GOI

inflammations, tuberculosis, malaria, and so on) and mortalities pattern in the country all suggested having a comprehensive primary healthcare system in the public sector. The country launched several disease control programmes at different points in time (Table 1.2), and their preventive care agendas are quite visible in Five-Year Plans, as well. (Table 1.3). A detailed description on policy/programme is provided in Gupta (2016).

Table 1.2 National Health Programmes in India

Year	Programme	Year	Programme
1952	National Family Planning Programme	2002	National Programme for Control of Blindness
1955	National Leprosy Control Programme	2003	Cigarettes and Other Tobacco products Act (COPTA)
1955–1962	Filaria (later became part of NVBDCP)	2003–2004	National Vector Borne Disease control programme (NVBDCP)
1958	National Programme on Malaria (later became part of NVBDCP)	2004	Integrated Disease Surveillance Project
1962	National TB Control Programme	2005	National Rural Health Mission/ Programme
1962	National Iodine Deficiency Disorders Control Programme (rechristened in 1992)	2005	National Programme on Janani Suraksha Yojna
1962–1963	Mid-Day Meal Programme, earlier initiated in 1923, 1946 and 1956	2005	Japanese Encephalitis (a part of NVBDCP)
1972	National Nutritional Anaemia Prophylaxis Programme	2005, 2012	National Program for Palliative Care
1972–1973	National Rural Drinking Water Programme	2006	National Programme for Rehabilitation of Persons with Disabilities
1975	Integrated Child Development Scheme	2006–2007	National Programme for Prevention and Control of Deafness

(Continued)

Table 1.2 (Continued)

Year	Programme	Year	Programme
1975	Vitamin A Prophylaxis Programme to prevent blindness	2006–2007	National Programme for Adolescent Girls
1975–1976	National Cancer Control Programme	2007	Initiative for Dengue and Chikungunya Fever (a part of NVBDCP)
1976	National Programme for Control of Blindness and Visual Impairment (NPCB&VI)	2007–2008	National Tobacco Control Programme
1977	Maternal and Child Health, updated several times	2007–2012	National Programme for Prevention and Management of Trauma and Burn Injuries
1977–1978	Drug DeAddiction Programme (modified in 1992–1993)	2008	National Programme for prevention and control of Cancer, Diabetes, CVD and Stroke
1982	National Mental Health Programme	2008	National Programme for Prevention and Control of Human Rabies
1983	National Leprosy Eradication Programme	2008	Rashtriya Swasthya Bima Yojana
1984	National Guinea Worm Eradication Programme	2008	Jan Aushady Kendra for Affordable Medicine for All
1985–1986	Universal Immunisation Programme	2008–2009	National Programme for Prevention and Control of Fluorosis
1992, 2003	National AIDS Control Programme; control of STIs/RTIs	2008–2009	National Programme for prevention and control of Fluorosis
1992	National AIDS control programme under NACO (modified in 1992, 1998, 2010 and 2012)	2008–2010	National Leptospirosis Control Programme (under NCDC)

Year	Programme	Year	Programme
1993	Directly Observed Treatment Short Course (DOTS)	2010	National Program for Prevention of Burn Injuries
1963–2000	National Nutrition Programmes (other prog. Applied NP Orisha 1963, Special Nutrition Programme (NP) 1970–1971, Balwadi NP 1970–1971, Tamil Nadu Integrated NP 1980, NP Adolescent Girl 2003, Mid-Day Meal Programme 2002, Antyodaya Anna Yozana 2000, Annapurna Scheme 2000)	2010	Indira Gandhi Matritva Sahyog Yojana
1994, 1996, 2011	Essential Medicines and Program of Rational use of Drugs	2010	Rajiv Gandhi Scheme for Empowerment to Adolescent Girls
1996–1997	Yaws Eradication Programme	2010–2011	IGMSY – a conditional maternity benefit scheme under ICDS
1996–1997	School Health Programme	2011	Janani Shishu Suraksha Karyyakaram
1997	Rashtriya Arogya Nidhi	2011–2012	National Programme for Health Care of Elderly
1997	Reproductive and Child Health Programme	2013	Navijaat Shishu Suraksha Karyakaram
1998–1999	National Program for Control & Treatment of Occupational Diseases	2013	Rashtriya Bal Swasthya Karyakaram
1999	National Oral Health Care Programme	2014	National Organ Transplant Programme (Act 1995, 2011)
2002	Kala Azar (a part of NVBDCP)	2014	National Urban Health Mission
		2018	Ayushman Bharat Programme

Source: Author's compilation for various government documents on health programmes, Ministry of Health and Family Welfare, Government of India; Gupta (2016)

Table 1.3 Policies and plans for health in India

Year	Health policy	Five-Year Plan/period	Area covered
1983	First National Health Policy	First FYP (1951–1956)	Provision of water supply and sanitation, malaria control, mobile health, MCH, health education, Self sufficiency in drugs and equipment, family planning and population control
1993	National Nutrition Policy	Second FYP (1956–1961)	Health protection of Rural Population including hospital service, medical education and research, dental service, nursing, indigenous system of medicine, control of communicable disease, WSS, nutrition, family planning, MCH care
1999	National Policy for Older Persons	Third FYP (1961–1966)	Drinking water, drainage and sewerage, rural sanitation, eradication of malaria and smallpox, FP
2000	National Population Policy	Fourth FYP (1969–1974)	FP, strengthening primary health sector, communicable disease, medical and paramedical personnel training, hospitals and dispensaries
2001	National Policy for the Empowerment of Women	Fifth FYP (1974–1979)	FPW, nutrition, malaria eradication, leprosy, blindness, filaria control, mid-day meal program, MCH
2002	National Policy on ISM And Homeopathy	Sixth FYP (1980–1985)	Rural health programme, promotive preventive and curative service, communicable disease, medical education and research, food adulteration, nutrition
2002	Second National Health Policy	Seventh FYP (1985–1990)	Rural health infrastructure; intersectoral coordination; community participation, education and training programme; urban health communicable disease; research for TB and leprosy; health for all by 2000
2002	National AIDS Prevention and Control Policy	Eighth FYP (1992–1997)	Urban health, secondary and tertiary care; containing population growth; MCH care; health personnel training; control of communicable diseases like vector borne, malaria, kala azar, leprosy, TB, etc.; decentralisation with area specific micro planning
2002	National Blood Policy	Ninth FYP (1997–2002)	Addressing CD and NCD, restructuring of CHC or PHC to promote access to primary care, development of HRH, health insurance, health personnel planning, involving people representative and voluntary organisations, engaging PRIs in planning and monitoring of health programme

Year	Health policy	Five-Year Plan/ period	Area covered
2003	National Charter for Children	Tenth FYP (2002–2007)	Reorganisation and restructuring of govt healthcare system; use of IT, HIMS, quality of care, monitoring and evaluation; participation of PRI and NGO in health promotion, education, PPE model, AIDS control programme, disease surveillance, accident and trauma services; environment and occupation health, production and quality of drugs, health system research and financing
2003	National Youth Policy	Eleventh FYP (2007–2012)	Reducing disparity in healthcare across regions and communities with special attention to vulnerable and marginalised sectors of society, implementation of NRHM, secondary and tertiary care to promote low cost and indigenous technology, use of e-health, implementing IPHS, AYUSH, HRH, extradition healthcare institutions, health system and biomedical research, health insurance-RSBY, decentralised governance, setting up of AIMS-like institutions, ensuring the supply of essential drugs
2017	Third National Health Policy	Twelfth FYP (2012–2017)	Moving towards UHC, transition of NRHM into NHM, re-prioritisation of primary health, access to free essential medicine, addressing inequity in access to health, treatment guidelines and protocols, MCH, universal immunisation coverage, FWP, decentralised planning, prevention and control of CD and NCD, NACO, AYUSH, disaster management, institutional delivery, publicly funded insurance, PPE models, IT in health

Source: Five-Year-Plan documents, Planning Commission, Government of India (now NITI Aayog) and National Health Policy 2017, Government of India;Gupta (2016)

A prominent policy discourse emerged at the first World Health Assembly of the World Health Organisation (WHO) held at Alma Ata in 1978. The discourse suggested that the persistence of the majority of the illnesses and untimely deaths of the time could often have been prevented and treated cost-effectively if adequate primary healthcare facilities had been available in the public system (WHO, 1978). At the conference, it was increasingly being realised that the health services in the so-called developing countries could not be perceived or oriented according to the Western industrial states and societies on several counts. The reasons for this were, first, that the Western system was one-sided and especially oriented to curative dimensions, while neglecting preventive and social medicine aspects. Second, the curative system was too expensive, and because of low fiscal capacity, the developing nations were not in a position to allocate the amount of funds required to replicate such a system. Third, the medical apparatuses of the industrial states were unaffordable and unfavourable for developing countries with regard to price and utility because difference in the pattern of disease prevalence. Fourth, their system could not directly fit into the developing nations, because of the lack of specialists (health personnel) who could handle the highly technical medicines and procedures. Fifth, the natural and scientific understanding of medicine in the West did not consider the traditional views concerning experiences of diseases that have spiritual background of the inhabitants, but were prevalent in the developing countries (WHO, 1978; Fisk, 2000).

The common consensus that emerged was that majority of prevalence of diseases in developing countries can be protected easily under the primary healthcare (PCH) system. The PHC approach emerged as a central concept for attaining the goal of 'health for all' (HFA) by 2000. This concept was heavily concerned with the principles of social justice, accessibility, appropriateness and acceptance of medical services, with consideration of the needs of people in the communities, their participation and orientation to the concept of health services. This strongly reaffirms that health is a state of complete physical, mental and social well-being – not merely the absence of disease or infirmity – and is a fundamental human right which the state should take prime responsibility to fulfil (WHO, 1978). It was also realised that health typically will be inefficiently allocated in a pure market system and in the absence of a reasonably well organised public healthcare system for all; people may be distressed by costly private healthcare. It adopted a holistic framework of comprehensive healthcare provision to achieve *health for all* through state intervention. For a better health system design, the need was felt for a more integrated and comprehensive health provision, comprising a three-tiered structure. Most of the participant nations, including India, signed and supported the HFA vision. India encompassed most of the HFA tenets (equity, universalism, comprehensiveness, government responsibility, community participation, etc.) in its First National Health Policy (NHP) announced in 1983, and considered expending primary healthcare across remotest part of the country.

However, it is important to note that India took very long (almost 35 years) after independence to announce its First National Health Policy in 1983. The policy, however, adopted a holistic approach on the principle that no one can be denied healthcare and it is the state responsibility to provide healthcare to the people. India sought for a more public investment to promote this primary health approach in the country. The country followed a population-based norm of expending a three-tier structure in the country. The current norms and resource requirements at primary, secondary and tertiary levels are elaborated in Figure 1.1 (GOI, 2011). The expansion of primary care facilities is also witnessed in rural areas, along with the implementation of several national health programmes for disease control under

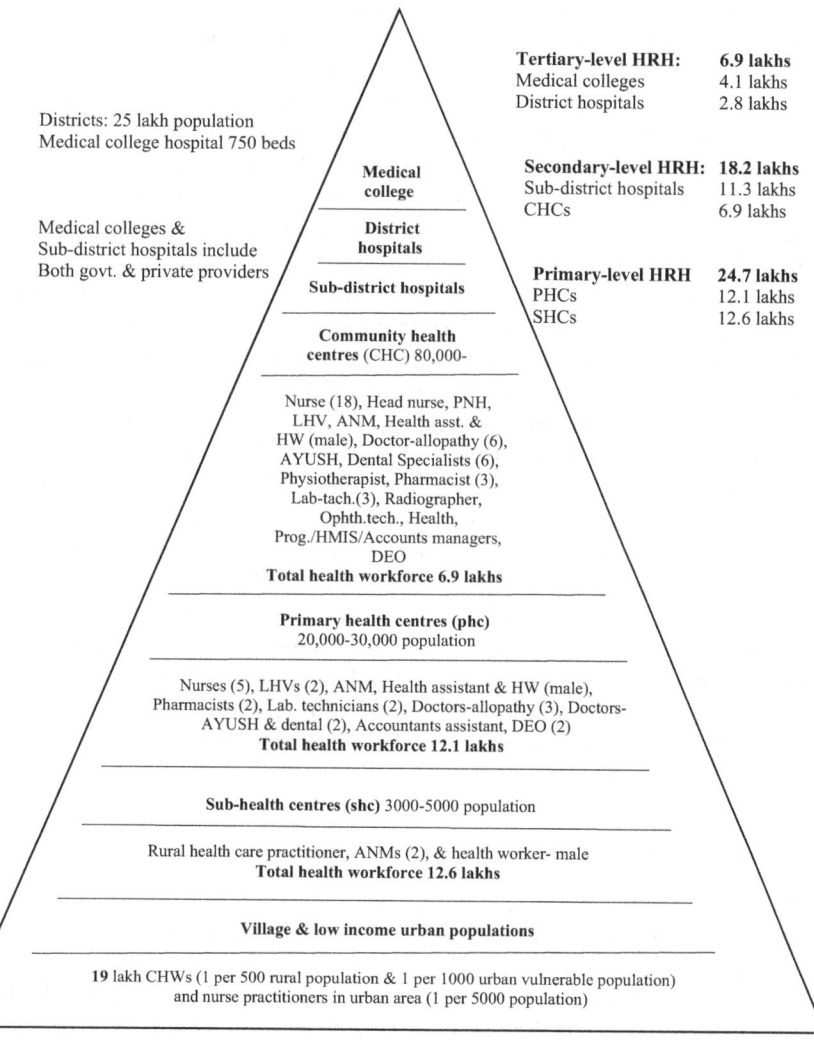

Figure 1.1 Requirements and norms at primary, secondary and tertiary levels

Source: GOI, 2011. High-Level Expert Group report on Universal Health Coverage for India, Planning Commission, Government of India (GOI). http://phmindia.org/wp-content/uploads/2015/09/Plg-Commission-HLEG-Report-on-Health-for-12th-Planrep_uhc0812.pdf

vertically designed and centrally monitored structure, as discussed in Table 1.2 and Table 1.3. However, it is interesting to note that the amount that was allocated to health was less than adequate to achieve the prescribed numbers of physical and human health infrastructure that can meet population requirements. The phenomena of rising public investment was short lived, ended by the late 1980s, even before the start of liberalisation period of the 1990s (Chapter 2). The health facilities were confronted with several problems, especially shortages and mismatches between human and physical infrastructure, lack of medicine and equipment, and other amenities at health centres (Chapter 3). However, the health services – even if of low quality and uneven in reach – were available free to the poor for use. Around the time of the First National Health Policy, the country observed effective containment of malaria which brought down the incidence from an estimated 75 million to less than 2 million, the eradication of smallpox and plague, the halving of maternal mortality, reduction in infant mortality from 160 per 1000 live births to about 105, containment of cholera and increase in longevity to almost 54 years from 32 years (NCMH, 2005). Services that are assumed to be there in the public system were not available in practice to meet population demand, as the system was confronted with several challenges.

The approaches to – as well as arguments about – treating health as a public good distorted over time. These are enforced by changing patterns of disease burden, growing population size and income of the country and individuals, and increases in awareness about health due to rise in literacy rate – and to a large extent, it is derived by technological changes and liberalisation initiatives across the globe. The phenomena of rise in non-communicable diseases (NCDs) become a reality for developing countries including India. The share of NCDs burden in the world increased from 53.67% in 1990 to 71.88% in 2017, and for India, it increased from 38.29% to 66.83% during the same period (Table 1.4). The developing countries, including India, could not devote adequate funds to the health sector to meet the growing health needs of the population. In the meantime, international agencies tried to develop a consensus for the greater role of the private sector and pushed the liberalisation agenda.

Enforcing market arguments: privatisation in healthcare

In the early 1990s, India was going through liberalisation and macroeconomic policy restructuring. One outcome of this restructuring was the implementation of structural adjustment programmes (SAPs) enforced by international agencies. The fiscal stringency induced by the structural adjustment measures affected the central – as well as state – finances in a big way. The SAPs enforced the central and state governments to restructure their expenditure pattern. The thrust of the SAPs was to reduce budget deficits either by increasing the revenue resources or by curtailing the expenditure – or both. Due to limited tax base, governments' revenue could not show

Table 1.4 Burden of diseases by causes: world and India

	World						India					
	1990		2005		2017*		1990		2005		2017*	
	Million	Percent	Million	Percent	Million	Percent	Million	Percent	Million	Percent	Million	Percent
Diarrhoea & common infectious diseases*	557.39	22.32	349.57	14.06	229.96	9.61	178.12	32.31	111.11	21.90	59.11	12.70
Neonatal disorders	277.79	11.12	238.13	9.58	185.78	7.77	77.01	13.97	61.72	12.17	44.39	9.54
Cardiovascular diseases	266.82	10.68	314.09	12.63	365.87	15.30	36.25	6.57	43.87	8.65	65.12	14.00
Cancers	159.58	6.39	191.75	7.71	233.51	9.76	13.59	2.46	17.58	3.47	26.48	5.69
Other NCDs	128.17	5.13	124.64	5.01	121.89	5.10	21.25	3.85	22.06	4.35	22.10	4.75
Unintentional injuries	126.21	5.05	115.16	4.63	105.94	4.43	23.69	4.30	23.85	4.70	23.23	4.99
Respiratory diseases	99.10	3.97	97.30	3.91	112.32	4.70	26.37	4.78	25.11	4.95	33.76	7.26
Malaria and neglected tropical diseases	92.88	3.72	92.11	3.71	62.28	2.60	15.01	2.72	10.00	1.97	6.82	1.47
Nutritional deficiencies	92.44	3.70	72.42	2.91	58.03	2.43	28.14	5.10	25.88	5.10	19.31	4.15
HIV/AIDS and tuberculosis*	84.18	3.37	161.35	6.49	101.13	4.23	27.16	4.93	30.52	6.02	19.72	4.24
Musculoskeletal disorders	83.70	3.35	111.42	4.48	138.72	5.80	11.69	2.12	16.26	3.21	21.83	4.69
Mental and substance use disorders	82.17	3.29	105.43	4.24	122.76	5.13	13.52	2.45	19.91	3.93	22.49	4.83
Diabetes, blood and endocrine diseases*	81.74	3.27	111.29	4.48	133.75	5.59	14.03	2.54	21.30	4.20	26.16	5.62
Transport injuries	75.54	3.02	79.71	3.21	75.33	3.15	9.33	1.69	12.06	2.38	13.09	2.81

(Continued)

Table 1.4 (Continued)

	World						India					
	1990		2005		2017*		1990		2005		2017*	
	Million	Percent	Million	Percent	Million	Percent	Million	Percent	Million	Percent	Million	Percent
Neurological disorders	68.94	2.76	89.16	3.59	111.17	4.65	10.71	1.94	13.94	2.75	17.64	3.79
Digestive diseases	67.39	2.70	76.21	3.07	85.29	3.57	10.91	1.98	13.40	2.64	15.48	3.33
Self-harm	36.32	1.45	36.28	1.46	34.01	1.42	8.92	1.62	10.13	2.00	10.47	2.25
Other communicable diseases*	32.53	1.30	29.69	1.19	23.47	0.98	7.98	1.45	9.40	1.85	2.14	0.46
Liver diseases	30.52	1.22	37.12	1.49	41.40	1.73	4.33	0.79	5.60	1.10	7.40	1.59
Interpersonal violence	23.12	0.93	26.49	1.07	26.00	1.09	2.65	0.48	2.85	0.56	2.73	0.59
Maternal disorders	19.86	0.80	16.28	0.65	11.80	0.49	6.81	1.24	4.91	0.97	2.84	0.61
Conflict and terrorism	7.93	0.32	4.49	0.18	10.10	0.42	2.50	0.45	2.83	0.56	1.12	0.24
Natural disasters	3.24	0.13	5.80	0.23	1.20	0.05	1.40	0.25	2.96	0.58	1.82	0.39
Overall non-communicable diseases	1340.49	53.67	1526.34	61.40	1719.26	71.88	211.14	38.29	253.71	50.02	310.92	66.83
Overall communicable diseases	1157.07	46.33	959.55	38.60	672.45	28.12	340.23	61.71	253.54	49.98	154.33	33.17
Total	2497.56	100.0	2485.89	100.0	2391.71	100.0	551.37	100.0	507.25	100.00	465.25	100.0

Note and source: in 2017, data for (*) diseases is reported for the year 2016; https://ourworldindata.org/burden-of-disease#:~:text=There%20has%20been%20a%20significant,infectious%20diseases%2C%20and%20neonatal%20disorders

any increment. Both central and several state governments went through the process of expenditure curtailment. In the restructuring process, a squeeze in social – largely in health – sector spending observed at national and state level. The sector was lacking of flow of budgetary resources (Chapter 2). The absence of a surveillance and epidemiological system resulted in poorly designed health interventions as well (NCMH, 2005).

On the top of that, in the beginning of the liberalisation phase, the World Bank published a report called 'Investing in Health' in 1993. The report (World Bank, 1993) stated that over the 40 years from 1950–1990, life expectancy of the world improved more than during the entire previous span of human history. In 1950, life expectancy in developing countries was 40 years; by 1990, it increased to 63 years. In 1950, 28 of every 100 children died before their fifth birthday; by 1990, the number had fallen to ten. Smallpox, which killed more than five million annually in the early 1950s, has been eradicated entirely. There was an effective containment of malaria, and eradication of smallpox and plague. The vaccines have drastically reduced the occurrence of measles and polio. Not only do these improvements translate into direct and significant gains in well-being, but they also reduced the economic burden imposed by unhealthy workers and sick or absent school children. The report argues that these successes have come about in part because of growing incomes and increasing education around the globe, and in part because of governments' efforts to expand health services. While it acknowledged the role of government's efforts in improving the health outcomes, it at the same time argued that public healthcare systems in developing nations are confronted with several challenges on efficiency and equity grounds. The report therefore insisted upon the limited role of government involvement in healthcare and insurance sector. The report rejected the idea of healthcare as a public good and insisted that healthcare is a matter of individuals and families, with their strikingly different health needs, to choose freely (Fisk, 2000). The report viewed healthcare as a private good and quite consistently proposed a strategy for spreading both private insurance and private delivery.

It argued that when a country develops, a section of its population becomes able and willing to spend its own money on healthcare. At such a point, the state, according to the World Bank, should not retain sole responsibility for a field like health. It should be shared with the private sector. The public sector would continue to have responsibility of healthcare for low income and public health matters. Beyond that, it would use its resources not to deliver healthcare but to make it possible for individuals to buy private insurance and care. It could return its obligatory fees for healthcare to individuals and add subsidies to those fees if they are insufficient for buying private insurance. As affluence spreads among citizens, such public sector stimulation of private insurance would create demand sufficient to call forth a brisk supply of private healthcare (World Bank, 1993; Fisk, 2000). This gives a notion of promoting privatisation in the health sector. Considering the fact of self-employment status and corporate and service sector emergence, it was argued that the middle-income population is growing; therefore, the insurance sector should be opened up for private players. With this effect, India opened up the health insurance sector for private players in 1999, setting the foreign direct investment (FDI) cap in health insurance at 26%. When the World Bank rejected the idea of free care, the health sector of India witnessed the introduction of user fees in public system from the late 1990s onwards (Ghosh, 2010). The reforms in the health sector in this phase were piecemeal but incremental, which led to extensive changes in the organisational structure, financing and delivery of healthcare services. As a result, a growth in private small clinics, medical centres, nursing homes and other informal for-profit and not-for-profit healthcare providers was observed during the time.

Neoliberal thinking further heavily tried to justify the rationale of public sector underfunding and privatisation in the beginning of the 2000s. This narrative comes from the World Bank's India-specific report entitled 'India: Raising the Sights: Better Health Systems for India's Poor' in 2001. The report mentioned that India's healthcare system is at a crossroads. Its ability to fight infant mortality, communicable diseases and malnutrition is being stretched. At the same time, it faces emerging demands for better service and more attention to chronic diseases of adulthood. India's underfunded public sector and extensive – but largely unaccountable – private sector cannot hope to meet the country's enormous, growing and shifting healthcare needs. If India continues on its present path, the mismatch between its health system and its health problems will become only more severe. The present moment is a decisive one because the government of India is now seeking to define a better health system for the country through the draft report 2001 of Second National Health Policy. The report highlights that country needs to promote private sector and then take advantage of capacity of the private sector in delivering better service for all regions and across socio-economic groups (World Bank, 2001). It further stressed that underfunding and the privatisation are actually defensible in the sense that the Indian economy has a potential to grow high and at faster rate, leading to increase in paying capacity of masses. Since the public system has largely been inefficient in meeting the population healthcare needs, there would not be any harm in marketising the healthcare sector. Such neoliberal arguments were made familiar to everyone who makes cut in public investment necessary. This was a neoliberal priority of opening up investment opportunities for private sector. This was a beginning of the crisis in Indian public healthcare: underfunding followed by privatisation (Chapter 7).

To realise the neoliberal strategy, India opened up the hospital sector for foreign players. In 2000, India approved 100% FDI in the hospital sector through an automatic route. The relaxation in import duties for importing medical equipment and technology were also extended during the 2000s. Granting long-term loans at low interest rates for private health institutions and confirmation of hospital sector with industry status in 2003–2004 budgets were other initiatives for encouraging the private (domestic and foreign) – especially the large and corporate-run – providers/enterprises to exploit the Indian hospital market (Chapter 7). The state was seen as facilitator to the private sector around and over time. An overall consensus emerged to support the private sector through subsidies and credits, and introducing public-private partnerships (PPPs) and insurance.

While citing achievements and failures, the government's own Second National Health Policy 2002 reported a limited success of health system 'in meeting the preventive and curative requirements of the general population'. About 13 of the total 17 goals of the previous health policy were not met, even in a spam of almost 20 years (Sen, 2012: 46). The report mentioned that while successes in communicable disease control are noticeable and mortality rates declined, inequality in access to healthcare has not reduced (Misra et al., 2003). The gap in health services access and outcomes between rural and urban areas and between the richer and poorer has even widened (Peters et al., 2002). There exist huge differences in health system performance and quality between the states. Within the states, the health system is grappling with an urban-rural dichotomy with concentration of facilities in urban areas while missing facilities in rural areas, leading to difference in health outcomes. The policy, however, complemented the role of the primary healthcare approach and sought more public investment in the healthcare sector, while not negating the larger role in service delivery of the private sector, which roughly provides three-fourths of outpatient and two-thirds of inpatient care treatments at the time.

The costly care of private sector over time resulted in enormously high (around 70%) out-of-pocket (OOP) health expenditure in the country (Hooda, 2017). This made health service inaccessible, particularly to poor, simply because they could not afford to pay at the time of healthcare needs and those who used services suffered financial hardship or even impoverishment, as they sold assets and/or borrow money because they had to pay. The high OOP brought out a new dimension in health sector. Now the country needs not only to address the health needs relating to burden of diseases and mortality, but has to devise policy that can address OOP burden, as well. Due to high OOP, the economic gradients of inequality in access to healthcare sharply worsened in the country. Under such a system, the rural and poor feel financially squeezed and experience difficulty in finding services they can afford. This generated a new requirement to find a way to provide financial protection. Financial protections mechanism were everywhere in the world around 2010, which brought out clearly under the renewed policy dialogue of achieving universal health coverage (UHC).

Diverting public funds from provisioning to coverage

When low-income people long felt financially squeezed and experiencing difficulty in accessing services they can afford, government – to address this issue – launched a public-funded health insurance scheme for the poor and informal worker called RSBY (Rashtriya Swasthya Bima Yojana) in 2008 when UHC was in discussion only. Some state-level funded health insurance experiments were even prevalent in the country since 2003.

The UHC debate across the globe around 2010 focused more on devising strategies to finance healthcare rather than providing the care. The world health reports suggested a road map for developing countries to adapt their financing systems to meet the requirements of universal health coverage (WHO, 2010, 2013). The reports highlight that UHC is important for addressing the equity, accessibility and affordability in developing countries. It advocated for an insurance-based health financing strategy to finance healthcare whereby all citizens are insured and can utilise healthcare services, regardless of whether they can afford it or not.

The government of India set up a High-Level Expert Group (HLEG) on UHC in 2010. The HLEG submitted its report to the then-Planning Commission in 2011 (GOI, 2011). While defining the UHC, the report upheld the principles of universality, equity and reflects that the state must be primarily and principally responsible for affordable, accountable and appropriate (promotive, preventive, curative and rehabilitative) health services for a UHC, and recommended to increase public investment in health between 2% to 3% of GDP. The report reflects that government being the guarantor and enablers – although not necessarily the only provider – of health and related services (GOI, 2011: 3), indicating that services can be provided through other mechanism say from private sector. Thereafter, the Planning Commission Steering Committee for the Twelfth Five-Year Plan, in its assessment report to the Prime Minister, criticised the HLEG for ignoring the well-established private sector and made it clear that given the major share of personnel, beds and patients, 'the private sector has to be partnered with national health goal' (Qadeer, 2013: 229).

In 2015, the government of India came out with a draft report of a Third National Health Policy. The draft report specified the role of comprehensive primary care provision in the public sector, while simultaneously supplemented the strategic purchase of secondary and tertiary care services from the private (and the public) sector to assure universal healthcare. These are incorporated in the final report of NHP 2017. The report highlighted that the current publicly (tax-based) financed national health insurance scheme would be aligned with this strategy, and that states would also be encouraged to do the same (GoI, 2017a). Recently, the government of India also launched a National Health Protection Scheme (called Pradhan Mantri Jan Arogya Yojana; PMJAY) under the Ayushman Bharat in 2018. It enhanced the size and scale of coverage which covers over 40% (10.74 crore families) of poor and vulnerable people of the country. This scheme called for providing an annual financial support of Rs. 5 lakh per family, almost 17 times higher than the coverage of pervious national scheme (RSBY) which offered Rs. 30,000 annually per family. The emerging government-funded health insurance (GFHI) scheme is almost entirely funded from public (tax) sources, whereby beneficiaries need not to pay any premium or registration fee. The GFHIs promise to cover below poverty line (BPL) families – in some cases, the informal community – and disadvantage groups under its preview with no contribution from beneficiaries (for details, see Chapter 8).

This brought out a major shift in policy dialogue which gives an intention to promote the purchasing of services through a financial protection package provided through government-funded health insurance. This begins an era when the state seems to ensure access to – but not necessarily the provision of – services, at the cost of public funds. The financing of insurance-based system entirely from public sources has led to an important shift in the fundamental nature of healthcare financing in the country. Until recently, public investment in healthcare was used for financing public health system for service provisioning; now, out of the total health budget, some (tax) funds will be diverted to finance the insurance-based system. That is, the currently promoted insurance-based system will be financed in the same way as the public health sector. The difference lies in the fact that the provisioning would now be shifted almost entirely to the private sector. To what extent changing financing nature affect the healthcare access and help in achieving the national goal of health is described in Chapter 8.

The Third National Health Policy of India 2017 also floated a new idea of strategic purchasing of health services from private players. The policy highlighted that strategic purchasing would ensure access to affordable and quality secondary and tertiary care services from private providers in healthcare services deficit areas. It highlights that private not-for-profit and for-profit hospitals would be empanelled, for comparable quality and standards of care. The policy also advocates a positive and proactive engagement with the private sector for critical gap filling towards achieving national goals. The policy recognises that there are many critical gaps in public health services which would be filled by strategic purchasing promoted through insurance. The strategic purchasing would play a stewardship role in directing private investment towards those areas and those services for which currently there are no providers or few providers. It advocates building synergy with not-for-profit organisations and the private sector, subject to availability of timely quality services, as per predefined norms in the collaborating organisation for critical gap filling. Under a heading, 'Align the growth of private healthcare sector with public health goals', the report clearly mentioned that India needs to influence the operation and growth of the private healthcare sector and medical technologies to ensure alignment with public health goals. Enable private sector contribution to make healthcare systems more effective, efficient, rational, safe, affordable and ethical. This is the first time when a policy full-heartedly advocated for promoting privatisation in the healthcare sector.

In addition, the NITI Aayog 2017 document and the 2020 budget of the government of India clearly stated to provide viability gap funding for setting up hospitals and other medical facilities independently and under the PPP model within the premises of public facility or elsewhere (GOI, 2017b, 2020). The government would facilitate the private players in land allotment, special window clearness and providing viability gap funding (VGF) for improving the financing viability and bankability of the project, and will be linked with GFHIs for coverage reimbursement of referred patients. Government also proposed to set up a VGF window for setting up medical facility in PPP mode in Tier-2 and Tier-3 cities, with a special emphasis in aspirational districts to address the shortage of qualified medical doctors, general practitioners and specialists. Thus, insurance-based financing over time became an integral part of health budgets and an instrument to promote privatisation in healthcare sector. How the private sector took the advantages of these initiatives and exploited the Indian healthcare market and helped in fulfilling the national health goal are some issues that needs to be studied. Chapter 7 is devoted to this.

In spite of these development that argues for private care and private and public insurance in health sector, several other efforts have also been attempted to improve the public sector efficiency to achieve national health goals.

Arguing for efficiency in the public system

State intervention has always been felt necessary to ensure equitable distribution of income and healthcare across the population to ensure equal opportunity in access and outcome, in contrast to the free market economy. Despite that, state intervention (in terms of resource allocation) has been less than adequate in the country, which led to inefficiency in utilisation whatever was the scanty amount allocated towards health sector. Advocates of health as a public good consistently argue for improving the health system performance via increasing the efficiency of resource utilisation. The pursuit of improving the performance of the public health system from an expenditure point of view in a country like India is imperative, because public funding – particularly in rural areas – is one of the single most important sources of health system funding. It is therefore necessary to ensure that funds allocated to the health sector are deployed effectively, and that such expenditure is in line with the local preferences. In conditions when tax and non-tax revenue sources are under stress, the effectiveness of every rupee that is spent becomes even more important. On the demand side, the high morbidity, undernourishment, burden of disease and ageing population on one side, and escalating healthcare costs from private sources on the other side, have added pressure to strategise the policies that improve the performance of health system. The two following fundamental arguments emerged for enhancing the efficiency of public system that hovered around institutional reforms and economic (resource) reforms.

Economic reforms: efficiency of resource allocation

The economic (resource) reforms revolve around allocation and distribution of public funding, specifically relating to underfunding and reprioritisation of health expenditure and efficiency in resource allocation. The size of public expenditure on health has immense importance for securing better health outcomes (Hooda, 2015). Inadequate allocation of public funds can slow down the progress in achieving many of the health outcomes, also reported in Second National Health Policy (Misra et al., 2003: 1). Thus, public intervention is imperative and public spending a necessity, and that any restriction on them would be devastating (Breman and Shelton, 2001; Maruthappu et al., 2015). However, resource allocation may distort the health outcomes if the public health policies are not well targeted in order to improve specific targets (Hu and Mendoza, 2010; GOI, 2002–07). For instance, the allocation of resources – particularly towards high-tech equipment or advanced hospitals – may have little effect on public health if morbidity indicators show the need for increased resources for primary care. Any concentration of health facilities in urban areas with facilities missing from rural areas compels the rural residents to travel longer distances than their urban counterparts to avail themselves of a health facility. Rural residents, then, many a time either postpone the care due to their low income or have to spend a higher share of their income on health and transportation. Because of this, not only do the rural poor face the double burden of poverty and ill health, the financial burden of ill health can push even the non-poor into poverty (Hooda, 2017). The biased provision of health services can be one of the reasons for persistence of the rural-urban gap in health outcomes (mortality, morbidity, undernourishment and burden of diseases are high in rural areas and twice as high among poorer segments of the society) (Hooda, 2015).

Furthermore, any mismatch or low or inadequate allocation of public funds on medicine, materials, supplies and equipment limits the health staff from performing better. Allocated funds may yield little benefit if complementary services are lacking, e.g. roads or transportation services to hospitals and clinics and easy access to water and sanitation (Wagstaff, 2002a, 2002b; Deolalikar, 2004). The allocation of funds towards water supply and sanitation (which is preventive in nature) generally have salubrious impact on both short-term and long-term healthy life in developing and poor countries and regions compared to the expenditures on medical, public health and family welfare (which are of both curative and preventive nature). Thus, along with the size, health outcomes can also be affected by allocation pattern of public funds within the health sector (Breman and Shelton, 2001; Gumber,

1997; Ensor et al., 2003). This needs to be looked into specially to identify the scope, if any, for improving the health system performance by changing the composition and restructuring of the public health spending.

In this direction, the National Rural Health Mission (NRHM, 2005) initiated some measures, along with increase in public health spending to 2–3% of GDP. It argues for providing funds for activities like selection and training of a new health cadre, upgradation of health facilities to first referral units, Indian Public Health Standards, constitution of patient welfare committees, untied funds for sub-centres to meet the immediate requirements (like medicine, water, equipment, etc.), new schemes as well as repackaging of earlier central schemes, rerouting the central fund through state health society and implementing agencies, and so on. All these are important aspects for increasing the efficiency of resource allocation (discussed in detail in Chapter 3). In addition, the allocation of public funds towards a particular sector has a political context. This is because in a democratic country like India, elected representative of different states must have ideological differences and prioritise health sector differently. How political/institutional factors could contribute towards reprioritisation in public spending is important.

Institutional reforms: decentralisation in service delivery

The idea about the role of institutions that strengthen the governance can be traced from the fundamental work of North (1990) on institutions and their possible channels that impact economic performance. North pointed out that institutions are everywhere, and ignoring them would lead to incompleteness of conclusions and policy implications. Scholars have pointed that inefficiencies are more in the context of management of public health services (and other sectors), which require a set of institutional reforms (Cassel, 1995). While referring to the case of absenteeism (35% in the world and 40% in the case of India) of health workers from health facilities, Chaudhury et al. (2006) indicated that the weak institutions for supplying public goods like health are a significant barrier to economic development. The idea of institutional economics/reforms is increasingly being applied to understand and accelerate the process of economic development, as well as for shaping the sector-specific outcomes from an efficiency point of view that influence the outcomes directly or indirectly via improving the efficacy of resource utilisation.

Among the various forms of institutions, the institution of federalism (decentralisation) has been advocated as a powerful means of improving the provision of public goods such as healthcare services and outcomes of the sector. It is argued that devolving power to local governments would improve service delivery, equity, accountability, effectiveness, efficiency and thereby utilisation of health services and health outcomes by bringing decision makers closer to the people and by enhancing the participation of the community in the decision making and implementation processes. The theoretical and empirical literature, however, presents mixed impacts (positive and negative) of local-level institutions in shaping the developmental and social outcomes. Pro-decentralisation advocates assume that decentralisation brings the government closer to the people, and that would increase the responsiveness of local officials to needs (Oates, 1994; Prud'homme, 1995). Their close relation with the local people enables them to know the local problems and needs, and they are therefore in a better position to establish the correct priorities than a central or regional government far away (World Bank, 2004).

While arguing about the relationship between decentralisation and efficiency of public services (Bossert and Beauvais, 2002; Litvack et al., 1998) argued that it is seen as a way of removing layers of bureaucracy or diseconomies of scale and of incorporating local information into decision-making processes. The idea behind productive efficiency is the proximity advantage of local officials to their constituents. As the distance barrier (between central and local citizens) could potentially hinder information flow between the citizens and local officials, the latter is placed in the best position to address their constituents' needs. Bardhan (1996) argued that not only do local governments have more and better information regarding their constituents, but they may be better able to enforce and coordinate policies and programmes, if a stable structure of government is in place. Being in close proximity to those in charge also enables citizens to better monitor the responsible parties' performance and hold them accountable.

The decentralisation passes responsibility and accountability to local bodies. It makes local governments work efficiently, flexibly and creatively by mobilising all the available resources to their localities to fulfil the targets. In health sector, decentralisation is expected to enhance the participation of local communities in decisions regarding health policy objectives, goals, strategies, planning, financing, implementation and monitoring, which are important to improve the health outcomes at the local level (Lieberman, 2002). It also promotes intersectoral coordination, increases accountability, reduces duplication and improves the implementation of health programmes (Litvack and Seddon, 1999; Lieberman, 2002). Decentralisation is expected to create an environment for decision makers to get appropriate and up-to-date information about the preferences and problems of the local people, an effective channel for the people to express their wants and priorities and a motivating environment for the local decision makers to respond to the local needs quickly and effectively (Khaleghian, 2003).

The discussion around benefits and risks of decentralisation reveals that the details and process of decentralisation are much more significant than mere establishment of decentralised institutions. Questions like which functions to centralise and which ones to decentralise, and in what form, become quite significant. Some responsibilities are better undertaken by the central government, while some can safely be delegated to local officials. We believe that the impact of institutions is contextual, as well as country specific. Therefore, one cannot isolate or generalise the factors underlying successful and unsuccessful decentralisation. The implications of decentralisation more or less depend on how the decentralisation is measured (Ebel and Yilmaz, 2002: 20) and how it has been implemented at the ground level. Thus, the issue is not whether or not to decentralise, but rather how to design and implement better decentralisation policies to achieve national and others health policy objectives. A well-designed and implemented decentralisation policy is expected to improve equity, efficiency, quality and coverage of healthcare services – and thereby, health outcomes.

India has been placing the strength of decentralisation in its development policy agendas since the time of independence. The direct democracy, however, was strongly mandated in the early 1990s through 73rd and 74th Constitution Amendment Acts (CAA). These Acts enabled the state legislatures to transfer, if they choose so, adequate powers and responsibilities to local bodies to enable them to prepare and implement schemes for economic development and social justice. The 73rd Act provided a viable way of transferring political,[1] fiscal and administrative powers to rural local bodies. This also made a provision of some mandated actions, like constitution of State Election Commission (SEC),[2] State Finance Commission (SFC),[3] District Planning Committee (DPC)[4] and Gram Sabha[5] to ensure an effective way and process of decentralisation in India. The responsibility on 29 functions,[6] under the Eleventh Schedule, is also sought to be entrusted to local Panchayat in planning and implementation of works of local significance (discussed in detail in Chapter 5). This Act, in a way, provides a formal instrument of *minimum* level of rural decentralised governance in India by enabling state legislative bodies to transfer functional, financial and functionaries (administrative) powers to local governments, along with delegation of political powers to ensure participation of people in grass-roots politics and policy. These decentralisation reforms are part of political reform process.

As part of health sector reform, the role of decentralisation and community participation in health policy making and implementation have been recommended since the Bhore Committee in 1946 to several other health committees/policies. Most of the initial initiatives failed to design and classify how to involve them in improving the health service delivery system. However, with the launch of National Rural Health Mission in 2005, such strategy became visible. The mission seeks to improve access to healthcare facilities, enable community ownership of services, strengthen public health systems, enhance the equity and accountability of the providers, and most importantly, strengthen and deepen the levels of decentralisation by increasing the resources available to the Panchayats (discussed in Chapter 5 and Chapter 6). While the responsibility of implementation of this programme rests with the state governments, the NRHM (now national health mission; NHM) seeks to empower the Panchayats to manage, control and be accountable for health services. The Panchayats are critical to the planning, implementation and monitoring of NRHM programme in the village. Village-level committees called Village Health and Sanitation Committee (VHSC, consisting of educated villagers, school principal, women, minority communities etc.) were entrusted with the planning and implementation of health programmes in the village to achieve equity and efficiency in healthcare use through decentralising services. The VHSC envisioned that local people will take leadership in health management of the health system and its related matter, and provided with an amount of Rs. 10,000 to help poor women during health emergencies/pregnancy and spread of diseases). This committee provided a significant mechanism for engendering inclusiveness in health planning. Under the mission, the interface between the community and public health system at the village level is entrusted through a female Accredited Social Health Activist (ASHA) for spreading awareness about the importance of basic facility and health programmes in the village and made accountable to Gram Sabha (a formal Panchayat meeting consisting of villagers, Panchayat representatives and health functionaries). Mission also introduced a cash incentive programme called Janani Suraksha Yojana (JSY) to promote institutional delivery along with some other committees called Rogi Kalyan Samiti (RKS) and Sakshar Mahila Samooh (SMS), etc., for planning and implementation of health programmes that involve community.

All these initiatives explain a sustained process of decentralisation that involve communities, local agents and local governments for effective delivery of healthcare services in rural India. We have postulated that the gain from these initiatives depends on how these initiatives have been implemented at ground level and helped in improving the health service delivery system in rural areas. These initiatives involve various dimensions of decentralisation, and participation by communities and local agents. The extent to which these dimensions help in improving healthcare service access and service delivery in rural India is discussed in greater detail in Part 2 of the book.

About the book

The preceding discussions reveal that the healthcare structure in India has an evolutionary and organic history. The basic feature of India's health system initially was set out on a principle that 'nobody should be denied access to health for his inability to pay' and the state should take primary responsibility to provide healthcare to the population. This publicly provided healthcare continued to be relevant and expanded. The states are seen finding innovative ways and new experiments to increase accountability and efficiency of resource utilisation via institutional (decentralisation delivery) and investment (resource) reforms. However, along with the effort of improving the functioning of public health system, the neoliberal thinking simultaneously heavily tried to justify the rationale of public sector underfunding and privatisation in the post-liberalisation phase. A desire and need have been articulated to encourage the private sector in the health service delivery and to partner it with national health goals. The market economy arguments have been enforced and facilitated over time.

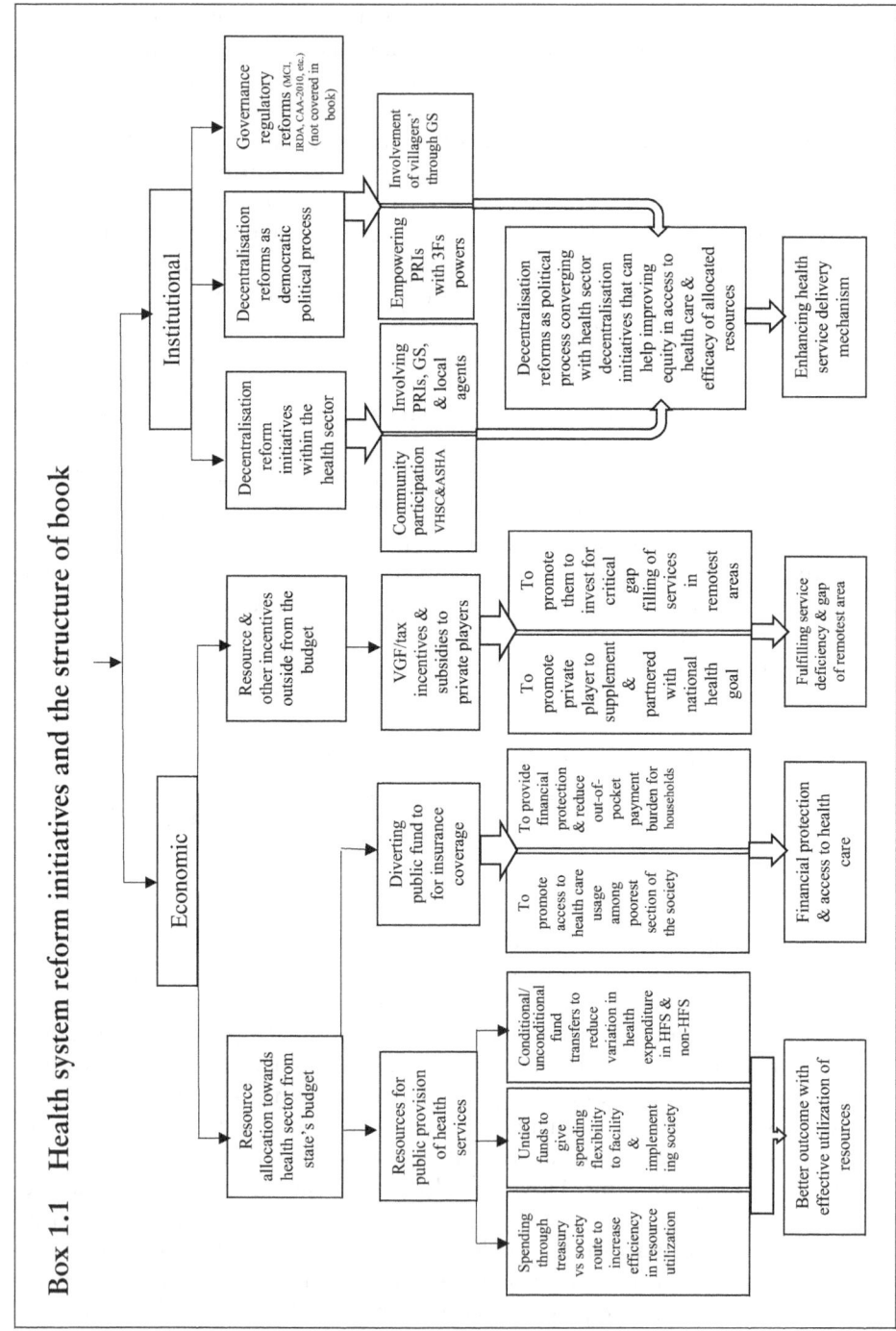

Box 1.1   Health system reform initiatives and the structure of book

Based on the aforementioned concerns, the study has tried to provide a deeper insight on all three aspects i.e., investment (resource) reforms (Part 1), institutional (decentralisation delivery) reforms (Part 2) and initiative towards promoting privatisation agenda for service access and delivery (Part 3). The evolutionary features of Indian health policies around these three aspects have been summarised in Box 1.1, which describes the overall structure and organisation of the book.

Part 1 provides a detailed analysis on resource allocation (to understand states' priories accorded to health), source of inefficiency in resource allocation and utilisation. Part 2 builds a case for improving the efficacy of allotted funds and delivery system through institutional reforms via ensuring decentralisation in governance and higher participation of local communities, elected governments and civil society in health policy making and service delivery. It discusses that institutions are important for shaping the sector-specific outcomes from an efficiency point of view, both directly and indirectly, via improving the efficacy of allotted funds in that sector. Part 3 discusses that in spite of having high asymmetric information and market failure in market-driven healthcare delivery system, the positive and proactive engagement of private sector for critical gap filling towards achieving national goals have been advocated. India has witnessed an important shift in healthcare financing with the introduction of pro-poor health insurance financed through public funds. It redefined the role of the state from being a provider to a financier of health services, which has the potential to profoundly affect the health sector. This section therefore discusses how the private sector has grown and has aligned its interests in fulfilling national health goals, and how and to what extent insurance-based financing has performed in providing financial protection to people.

Emerging challenges and current developments

Policy makers, public health experts and governmental and non-governmental institutions across the world – including India – have been trying to find ways to address the devastation caused by the current COVID-19 pandemic. Some countries showed an early alertness and undertook preventive measures (including testing, tracing, social distancing, hand hygiene and use of masks) to curb the spread of virus, along with a varied forms of lockdown. Amongst others, testing, tracing and treatment (including vaccination) are crucial aspects that describe the functioning of a country's health system. The success, to a large extent, is found to depend on how a nation has designed its health system and which type of distinct features and components its system has, namely, financing, organisation of service delivery, payment mechanism, regulatory aspects, etc. The market-driven healthcare system which gets financed through out-of-pocket payment (India) or through insurance (United States) could not outperform well. Systems that have efficient decentralised service delivery mechanisms, with equitably (rural-urban setting) distributed physical and human infrastructure around primary, secondary and tertiary care, were found to perform well; several global health experts cited the case of Kerala in India, which could engage widely-spread primary healthcare workers in contact tracing. Other countries' examples are also prevalent. In this context, the book argues for the need to strengthen the economic (resource) as well as the institutional reforms for improving the accountability, efficacy of allotted funds and service delivery systems which have become significant in the current context. The market-driven system has failed to deliver affordable and equitable care so far. The Indian private health sector has remained silent in helping the fight against the COVID-19 pandemic in offering affordable treatments. The virus has taught us that a more inclusive, equitable and accountable system guided by decentralised and multisectoral decision-making approaches is important. This crisis has thrown a unique opportunity before the global community to re-imagine and transform its health systems. This has also amplified long-standing systemic and structural problem in the Indian healthcare system. In this direction, the book is a timely intervention that discusses approaches towards reforming the health sector and will be useful for policy makers. The limitations, if any, have been reported in respective chapters.

Notes

1 Under this Act, from political standpoint, there is a provision of three tiers of Panchayats, namely, at village, intermediate and district levels. This Act not only gave discretionary political power to states to devolve power to Panchayati Raj Institutions (PRIs), but also sought to protect the political rights of hitherto neglected groups such as schedule castes, tribes and women by providing them reservation in politics. This involves the provisions for greater participation of backward and deprived sections of the society in decision making.
2 The SEC helps to ensure improved democracy by ensuring regular, free and fair elections at the local level every five years.
3 The SFC is constituted, every five years, to govern the distribution and devolution of financial resources so as to improve the financial position of the Panchayats across the districts within a state.
4 The DPC involves in planning processes and the plans of the Panchayats and Urban Local Bodies in a district will consolidated by DPCs. All Panchayats are to engage in (economic development and social justice) planning processes under the mandatory action of Constitution. Plans of the Panchayats and Urban Local Bodies in a district are to be consolidated by the District Planning Committees (DPCs). If the Constitutional mandate were to be operationalizing, minimally, such bodies should be formed and appropriately resourced.
5 The Gram Sabha, or village council, has been envisioned as the foundation of the Panchayati Raj system, as it ensures community participation.
6 The functions range from drinking water, agriculture, poverty alleviation programmes, health and family welfare, education, libraries and cultural activities, maintenance of community assets, etc.

References

Bardhan, P. 1996. Decentralized Development. *Indian Economic Review*, Vol. XXXI, No. 2, pp. 139–156.

Bhore Committee. 1946. *The Report of Health Survey and Development Committee (Bhore Committee) 1946*, vols.1, 2 and 3. Government of India, Kolkata. https://www.nhp. gov.in/bhore-committee-1946_pg

Bossert, T., and Beauvais, J. C. 2002. Decentralization of Health Systems in Ghana, Zambia, Uganda and the Philippines: A Comparative Analysis of Decision Space. *Health Policy and Planning*, Vol. 17, No. 1, pp. 14–31.

Breman, A., and Shelton, C. 2001. *Structural Adjustment and Health: A Literature Review of the Debate, Its Role-players and Presented Empirical Evidence*. www. eldis.org/document/A29545

Cassel, A. 1995. Health Sector Reform: Key Issues in Less Developed Countries. *Journal of Health and Population*, National Institute of Health and Family Welfare (NIHFW), New Delhi, Vol. 7, No. 3, pp. 329–347.

Chaudhury, N., Hammer, J., Kremer, M., Muralidharan, K., and Rogers, F. H. 2006. Missing in Action: Teacher and Health Worker Absence in Developing Countries. *Journal of Economic Perspectives*, Vol. 20, No. 1, pp. 91–116.

Deolalikar, A. 2004. *Attaining the Millennium Development Goals in India: Role of Public Policy and Services Delivery*. World Bank, Washington, DC.

Ebel, R., and Yilmaz, S. 2002. *On the Measurement and Impact of Fiscal Decentralisation*. Policy Research Working Paper 2809, Economic Policy and Poverty Reduction Division, World Bank Institute, The World Bank. https://doi.org/10.1596/1813-9450-2809

Ensor, T., Ali, L., Hossain, A., and Ferdousi, S. 2003. Projecting the Cost of Essential Services in Bangladesh. *The International Journal of Health Planning and Management*, Vol. 18, No. 2, pp. 137–149. https://doi.org/10.1002/hpm.701

Fisk, M. 2000. Neoliberalism and the Slow Death of Public Healthcare in Mexico. *Journal of Socialism and Democracy*, Vol. 14, No. 1, pp. 63–84.

Ghosh, S. 2010. *Catastrophic Payments and Impoverishment Due to Out-of-pocket Health Spending: The Effects of Recent Health Sector Reforms in India*. Asia Health Policy Program, Working Paper No. 15, July, SSRN at https://papers.ssrn.com/sol3/papers.cfm?abstract_id=1658573

GOI. 1951. *Census of India-1951*. Registrar General of India, Government of India (GOI).

GOI. 2002–07. *Tenth Plan Document (2002–07), Planning Commission*. Government of India, New Delhi.

GOI. 2005. *National Rural Health Mission Document*. Ministry of Health and Family Welfare, Government of India.

GOI. 2011. *High Level Expert Group* (HLEG) *Report on Universal Health Coverage for India: Instituted by Planning Commission of India*. Government of India, New Delhi. http://planningcommission. nic. in/reports/genrep/rep_uhc0812.pdf

GOI. 2017a. *National Health Policy, Ministry of Health and Family Welfare*. Government of India. https://mohfw.gov.in/sites/default/files/9147562941489753121.pdf

GOI. 2017b. *NITI Aayog Draft Guidelines on Public Private Partnership for NCDs in District Hospitals-2017*. Government of India. https://niti.gov.in/writereaddata/files/document_publication/Draft%20Guidelines%20on%20PPP%20in%20NCDs_0.pdf

GOI. 2020. *Budget Speech*. Union Government, GOI.

Gumber, A. 1997. Burden of Diseases and Cost of Ill Health in India: Setting Priorities for Health Interventions During the Ninth Plan. Margin. *National Council of Applied Research*, Vol. 29, No. 2.

Gupta, R. P. 2016. *Health Care Reforms in India: Making up for the Lost Decades*. Elsevier, India.

Hooda, S. K. 2015. Government Spending on Health in India: Some Hopes and Fears of Policy Changes. *Journal of Health Management*, Vol. 17, No. 4, pp. 458-486.

Hooda, S. K. 2017, April 22. Health Payments and Household Well-being: How Effective Are Health Policy Interventions? *Economic & Political Weekly*, Vol. LII, No. 16, pp. 54–65.

Hsiao, W. C. 2003. *What Is a Health System? Why Should We Care?* www.mediastudies.fpzg.hr/_download/repository/Hsiao2003.pdf

Hu, B., and Mendoza, R. U. 2010, April. Public Spending, Governance and Child Health Outcomes: Revisiting the Links. *Journal of Human Development and Capabilities*, UNICEF, Policy and Practice, Vol. 14, No. 2, pp. 285–311.

Khaleghian, P. 2003. *Decentralisation and Public Services: The Case of Immunization*. World Bank Policy Research Paper, No. 2989, Public Service, Development Research Group, The World Bank, March.

Lieberman, S. 2002. *Decentralisation and Health in the Philippines and Indonesia: An Interim Report*. World Bank, Washington, DC.

Litvack, J., Ahmad, J., and Bird, R. 1998, September. *Rethinking Decentralisation in Developing Countries*. World Bank Sector Studies Series. World Bank, Washington, DC.

Litvack, J., and Seddon, J. 1999. *Decentralization Briefing Notes*. World Bank Institute, WP No. 37142, World Bank, Washington, DC.

Maruthappu, M., Bonnie Ng, Ka Ying, Williams, C., Atun, R., and Zeltner, T. 2015, April. Government Health Care Spending and Child Mortality. *American Academic of Pediatrics, Pediatrics*, Vol. 135, No. 4, pp. e887–e894. https://doi.org/10.1542/peds.2014-1600

Misra, R., Chatterjee, R., and Rao, K. S. 2003. *India Health Report*. Oxford University Press, New Delhi.

NCMH. 2005. *Report of the National Commission on Macroeconomics and Health*. National Commission on Macroeconomics and Health (NCMH), Ministry of Health & Family Welfare, Government of India, New Delhi.

North, D. C. 1990. *Institutions, Institutional Change and Economic Performance*. Cambridge University Press, Cambridge.

Oates, W. 1994. Federalism and Government Finance. In J. Quigley and E. Smolensky (Eds.), *Modern Public Finance* (Chapter 5). Harvard University Press, Cambridge, MA, pp. 126–151.

Ourworldindata. n.d. https://ourworldindata.org/burden-of-disease#:~:text=There%20has%20been%20a%20significant,infectious%20diseases%2C%20and%20neonatal%20disorders

Peters, D., Yazbeck, A., Sharma, R., Ramana, G., Pritchett, L., and Wagstaff, A. 2002. *Better Health Systems for India's Poor*. Human Development Network, World Bank, Washington, DC.

Prud'homme, R. 1995. *On the Dangers of Decentralization*. Policy Research Working Paper No.1252. World Bank, Washington, DC.

Qadeer, I. 2013. Universal Health Care in India: Panacea for Whom? *Indian Journal of Public Health*, Vol. 57, No. 4, pp. 225–230.

Rao, K. S. 2017. *Do We Care?: India's Health System*. Oxford University Press, Oxford.

Sen, Gita. 2012. Universal Health Coverage in India: A Long and Winding Road. *Economic & Political Weekly*, Vol. 47, No. 8, pp. 45–52.

Wagstaff, A. 2002a. Inequality Aversion, Health Inequalities, and Health Achievement. *Journal of Health Economics*, Vol. 21, No. 4, pp. 627–641.

Wagstaff, A. 2002b. Poverty and Health Sector Inequalities. *Bulletin of the World Health Organization*, Vol. 80, No. 2, pp. 97–105.

WHO. 1978. *Primary Health Care, Report of the International Conference on Primary Health Care*, Alma Ata, USSR, 6–12 September 1978. https://apps.who. int/iris/handle/10665/39228.

WHO. 2010. *The World Health Report: Health System Financing: The Path to Universal Coverage*. World Health Organization, Geneva.

WHO. 2013. *World Health Report 2013: Research for Universal Health Coverage*. World Health Organization, Geneva.

World Bank. 1993. *World Development Report: Investing in Health*. World Bank, Washington, DC.

World Bank. 2001. *India: Raising the Sights: Better Health Systems for India's Poor*. HNP Unit-India, Report No. 22304. World Bank, Washington, DC.

World Bank. 2004. *World Development Report 2004: Making Services Work for Poor People*. World Bank, Washington, DC.

Zodpey, S. P., and Negandhi, P. H. 2018. Tracking India's Progress in Health Sector after 70 Years of Independence. *Indian Journal of Public Health*, Vol. 62, pp. 1–3. www.ijph.in/article.asp?issn=0019-557X;year=2018;volume=62;issue=1;spage=1;epage=3;aulast=Zodpey

Part 1

The state as a provider of healthcare services

An efficient healthcare system is essential for improving well-being of people and reducing burden of diseases and overall growth of the country. This requires adequate investment, but a pertinent question is that who should invest in health. A theoretical construct argues that intervention of the state in healthcare leads to increases in social welfare through better outcomes, greater equity and more consumer satisfaction. Intervention of the state is important in areas where private players fail to provide adequate services; it becomes important in situations of market failure, and it becomes crucial in contexts when the elites and other powerful groups corner greater gains of resources because of uneven distribution of social and economic power. Intervention of the state is necessary to ensure equitable distribution of income and healthcare across the population by ensuring equal opportunity in access and outcomes in contrast to the free market economy.

Since independence, India has tried to build its healthcare system with the principle that 'nobody should be denied access to health services for his inability to pay' (Bhore Committee, 1946: 17) and that the state should take primary responsibility to provide healthcare to all. India has constituted several committees to suggest a robust health system and has produced three national-level health policies to strengthen the system for meeting the growing healthcare needs of the population.

Items like health and sanitation, hospitals and dispensaries are placed under the State List of the Constitution of India. The central government, however, intervenes directly in establishing major hospitals to assist medical education and research in the states and indirectly through fund transfer under central planning and centrally sponsored schemes. Thus, major responsibility of resource allocation towards health is with the state. Given the federal nature of the country, states must have ideological differences and prioritise their health sectors differently under different macroeconomic restructuring and other policy-changing scenarios. Therefore, Chapter 2 is devoted to exploring the pattern of healthcare financing, size of public funds allocated, (in)adequacy of funds if any, status of spending commitments of states and central governments and their achievements, and the effect of

DOI: 10.4324/9781032108438-2

macroeconomic conditions and health policy changes in influencing the level of public funds allocated towards health.

No doubt, the size of public expenditure has immense importance; any inadequacy of public funding can slow down the progress in achieving many of the health outcomes. The resource allocation, however, may distort the health outcomes if the public health policies are not well targeted in order to improve specific targets. For instance, allocation of resources particularly towards high-tech equipment or advanced hospitals may have little effect on public health if morbidity indicators show the need for increased resources for primary care. Any concentration of health facilities in urban areas with missing corresponding facilities from rural areas compels the rural residents to travel longer distances than their urban counterparts to avail themselves of health facilities, which can have long-lasting implications for payments, accessibility and postponement of the care. Any mismatch or low/inadequate allocation of public funds on medicine, material, supply and equipment limit the health staff to perform better rendering the system inefficiency. Allocated funds may yield little benefit if complementary services are lacking e.g., roads or transportation services to hospitals and clinics and easy access to water and sanitation which have salubrious impact on both short-term and long-term healthy life, especially in under-developed regions compared to the expenditure on medical, public health and family welfare (which have both curative and preventive nature).

Such types of inaccessibility, inappropriateness and inefficiency are likely to deny treatments and health improvement to patients who would otherwise have received if resources had been better placed and used. Such types of inefficiencies in economic terminology signifies wasted resources and means a lot for a developing country like India. The available low fiscal space with the state also adds pressure for increasing the accountability and efficiency of resource use. The elimination of inefficiency from any system acts as a source of finance, as it is equivalent to an increase in the resource availability. The pursuit of improving the performance of the public health system from an expenditure point of view in a country like India is imperative, because public funding – particularly in rural areas – is the most important source of health system funding. It is therefore necessary to ensure that the allocated funds to the health sector are deployed effectively and that such expenditures are in line with the local preferences. In conditions when tax and non-tax revenue sources are under stress, the effectiveness of every rupee that is spent becomes even more important.

The Ninth Five-Year Plan of India for the first time envisioned the expansion and improvement of health services to meet the increasing healthcare needs of the population. It felt the need to improve the health status of the population by optimising coverage and quality of care by identifying and rectifying critical gaps in infrastructure, personnel, equipment, essential diagnostics and drugs. It envisions the need to improve functional efficiency of the healthcare system, though no specific targets were set. Further, in 2005, the government of India launched the National Rural of Health Mission, which proposed several new provisions for improving the efficacy of both rural and urban health systems (the latter in 2013 with the implementation of National Health Mission; NHM). The mission sets the objectives to devolve more resources in priority states/areas and provide untied funds and more spending autonomy to primary healthcare centres, rerouting and implementing the central funds through state implementing agencies. The diversion in fund allocation from treasury route to society route was made to increase the resource utilisation without any delay and to give more power to decentralised implementing agencies. These provisions were made to improve the performance/efficiency in primary healthcare system.

Considering the fact that healthcare outcomes can be affected by size, as well as by allocation pattern of public funds within the sector, an in-depth analysis of source of inefficiency and allocation pattern of public funds is provided in Chapter 3, specially to identify the scope for improving healthcare system performance via changing the composition and restructuring of public health spending. A detailed discussion is included of NRHM/NHM funding and new provisions, especially to highlight the nature/types of hopes and fears such policy changes have brought out.

2 Investing in health
Health policies and expenditure priorities[1]

An efficient healthcare system contributes to enhanced quality of life, well-being of people and reduction of the burden of diseases, which in turn increases productivity and growth of a country (NCMH, 2005). The poor status of human health causes capability deprivation and leads to the world's poverty and unemployment (Sen, 1999), while better human health increases productivity and enhances the ability of individuals to earn more income. Thus, investing in health is integral to human, as well as economic, development of a country. However, there is a considerable debate around who should invest in health. The theoretical construct argues that health is a public/merit good, and therefore cannot be left to the market from an efficiency point of view. The healthcare market is inherently imperfect on account of asymmetry of information, uncertainty and existence of externalities (Arrow, 1963; Kethineni, 1991), which enhances the vulnerability of patients. Markets do not deliver care to low-paying individuals on account of non-profitability and low returns on investment. Experiences from the developing world, particularly from newly independent (from colonial rule) Third World countries (including India) have shown that private players either provide costly care or do not deliver basic healthcare in remote areas. The inherited historical pattern of health system in these countries is found to be grossly biased towards urban and curative care services, which is not fit to cater to or serve the needs of the general population (Hall and Taylor, 2003). Generally, it is argued that public intervention in social sectors like health leads to increase in social welfare through better outcomes, greater equity and more consumer satisfaction (World Bank, 1993; Getzen, 2004). The intervention of the state becomes significant in areas where private players fail to provide adequate services; it becomes important in situations of market failure, and it becomes crucial in contexts where the elites and other powerful groups corner greater gains of resources because of uneven distribution of social and economic power. State intervention (here we mean resource allocation by the state) is necessary to ensure equitable distribution of income and healthcare across the population by ensuring equal opportunity in access and outcome in contrast to the free market economy.

DOI: 10.4324/9781032108438-3

When it comes to the approaches to finance healthcare, the world has followed a much diversified approach to strengthen healthcare systems. Some spend higher amounts of public funds than others, while some rely more on the private sector for service delivery. The developed nations, in most cases, spend a high amount on health out of their total budget, as a share of GDP and in per capita terms, when compared to developing economies (Table 2.1). The health sector in low-developed economies generally suffers from an underfunding problem, along with a disproportionally high disease burden, as reported in Chapter 1. The World Health Report 2019 also documented the persistence of high levels of maternal mortality (over 90% of all maternal deaths) in these economies (WHO, 2019); consequently, their health systems also suffer from underfunding problems – and perhaps is one of the reasons for low outcome of their health sectors. The growth in health expenditure in these countries, including India, is highly vulnerable to their political and economic contexts, as discussed later in this chapter.

India is a federal country. The predominant responsibilities of the health sector are accorded to the state governments. Items like public health and sanitation, hospitals and dispensaries are placed under the State List in the 7th Schedule of the Constitution of India. The central government, however, can intervene directly in establishing major hospitals to assist medical education and research in the states and indirectly through central plan and centrally sponsored schemes – note that most of the CSS directed at augmenting health services are (almost) 100% financed by the centre and routed through the state budget; there are some central schemes where central component are 88%, 75% and 50% – that are implemented through state budgets. Since the allocation of public spending towards health is state specific in India, it has political context, as well. This is because in a democratic country like India, elected representatives of different states must have ideological differences and prioritise the health sector differently. Keeping these views in advance, this chapter explores how the healthcare sector is financed in India – specifically the size of public funds allocated towards health by central and state governments, whether allocated amounts are adequate to meet required levels of basic services and how political context and priority, macroeconomic conditions and health policy changes have affected the health spending, along with the historical account of health spending commitments and achievements.

At the outset, the size of public expenditure on healthcare is compared with the spending of international and neighbouring countries. It is then compared with health spending commitments made in various policy documents, especially to understand whether government's commitments are based on unmet healthcare needs of population. The health expenditure is presented as a share of total budget of central and state governments separately, in real per capita terms (at 2004–2005 prices), as a ratio of GDP and gross state domestic product (GSDP). This helps to understand variation and rate of growth of health expenditure (HE), especially to see whether HE is growing faster than GDP and/or faster than population growth and how it has been prioritised in the government budget. Analysing health expenditure around these three measure is important because Wagner's Law in 19th century narrated a tendency that with the increase in growth of an economy, the size of government grows, which in turn results in greater government spending on various sectors, including health. Health expenditure as a share of government budget tells how the sector is reprioritised every year when government size increases, and whether the growing share can meet the population demand; then per capita terms became important. The impact of different health policies and macroeconomic conditions is analysed by dividing the study period into different sub-periods. The sub-periods are identified by analysing the health expenditure trends and a break is given at the major turning point in health expenditure (see the following section for details).

The results are presented for major states of India, which are at some places classified as low-high income, high-focused and non–high-focused states as categorised under the National Rural Health Mission 2005.

Size of health expenditure

A prominent debate within the healthcare sector hovered around the size and allocation pattern of public expenditure. Internationally, it is suggested that every country should spend at least 5% of its GDP on health (Savedoff, 2007: 963). The quantified goals of spending, however, are not based on much solid analysis. While, based on international comparisons and immense unmet needs, one could argue that government should spend more on health than it has in the past, setting a specific goal for government spending should really be based on an analysis of what the government wants to achieve with its spending. A low level of public spending is a reflection of government failure in providing a reasonable level of health facilities. For instance, bed: population ratio (hospital beds per 10,000 people) varies between as low as 21:10,000 ratios in developing nations, while as high as 50:10,000 ratios in advanced (OECD) nations (HDR, 2019). This ratio is 7:10,000 for India, while world average is 28:10,000. India has 7.8 number of physician per 10,000 population, well below the world average of 14.9 physicians and 28.9 physicians in OECD and 11.5 physicians in developing countries. When comes to the bed: population in the public sector it is less than one in India. This indicates the necessity of more spending in health sector.

The global health expenditure statistics reveal a many-fold variation in per capita health expenditure. The per capita public expenditure on health varies more than 100-fold, ranges between less than I$27 per capita to well over I$3556 per capita and ranges between 1% and 8% as a share of GDP and 3% to 22% as a share of total budgetary spending (Table 2.1). The size of public spending on health in India is reported as around 1.17% of GDP, as per National Health Profile 2019 (GOI, 2019), while it was reported to be around 0.96% of GDP in WHO-NHA data in 2017 (Table 2.1). India's spending is almost one of the lowest even amongst the Southeast Asian countries and low-income countries (GOI, 2019). Being a low level of per capita income, neighbouring Sri Lanka and Bangladesh spend more public fund on health than India (Table 2.1).

India's spending on health is grossly less than the internationally recommended level, and even lower than that of neighbouring countries, which presents an inadequate and dismal state of a public health system to meet the population's health needs. This certainly encourages the people, especially the poor and underprivileged, to seek care from the private sector, which in turn results in high out-of-pocket (OOP) burden. The OOP burden in India is one of the highest in the world, with about 70% of health expenditure financed from households' own pockets (HLEG, 2011). The high OOP expenses not only push non-poor into poverty (Wagstaff and Doorslaer, 2003), but adversely affect access to care and health outcomes. India, a highly populated country – has always been off the track in achieving most of its health targets set by international (MDGs) and national agencies (discussed in following sections). Some of the health outcomes – such as infant, child and maternal mortality rates – are even worse than some of the developing and neighbouring countries. In 2018, the infant mortality rate (IMR) in India was recorded at around 34.6 per 1000 live births, whereas Sri Lanka's IMR was 8 per 1000 live births (Table 2.1). The life expectancy at birth (about 69) of an average Indian is at least 14 years less than those in developed countries, and even lower than the neighbouring Sri Lanka's 76.8 years (Table 2.1). Almost half of Indian children suffer from malnutrition (UNICEF, 2019), and this situation in some places is even worse than sub-Saharan Africa. More than 50% of women suffer from anaemia (NFHS, 2016). The poor-rich and rural-urban gaps in health outcomes still persist.

Financing health expenditure

National Health Account (NHA) of India provides a detailed analysis of how the health sector is financed. Figure 2.1 provides an interesting insight into how the current health expenditure is distributed across financing sources, financing schemes, providers and healthcare functions. The NHS

Table 2.1 Comparing health expenditure across select countries

HDI index 2019 #	Country	Total exp. on health as % of GDP; WHS-2015	Per capita total exp on health (PPP I$) WHS-2015	Per capita govt exp. on health (PPP I$) WHS-2015	Govt. exp.on health as % of GDP 2017*	Govt exp. on health % to total govt. exp. WHS-2020	Health indicators 2018 #			GNI per capita (PPP-US$) 2018 #
							Life expectancy at birth (years)	IMR per 1000 live births	MMR per one lakh live births	
4	Germany	11.3	4635	3556	8.73	19.9	81.2	3.2	6	46946
6	Australia	8.9	3855	2583	6.34	17.8	83.3	3.1	6	44097
13	Canada	10.9	4610	3229	7.79	19.3	82.3	4.3	7	43602
15	UK	9.3	3235	2716	7.65	18.7	81.2	3.7	9	39507
15	United States	17.0	8845	4153	8.56	22.5	78.9	5.6	14	56140
26	France	11.6	4213	3259	8.72	15.5	82.5	3.9	8	40511
61	Malaysia	4.0	894	494	1.95	8.9	76.0	7.1	40	27227
71	Sri Lanka	3.1	270	105	1.64	8.5	76.8	8.0	30	11611
76	Mexico	6.1	1062	550	2.84	11.0	75.0	12.4	38	17628
77	Thailand	4.5	630	500	2.85	15.0	76.9	10.5	20	16129
79	Brazil	9.5	1388	659	3.96	10.3	75.7	13.5	20	14068
85	China	5.4	578	323	2.92	9.1	76.7	8.5	27	16127
111	Indonesia	3.0	273	108	1.45	8.7	71.5	22.2	126	11256
129	India	3.8	196	60	0.96	3.4	69.4	34.6	174	6829
135	Bangladesh	3.5	85	27	0.38	3.0	72.3	28.2	176	4057
147	Nepal	5.5	118	47	1.24	4.5	70.5	28.4	258	2748
152	Pakistan	2.8	122	45	0.92	4.3	67.1	64.2	178	5190

Source: World Health Statistics (2015–2020) and #-Human Development Report (2018, 2019); *-https://apps.who.int/nha/database/ViewData/Indicators/en

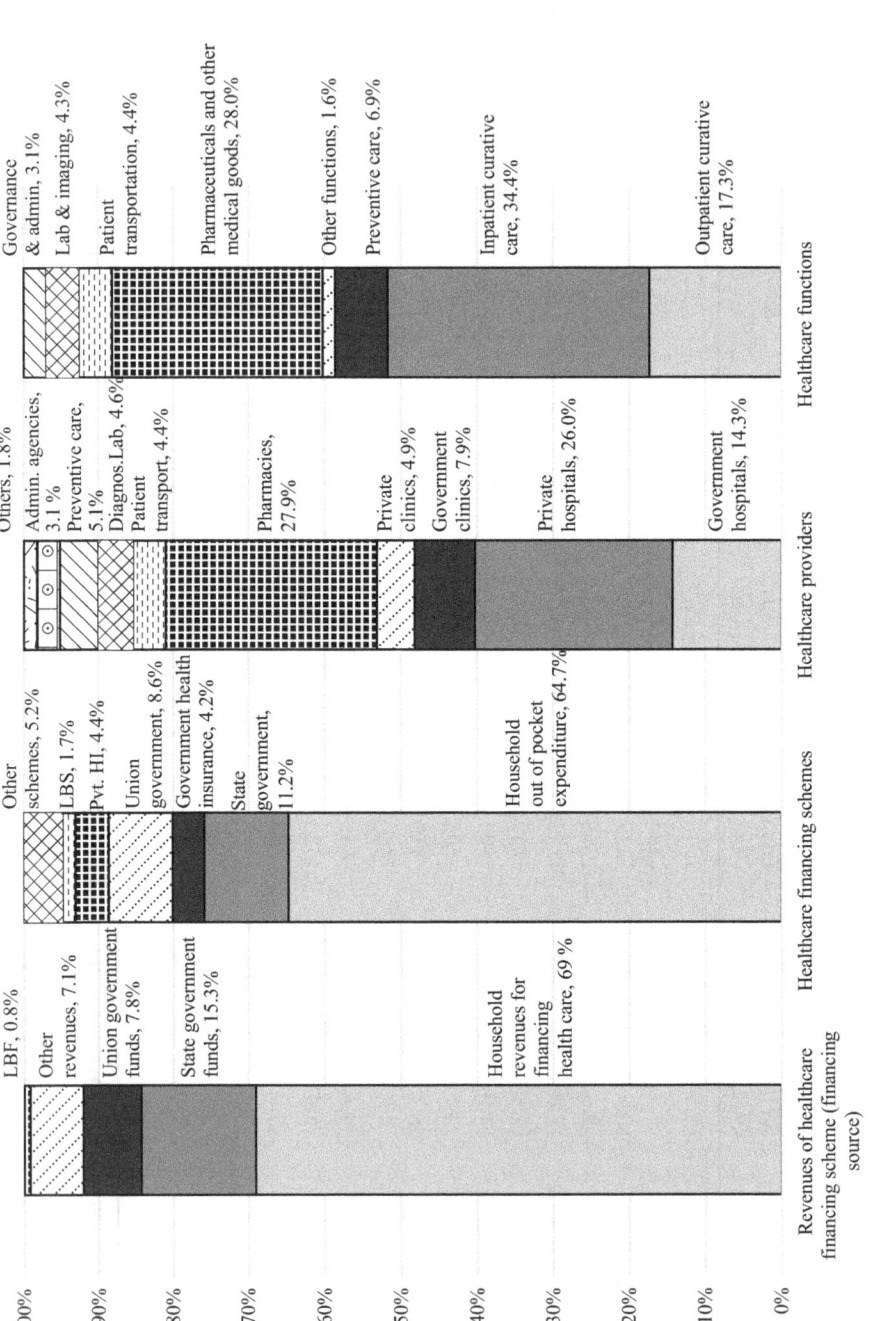

Figure 2.1 Distribution of current health expenditure by sources: 2015–2016

Note: LBS-Local Bodies Schemes; HI-Health Insurance; LBF- Local Bodies Funds

Source: NHA (2018). National Health Account for India: 2015–2016, NHSRC, Ministry of Health and Family Welfare, Government of India

reported that out of the total health expenditure (THE; 3.84% of GDP, and Rs. 4116 in per capita terms), a major share is financed through households' OOP expenditures. Government health expenditure constitutes 30.6% of THE, which accounts to be 1.18% of GDP and Rs. 1261 in per capita terms (NHA, 2018). Given the three-tier federal structure of government within the total government health spending, share of state governments constitutes around 64% while union government share is 35%. The share of spending of local governments – which were envisioned the delegation and devolution of some health-related functions under 73rd and 74th Constitutional Amendments 1992–1993 – remained almost negligible (Figure 2.1), indicating state governments have the predominant responsibility of health. The contribution of firm, NGOs, insurance and external sources is also very marginal (Figure 2.1).

Of the total health expenditure, the current health expenditure is accounted to be around 93.7% (Rs. 4,95,190 crores), whereas capital expenditures constitute a meagre share of around 6.3% and Rs. 33,294 crores (NHA, 2018).

Health policies and expenditure priorities

To understand the political economy of state priority in the healthcare sector, this section assesses the investment commitments made over time and how much effort is put forwards to achieve them. The commitments made under any specific health policy are highlighted. The historical account suggests that commitments of resource allocations and provisioning of health services made under various health policy reforms have always left much to be desired in India. The foremost committee on health in India (Bhore Committee, 1946) was constituted to recommend the design and structure of healthcare provisioning in the country. The committee put forth a principle that 'nobody should be denied access to health services for his inability to pay' (17) and recommended to achieve certain numbers of population-based health centres. The focus was given to achieve primary healthcare. The minimum level of health infrastructure recommended by the committee was not fulfilled even in 2010 (Table 2.2) and thereafter. After independence, the government of India formulated a plan under the Community Development Programme (1951–1955) to achieve a certain level of health infrastructure, particularly the number of primary health centres (PHCs) on population basis. India also could not achieve these targets. In order to improve the quality of existing facilities, the government specified that the existing health centres must achieve Indian Public Health Standard (IPHS). As per guidelines, there should be 4–6 beds and 30 beds in each primary health centre (PHC) and community health centre (CHC), respectively. As per Rural Health Statistics 2019, a shortfall of 81.8% specialists was recorded in CHCs in the year 2019. Only 3.39% of the sub-centres, 8.26% of PHCs and 21.8% of CHCs in the rural areas were found to be functioning as per IPHS norms in 2019 (RHS, 2019).

Table 2.2 Commitments vs. achievements in the health sector since independence

Policy initiatives	Commitments	Achievements/Failure/ Existing position		Remarks
Bhore Committee, 1946	PHC with 75 beds for each 10,000–20,000 population	% of PHC with 4–6 beds (as on March 2010) = 59.3% % of CHC with at least 30 beds (as on 2010) = 71.8%		Not achieved
Community Development Programme, 1951–1955	One PHC per one lakh population	One PHC per 5.5 lakh population, 2010		Not achieved
Alma Ata Deceleration, 1978 and First National Health Policy, 1983: Strategy to achieve 'Health for All by the year 2000 AD'	To achieve the target of	Existed in 2000–2001	Requirement in 2000–2001	
	One PHC per 20, 000–30,000 population	22842	24717	Not achieved
	One Sub-Centre per 30,00–50,00 population	137311	148303	Not achieved
	One Community Health Centre per 100,000 population	3043	7415	Not achieved
Second National Health Policy, 2002	Increase government spending in healthcare from existing 0.9% to 2% by 2010	Public expenditure on health recorded 1.09% of GDP in 2010		Not achieved
	Increase share of central grants to constitute states at least 25% of total health spending by 2010	Centre:State ratio in 2010 was 29:71		Achieved
	Increase the state sector health spending from 5.5% to 7% of the budget by 2005 and to 8% of the budget by 2010	State spending on health out of total expenditure was recorded 6.67% in 2005 and about 6.41% in 2010		Not achieved
National Rural Health Mission, 2005	Increase the government spending in healthcare (from its around 1% level) to 2–3% of GDP by 2012, the end of the Eleventh Five-Year Plan	It is recorded around 1.2% of GDP at the end of the Eleventh Five-Year Plan and even after adding water supply and sanitation expenditure it hovered around 1.6% of GDP, which is less than the commitment		Not achieved

Policy initiatives	Commitments	Achievements/Failure/ Existing position	Remarks
National Commission of Macroeconomic and Health of India, 2005	NCMH estimated the required level of resource that need to be spend by every state governments to meet the adequate level of basic health services, with the targets to be achieved by the end of 2009–2010	The prescribed level of health spending could not be achieved by most of the state governments	Not achieved by many states
Universal Health Coverage Report, 2012	Increase spending by the government (centre and states) in healthcare from its current level 1.2% of GDP to 2.5% by the end of the Twelfth Five-Year plan, and to at least 3% of GDP by 2022	Past experiences show that the health expenditure 2.5% of GDP looks unrealistic to achieve	Not achieved
National Health Policy, 2017	Increase the government expenditure on health from the existing 1.15% of GDP to 2.5 % of GDP by 2025	The recent growth rate in health expenditure of the government reveals that it would be difficult to achieve the 2.5% target by 2025	Seems unfeasible to achieve

Source: Author's calculations, using relevant policy documents

India constituted almost 25 different committees on health within the first three decades following independence: the Sokhey Sub-committee (1948), Mudaliar (1962), Chaddha (1963), Kartar Singh (1974) and Srivastava (1975) Committees and Indian Council of Medical Research–Indian Council of Social Science Research (ICMR–ICSSR 1980) Joint Panel, to name a few (see Chapter 1 for details). All these committees stressed the need for a more integrated and comprehensive (preventive and curative) health system in the public sector with a three-tiered structure: primary, secondary and tertiary. In between, the world's first health assembly held at Alma Ata in 1978 defined health as a fundamental human right and adopted a holistic framework to achieve 'health for all by 2000' through provisioning of comprehensive primary healthcare. This sought for greater public investment to ensure *health for all* within the specific time.

India became signatory to the Alma Ata Declaration and encompasses most of its tenets (such as equity, universalism, comprehensiveness, government responsibility, and community participation) in health policy, but India took around three and a half decades after independence to bring out its First National Health Policy (NHP) in 1983. This casts doubt on the seriousness of the government towards the healthcare sector. The policy was committed to achieve *health for all* by 2000. This would be achieved through the introduction of certain number of CHCs, PHCs and SCs across the most remote parts of the country. The prescribed amounts of physical and human health infrastructure could not be achieved by 2000 – the year by which these should have been achieved. The existing numbers of CHCs, PHCs and SCs in the year 2001 were lagging significantly behind the required provision of health infrastructure (Table 2.2). Despite these unsatisfactory achievements, the Indian public healthcare system was known to be quite effective until the mid-1980s, before the economic reforms. This was a time (between late 1970s and early 1980s) when budgetary allocation towards the healthcare sector showed an increasing trend. The public health system was noticed to be effective in later periods of the mid-1980s in some Indian states such as Andhra Pradesh, Karnataka and Kerala (Bhatia et al., 2006). Health services, even though of low quality and uneven in reach, were available to the poor.

The idea of *health for all* through primary healthcare was complemented by the National Population Policy 2000 and India's Second National Health Policy 2002. Second NHP, however, acknowledged that the performance of Indian healthcare system was not satisfactory and that 13 of the 17 goals of the previous policy had not been met. The health system was critiqued on several grounds: a) the limitations of a system centred around vertical programmes; b) rural-urban disparities in health infrastructure; c) shortage of medical personnel at health centres and doctors at hospitals; d) absence of legislation on minimum standards for private medical establishments; e) decline in the number of drugs on the price-controlled list from more than 300 in the 1970s to around 30 in the mid-1980s; and f) absence of mechanisms for decentralisation of service delivery, etc. In order to address some of these issues, Second NHP made commitment to increase public spending in health from the existing 0.9% to 2% of GDP, and state spending from the existing 5.5% level to 8% as a share of their total budgetary spending (Table 2.2), which were to be achieved by 2010. The evaluation suggests that government health spending in the year 2010 was about 1.09% of GDP and share of state spending was 6.85% out of their total budgetary spending, indicating less spending than the commitments.

In order to bridge rural-urban health outcome gaps and achieve some of the Millennium Development Goals for health, the government of India launched the National Rural Health Mission (NRHM) in 2005. The mission stressed the improvement in service delivery through strengthening the public healthcare system. The mission committed to increase the government spending on health about 2–3% of GDP by 2012, the end of the Eleventh Five-Year Plan. Government health spending, however, recorded around 1.2% of GDP at the end of the 11th FYP (Table 2.2). This indicates that the targets of NRHM were not achieved. Even after adding the expenditure on complementary (water supply and sanitation) services, the total spending hovered around 1.6% of GDP, an amount less than the committed level. This reflects less priority on the healthcare sector by both centre and state governments. This resulted in shortage of physical and human healthcare infrastructure, along with poor availability of medicines and equipment in hospitals and healthcare centres – that is, even the services that were assumed to be there in the public healthcare system were not available in practice.

In 2005, the National Commission of Macro-Economics and Health of India (NCMH, 2005) estimated the required level of resources that needed to be spend by every state government to meet the adequate level of basic health services in the country. The targets were to be achieved by the end of 2009–2010. An analysis of the required level of resources against the actual allocation of resources shows that most of the state governments could not achieve the prescribed level of healthcare spending. There exists a significant gap between required resources and actual spending in most of the states, except for Himachal Pradesh (Figure 2.2). The gaps in resource requirements surprisingly recorded much higher in some of the richer states like Punjab and Maharashtra, as well as in some low-income states like Bihar, Orissa, Rajasthan and Uttar Pradesh (Figure 2.2).

In 2011, India constituted a high-level expert group on universal health coverage. The HLEG proposed to increase government spending (central

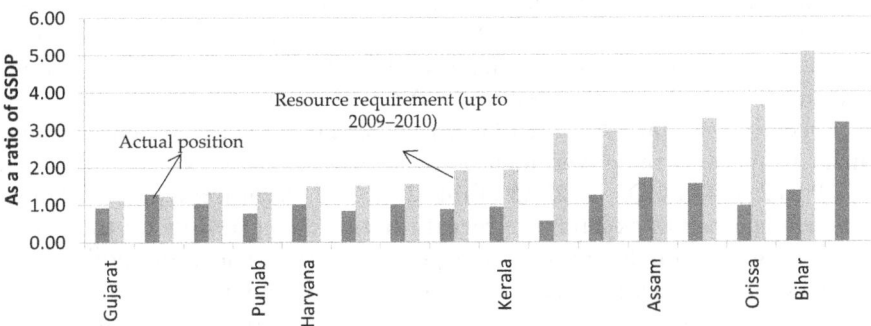

Figure 2.2 State-level resource requirements vs. actual spending on health

Note: The actual expenditure includes medical, public health, family welfare, water supply, sanitation and NRHM allocation for the year 2010–2011. For resource requirements see NCMH background paper, Rao, M.G., Choudhury and Anand M. 2005, pp. 297–317.

Source: NRHM expenditure statements, Government of India; https://nhm.gov.in/images/pdf/FMG/FMG_RTI/Central_Release_State_Share_Credited_and_Expenditure_undr_NHM.pdf

Table 2.3 Projected levels and share of public-private and centre-state health expenditures, 2011–2022

	2011–2012	2016–2017	2021–2022
Total health expenditure as % of GDP*	4.5	4.5	4.5
Total public expenditure on health as % of GDP	1.2	2.5	3.0
Total private expenditure on health as % of GDP	3.3	2.1	1.5
Per Capita Total Health Expenditure (Rs. 2009–2010 prices)	2500	3725	5175
Per capita private spending (Rs. 2009–2010 prices)	1825	1750	1725
Per capita public spending (Rs. 2009–2010 prices)	675	1975	3450
– Of which share of Centre (1/3) (Rs.)	225	658	1150
– Of which share of States (2/3) (Rs.)	450	1317	2300

Source: GOI (2011: 100, 106)

and state combined) in healthcare from the current level of 1.2% of GDP to at least 2.5% by the end of the Twelfth Five-Year Plan and to at least 3% of GDP by 2022. In per capita terms, the public expenditure on health (at 2009–2010 prices) should reach from Rs. 675 in 2011–2012 to Rs. 1975 in 2016–2017. The National Health Profile 2019 reflects that per capita public expenditure on health in nominal terms has gone up from Rs. 621 in 2009–2010 to Rs. 1657 in 2017–2018; if one take it in real terms, per capita spending would be little less. The projection of per capita public health expenditure is Rs. 3450 by 2021–2022 (Table 2.3), given the COVID-19 pandemic situation, it seems difficult to achieve, as a major share of public expenditure has been allocated for COVID-19 vaccination.

Recently, the Third National Health Policy 2017 made a similar commitment to increase the government expenditure from the existing 1.15% of GDP to 2.5% of GDP by 2025 (Table 2.2). The recent trend growth rate in government health expenditure reveals that it would be difficult to achieve 2.5% target within the specified time period by 2025. The health policy commitments in the past have largely been abortive in India.

Overall assessment around commitments made and achievements reflects that despite having high burden of preventable morbidities and mortalities in many of the states, no major lesson has been learnt. The PHC approach never been implemented effectively. The goal of *health for all by 2000* could not be met and spending commitments have never been fulfilled. To date, the government almost failed in serving and delivering adequate levels of health services to the population.

Historical trends and macroeconomic conditions

A historical pattern of health spending under different macroeconomic conditions and health policy changes scenarios that the country might have gone through is presented here. Besides the several health policy changes, India has gone through different changes at macroeconomic fronts over time, which might have influenced central and state finances and its composition in a big way. The Figure 2.3 has documented the adverse macroeconomic conditions started in early 1990 (the period of early stress of fiscal crisis), the fiscal crisis in 1991 and the international financial crisis in 2008–2009, along with the other policies changes like the 5th and 6th Pay Commissions recommendations in 1996–1997, 2006–2007 and 2016–2017, and Fiscal Responsibility and Budget Management Act, 2003, etc.

Analysis from the period of 1972–2020 shows high fluctuations in state spending (Figure 2.3). During the period, expenditure on water supply and sanitation (WSS) up to 1984–1985 was clubbed with the expenditure heads of medical and public health and family welfare (HFW). The expenditure on these components during the time therefore shows an increasing trend

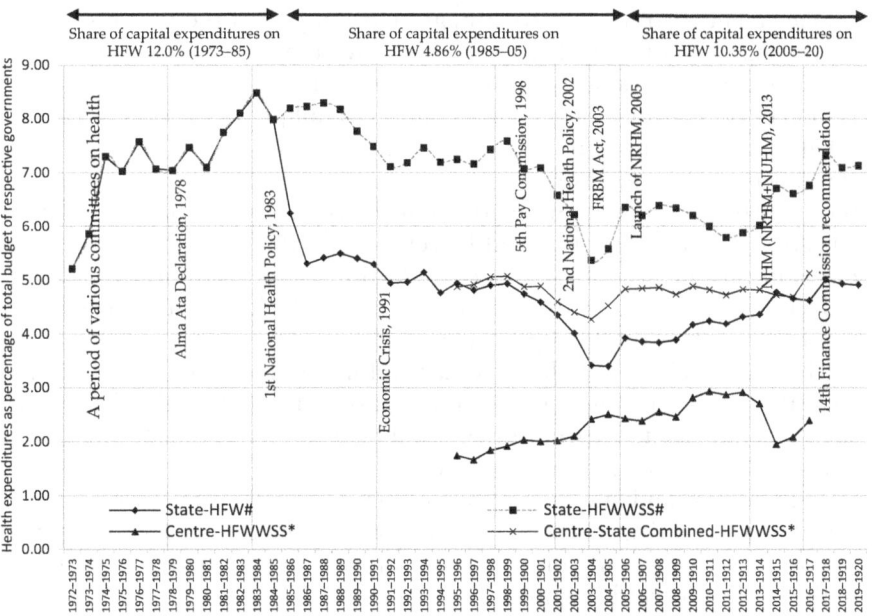

Figure 2.3 Trends in central and state government expenditures on health under policy changes scenario

Note: HFW – expenditure on medical, public health and family welfare; HFWSS – expenditure on HFW and water supply and sanitation; state – indicates 31 states of India

Source: Designed using data from (#) ww.epwrfits.in and (*) Indian Public Finance Statistics, Department of Economics Affair, Government of India, various years, https://dea.gov.in/indian-public-finance-statistics

from 5.2% to 8.5% of the total budget. After separating out of HFW expenditure from total HFW and WSS since 1985–1986, budgetary expenditure on HFW was reported to be low. Different macroeconomic conditions and other policy changes have also impacted the state spending on health (HFW) significantly (Figure 2.3). Health spending affect adversely even before the fiscal crises start in 1991 and it hit badly during the crisis time. The share of state health spending in total budgetary spending of all state governments dropped at least by 1 percentage point between 1985–1986 to 1990–1991. It dropped over 1 percentage point since then to the Second National Health Policy announcement in 2002. The share of states' health spending observed a slight increase when recommendations of the 5th Pay Commission were implemented in 1998. This can be attributed largely to increases in the salary bill due to the implementation of the pay commission, as the share of capital expenditure during the period was one of the lowest in all states.

The Second National Health Policy 2002 imposed on the states that budgetary spending on health should increase to 8% by 2010. However, no sign of increment in state health expenditure is observed after the policy announcement. The implementation of Fiscal Responsibility and Budget Management (FRBM) Act 2003 might have impacted the health spending. As the mandate of FRBM Act was to enforce the central and state governments to reduce fiscal and revenue deficits, either by increasing the revenue resources or by restructuring or curtailing overall public expenditures (GOI, 2004). Given the federal nature of the country, increase in tax revenue of states was not so easy, as most of the revenue generating capacities are with the central government. State governments therefore adopted expenditure curtailment route, and the health sector bears the brunt of this expenditure curtailment process. The average healthcare expenditures of all states reduced significantly at that particular time, which was recorded around 3.4% out of their total budget (Figure 2.3).

The year 2005 came with a landmark reform in the health sector when the central government implemented the National Rural Health Mission. The share of state health expenditure in total budgetary spending of both centre and state government increased thereafter. Again, a little setback is observed in both central and states' healthcare spending at the time of the international financial crisis in 2008–2009; otherwise, one can see a consistent rise in government spending on health out of their overall budgetary spending in the NRHM period (Figure 2.3).

These changes influenced the central and state finances and health spending differently. The share of central government spending on health as a ratio of total budgetary spending of central government increased marginal from 1.74% in 1991 to 2.91% in 2014 (Figure 2.3). One significant twist in central health spending is observed after 2014–2015 and 2015–2016 and in some later years in state health spending, as well. This is largely due to change in the fiscal transfer strategy from the centre to states.

In India, due to the federal structure nature of the country, the central government has a history to devolve central funds to state governments through the Finance Commission, erstwhile Planning Commission and Central Ministries. The funds are generally transferred in tied (through Centrally Sponsored Schemes; CSS) and untied form. The transfer through Finance Commission has always been a major source of federal devolution to states (FFC, 2015). Unlike the earlier 13th FC, the 14th FC recommended to increase the share of states in total divisible pool of taxes from 32% to 42%, which is largely untied in nature. The objective behind increase in untied funds was to give more autonomy to states to decide their expenditure priorities. The tied transfers are generally conditional, which requires 'matching contribution' from states (Choudhury et al., 2016: 2). Such grant would remain unutilised if a state – due to low fiscal flexibility – is unable to provide matching funds. Therefore, FFC recommended increase in the devolution of untied resource to states. A review of few studies (Choudhury et al., 2016) reflected a net gain in overall state resources following the FFC recommendations. Thus, this policy change (FC recommendation) has accorded more fiscal autonomy to states. However, it is quite likely that the centre withdrew some of the transfers from CSS specifically to reduce overall tied transfers to states.

Following the FC recommendations, states have been accorded more autonomy. How states have prioritised their expenditure towards the healthcare sector and what has been the trend in central spending on health sector is reported in Figure 2.3. The share of central government expenditure on healthcare out of its total budget expenditure decreased following the recommendation of FFC, an indication of reduction in tied funds allocation to states towards health sector. Another study has also observed a negative growth in central tied nature of transfer to health from 13th FC to 14th FC in both EAG and non-EAG states of India (Das, 2016). Since the states had more fiscal autonomy and therefore were supposed to give more priority to health sector, their expenditures on health out of their total budgetary spending declined marginally after the FFC recommendations. There is a slight rise in state spending towards health in the first year of FFC, but a sharp dip in central health spending from 2014 onwards (Figure 2.3).

The priority of individual states to health sector at the times of the Second (2002) and Third (2017) National Health Policies reflects that health expenditures in most of the states as a percentage of their total budgets increased. However, West Bengal and Jharkhand showed no incremental growth (Figure 2.4). The HFS shows higher increments in allocation of public funds to the healthcare sector than the non-HFS. Some of the high-income states like Punjab, Maharashtra and Haryana show a marginal increment in health budget. The state health spending as a ratio of GSDP of the state show an interesting picture. The share of state health spending in GSDP increased in HFS, while no increment in case of Non-HFS. Their expenditure rather declined marginally. The increment in health expenditure as a ratio of GSDP is observed in most of the HFS like Uttar Pradesh, Rajasthan,

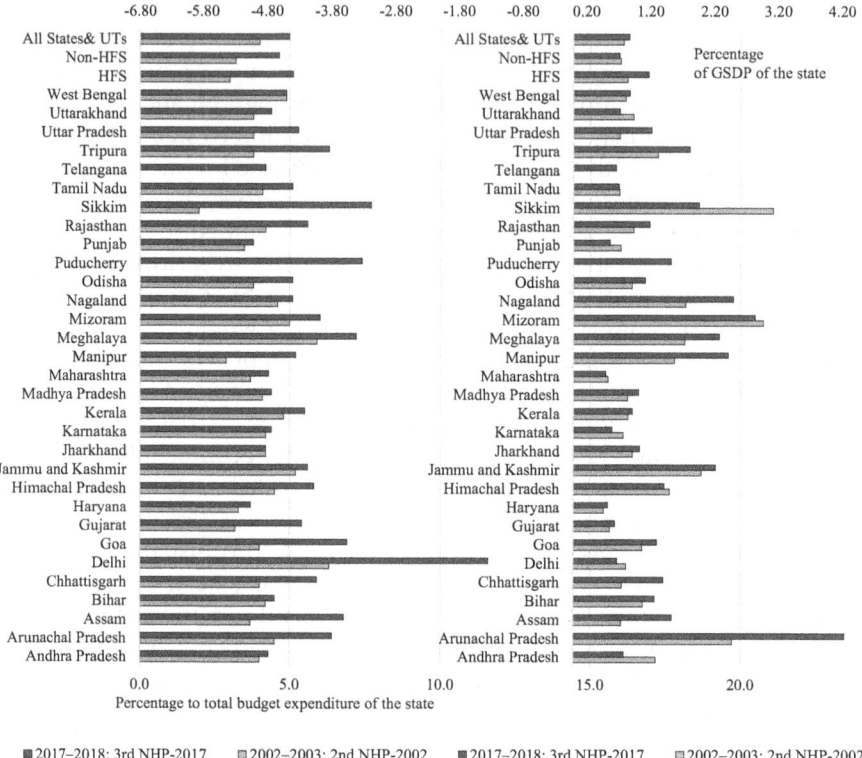

Figure 2.4 Healthcare spending of states during two National Health Policy years
Source: Designed using data from ww.epwrfits.in

Orissa, Chhatisgarh, Bihar, Assam and Madhya Pradesh, while it declined in Uttrakhand. Most of the Northeast states observed a higher increment. Amongst the non-HFS, states like Tamil Nadu, Maharashtra, Karnataka, Andhara Pradesh and Delhi experienced a decline in health expenditure as percentage of GSDP. Delhi observed the highest increment in health expenditure out of their total budget, while it experienced a decline as percentage of GSDP (Figure 2.4).

Variation in health expenditure

There is a wide variation in per capita health spending of individual states, indicating varied priorities by individual states. The variation in per capita health expenditure across major (HFS plus non-HFS) states of India increased from a coefficient value of 47% in the first sub-period 1872–1883 to 52.4% before the year of NHRM implementation. In the first five years

Table 2.4 Variation in real per capita public expenditure on health (in rupees)

	1985–1986 to 1996–1997	1997–1998 to 2004–2005	2005–06 to 2014–2015	2015–2016 to 2018–2019
HFS	0.22	0.22	0.39	0.34
Non-HFS	0.42	0.44	0.39	0.41
HFS plus non-HFS	0.43	0.47	0.45	0.41
Northeast states	0.58	0.44	0.38	0.39
All states	0.79	0.72	0.74	0.67

Source: Estimated using data from epwrfits

Note: The government expenditure on medical, public health and family welfare is reported. Real expenditure is at 2004–2005 Prices. State-wise per capita expenditure is reported in Table 2.4.

of NRHM, the value of coefficient of variation even further increased to 57.4%; however, it declined later (Table 2.4). The variation in per capita health spending of HFS remained lower than the spending of non-HFS. The variation in health expenditure themselves is not a matter for concern if it is due to the exercising of preferences by individual states on the basis of prevailing disease or mortality rate in the state. It became problematic when states with high prevalence of disease and/or mortality rates and states with high level of income allocate few funds in the healthcare sector. Given the high shortage of physical and human infrastructure compared to the required level, spending less on healthcare means these states are shying away from fulfilling the commitment of 'Right to Health' for their citizens and have placed a low priority on healthcare.

The average per capita health spending of HFS found to be lower than the spending of non-HFS. In the recent period, per capita health spending of Rajasthan, Chhatisgarh and Uttrakhand were higher than some of the high-income states like Maharashtra, Gujarat and Haryana (Table 2.5). Health spending remained consistently low in some low-income states like Bihar, Jharkhand, Madhya Pradesh and Uttar Pradesh, even after providing more fiscal autonomy to them under the FFC period, while some other low-income states like Orissa, Chhatisgarh, Rajasthan and Uttrakhand accorded high priority to healthcare after FFC recommendations.

The per capita health expenditure of individual states reflects that they dealt differently with the health sector under different macroeconomic and health policy–changing scenarios. The impact of these changes on government health expenditure is captured by dividing the whole study period into different sub-periods. The growth rates in per capita health expenditure across states in different sub-periods is estimated using an appropriate technique called 'kinked exponential growth model' technique.[2]

The growth rate in per capita state health spending suggests that in first sub-period (1972–1973 to 1984–1985), most of the states recorded positive growth rate except for Northeast states. In the second sub-period (1985–1986 to 1996–1997), except for three states (Bihar, Delhi and Karnataka) many states recorded negative growth rate in per capita health expenditure. A significantly negative growth rate is observed in Haryana, Maharashatra and Northeast states (Table 2.5). The fiscal stringency induced by the structural adjustment measures affected the central as well as state finances in a big way. The thrust of structural adjustment programmes (SAP) was to reduce the budgetary deficit either by increasing the revenue resources or curtailing the expenditure, or both. Because of limited base of tax structure, the revenue of both central and state governments did not show any increment and showed similar trends in revenue/GDP ratio during the period. It reveals from the literature that most of the Indian states gone through the process of expenditure curtailment (Breman and Shelton, 2001). The impact of curtailing in total expenditure of state governments resulted in adverse impact in the healthcare sector.

Between 1997–1998 and 2004–2005, the growth rate in healthcare expenditure is recorded as negative in nine states, while only three states recorded positive significant growth in health expenditure. This period experienced the implementation of 5th Pay Commission, second generation economic reforms, and announcement of the Second National Health Policy (GOI, 2002), which must have positive impact on health expenditure, but at the same time, FRBM Act 2003 must have imposed adverse repercussions on expenditures. The lower growth in health expenditures is witnessed in most of the high fiscal stringency (identified through fiscal deficit to GDP ratio) states (RBI, 2016). That is, deteriorating fiscal position of a particularly state destabilised the spending pattern in India. Some of the Indian states, even during fiscal stringency, continued its commitment to improve the overall health of the society by maintaining positive growth rates in health expenditure.

In the fourth phase (2005–2006 to 2014–2015), the government of India initiated healthcare sector reform and introduced the National Rural Health Mission in 2005. NRHM made a commitment to increase in public spending to 2–3% of GDP. Growth rates estimation in health expenditure show that in the first decade of NRHM implementation, most of the Indian states recorded positive and significant growth rates. NRHM initiatives have been able to maintain positive growth rates in healthcare expenditures, but achievement of 2–3% of GDP spending on healthcare remained a distance dream. In the last four years of NRHM/NHM (2015–16 to 2018–2019), a period when states were accorded high fiscal autonomy through FFC recommendations, most state recorded positive and significant growth rate, but Delhi, Punjab, Uttar Pradesh and Uttrakhand recorded positive but insignificant growth, while Andhra Pradesh recorded negative growth in per capita health expenditure (Table 2.5).

Table 2.5 Change in growth of real per capita public expenditure on health

State	Kink exponential growth estimation						Real PC expenditure			
	1972–1973 to 1984–1985	1985–1986 to 1996–1997	1997–1998 to 2004–2005	2005–2006 to 2014–2015	2015–2016 to 2018–2019	Adj. R2	1985–1986 to 1996–1997	1997–1998 to 2004–2005	2005–2006 to 2014–2015	2015–2016 to 2018–2019
Andhra Pradesh	0.059***	-0.017**	0.103***	0.084***	-0.043	0.960	138	203	507	587
Assam	0.050***	-0.013*	0.002	0.086***	0.171***	0.900	165	145	252	505
Bihar	0.057***	0.027**	-0.021	0.044***	0.182***	0.860	89	100	118	232
Chhattisgarh			0.150**	0.090***	0.207**	0.9		122	232	606
Delhi		0.265***	0.062***	0.072***	0.050	0.96	256	451	894	1307
Gujarat	0.037**	0.008	0.003	0.114***	0.095*	0.92	149	196	336	664
Haryana	0.056***	-0.032***	0.031**	0.077***	0.142***	0.9	160	174	278	563
Himachal Pradesh	0.070***	-0.012	0.046**	0.047**	0.151**	0.86	398	536	767	1392
Jharkhand			0.144*	0.008	0.211**	0.68		157	249	432
Karnataka	0.030***	0.024***	0.021**	0.068***	0.117***	0.96	150	214	311	559
Kerala	0.019**	0.004	0.043***	0.083***	0.113**	0.95	192	255	458	824
Madhya Pradesh	0.036**	0.015	-0.002	0.075***	0.104**	0.85	114	150	202	375
Maharashtra	0.044***	-0.022***	0.036***	0.070***	0.102**	0.92	168	189	293	498
Orissa	0.042***	-0.015*	0.014	0.076***	0.223***	0.89	123	144	200	539
Punjab	0.052***	0.002	0.009	0.049***	0.076**	0.89	206	260	301	479

(Continued)

Table 2.5 (Continued)

State	Kink exponential growth estimation						Real PC expenditure			
	1972–1973 to 1984–1985	1985–1986 to 1996–1997	1997–1998 to 2004–2005	2005–2006 to 2014–2015	2015–2016 to 2018–2019	Adj. R2	1985–1986 to 1996–1997	1997–1998 to 2004–2005	2005–2006 to 2014–2015	2015–2016 to 2018–2019
Rajasthan	0.025*	-0.002	0.016	0.071***	0.154**	0.81	146	184	260	546
Tamil Nadu	0.041***	0.007	0.019	0.088***	0.080**	0.92	172	219	370	652
Telangana					0.180**	0.96			355	634
Uttar Pradesh	0.076**	-0.038*	0.078**	0.069**	0.091	0.62	105	108	214	353
Uttarakhand			0.352***	0.063**	0.093	0.88		196	475	795
West Bengal	0.034***	0.010	0.031**	0.051***	0.085**	0.92	128	182	238	393
HFS	0.049***	-0.002	0.024**	0.069***	0.142***	0.94	113	130	209	406
Non-HFS	0.042***	-0.0019	0.040***	0.075***	0.083***	0.97	161	216	356	609
HFS + non-HFS	0.044***	0.00022	0.031***	0.072***	0.107***	0.96	138	175	282	510
NE States	0.038***	0.00021	0.047**	0.081***	0.065	0.9	312	448	801	1301
All States	0.045***	0.001	0.032***	0.073***	0.107***	0.96	140	178	288	520

Note: ***; ** and * are 1%, 5%, and 10% significance level; real income at 2004–2005 prices

Source: See Table 2.3

Conclusion

Healthcare spending in India is generally dominated by private out-of-pocket spending, with 70% share in total health spending. India's public expenditure on healthcare found lower than the international standard of spending, as well as lower than required levels of resources that could provide basic health facility across states. Since independence, India has made several commitments to spend high amounts on healthcare, but analysis shows that neither the centre nor the state governments have ever fulfilled their commitment of spending. This has resulted in inadequate provision of health facility in the country, e.g., bed-to-population ratio in India is 1:1000 compared to the 7:1000 in developed nations.

Health expenditure affected highly under adverse macroeconomic conditions. The growth in per capita health expenditure in some low-income states remained negative. Some of the high-income states could also not maintain significant positive growth rate in health expenditures. There also exists a high interstate variable in per capita health expenditures in India.

Overall, India and its states are found to be shying away from fulfilling their constitutional commitment of a 'right to health' for their citizens. Given the low level and the declining and fluctuating behaviour of health expenditure of almost four decades, it is not surprising that the healthcare sector performance in improving healthcare outcomes is not satisfactory. The failing nature of better healthcare outcomes, however, can easily be reversed with a high level of public funds allocation, for which India needs to double or triple its health spending from its existing level.

Notes

1 This chapter draws some inferences and data from my previously published work originally published in S. K. Hooda. 2015. Government Spending on Health in India: Some Hopes and Fears of Policy Changes. *Journal of Health Management*, Vol. 17, No. 4, pp. 458–486 Copyright 2015 © Indian Institute of Health Management Research. All rights reserved. Reproduced with the permission of the copyright holders and the publishers, SAGE Publications India Pvt. Ltd, New Delhi.
2 The kinked exponential growth model (Boyce, 1986) is preferred over the conventional growth rate estimation models primarily because this model makes use of entire time series information even while estimating the growth rate for a sub-period in the series. That is, this model allows us to incorporate all phases at a time simultaneously without distorting the statistical properties of the coefficients. An estimation of growth rate for a sub-period, which includes few observations, provides misleading result. This model removes such types of inconsistency by taking exponential trend function. The advantage of this model is that sample size and degrees of freedom can be increased by combining the sub-periods. The increase in sample size is definitely an advantage when the sub-period estimation is based on a very small sample size. The generalized kinked exponential growth model is as follows:

$$Y_t = \alpha_1 + \beta_1(D_{1t} + \sum_{j=2}^{m} D_j k_1) + \beta_2(D_{2t} - \sum_{j=2}^{m} D_j k_1 + \sum_{j=3}^{m} D_j k_2) + \ldots$$

$$+\beta_i(D_{it} - \sum_{j=i}^{m} D_j k_{i-1} + \sum_{j=i+1}^{m} D_j k_i) + \ldots + \beta_m(D_{mt} - D_m k_{m-1}) + u_t$$

Where, Y = real per capita public expenditure on health; D = dummies; K = break (kink) points; B's = coefficients of estimated growth rate; j = is jth sub period; Dj = is a dummy variable which takes the value 1 in the jth sub-period and 0 otherwise and t is renormalized so that it is 0 at the break point. This model can be estimated using ordinary least square (OLS) method with one, two and multiple kink points. The growth rates in health expenditure are estimated by taking into account the sub-periods.

References

Arrow, K. J. 1963. Uncertainty and the Welfare Economics of Medical Care. *The American Economic Review*, Vol. 53, No. 5, pp. 941–973.

Bhatia, M. R., Yesudian, C. A. K., Gorter, A., and Thankappan, K. R. 2006. Demand Side Financing for Reproductive and Child Health Services in India. *Economic & Political Weekly*, Vol. 41, No. 3, pp. 279–284.

Bhore Committee. 1946. *The Report of Health Survey and Development Committee 1946*, vols.2. Government of India, Kolkata. https://www.nhp. gov.in/bhore-committee-1946_pg

Boyce, J. K. 1986. Kinked Exponential Models for Growth Rate Estimation. *Oxford Bulletin of Economics and Statistics*, Vol. 48, No. 4, pp. 385–391.

Breman, A., and Shelton, C. 2001. *Structure Adjustment and Health: A Literature Review of the Debate, Its Role-players and Presented Empirical Evidence*. Working Paper WG6:6, June. Commission on Macroeconomics and Health (CMH). http://library.cphs.chula.ac.th/Ebooks/HealthCareFinancing/WorkingPaper_WG6/WG6_6.pdf

Choudhury, M., Mohanty, R. K., and Dubey, J. D. 2016. *Impact of the Recommendations of the 14th FC: Central Transfers and Social Sector Expenditures in the 1st Year*. National Institute of Public Finance and Policy WP No. 183, November, New Delhi.

Das, N. 2016. *Federal Fiscal Transfers on Health: Implications of Fourteenth Finance Commission Recommendations at Subnational Level*. MPRA Paper No. 79627. https://mpra.ub.uni-muenchen.de/79627/

Fourteenth Finance Commission. 2015. *Report of the Fourteenth Finance Commission, 2015*. Fourteenth Finance Commission of India, Government of India.

Getzen, T. E. 2004. *Health Economics: Fundamentals and Flow of Funds*, 2nd Edition (Chapter 14). John Wiley & Sons, Inc., pp. 284–303. https://bcs.wiley.com/he-bcs/Books?action=index&itemId=0471432032&itemTypeId=BKS&bcsId=2364

Government of India. n.d. *NRHM Expenditure Statement*. Ministry of Health and Family Welfare, Government of India, New Delhi.

Government of India. 2002. *Second National Health Policy 2002*. Ministry of Health and Family Welfare Government of India, New Delhi.

Government of India. 2004. *Report of the Task Force on Implementation of the Fiscal Responsibility and Budget Management Act, 2003*. Ministry of Finance, Government of India, New Delhi.

Government of India. 2005. *Mission documents of the National Rural Health Mission (NRHM)*. Government of India, New Delhi. http://mohfw.nic.in/nrhm.html

Government of India. 2011. *High Level Expert Group Report on Universal Health Coverage for India*. Planning Commission, Government of India (GOI), New Delhi. http://planningcommission.nic.in/reports/genrep/rep_uhc2111.pdf

Government of India. 2016. *National Health and Family Survey-4*. Ministry of Health and Family Welfare, Government of India, New Delhi.

Government of India. 2017. Third *National Health Policy 2017*. Ministry of Health and Family Welfare Government of India, New Delhi.

Government of India. 2019. *National Health Profile*. Ministry of Health and Family Welfare Government of India, New Delhi.

Hall, J. J., and Taylor, R. 2003, January. Health for all beyond 2000: The Demise of the Alma Ata Declaration and Primary Health Care in Developing Countries. *Medical Journal Australia*, Vol. 178, No. 1, pp. 17–20.

HDR. 2018, 2019. *Human Development Report*. United Nation Development Programmes. http://hdr.undp.org/en/global-reports

HRS. 2006–19. *Bulletin on Rural Health Statistics in India*. Ministry of Health and Family Welfare. Government of India, New Delhi.

Kethineni, V. 1991, October 19. Political Economy of State Intervention in Health Care. *Economic and Political Weekly*, Vol. 26, No. 42, pp. 2427–2433.

Misra, R., Chatterjee, R., and Rao, K. S. 2003. *India Health Report*. Oxford University Press, New Delhi.

NCMH. 2005. *Report of the National Commission on Macroeconomics and Health*. National Commission on Macroeconomics and Health (NCMH), Ministry of Health & Family Welfare, Government of India, New Delhi.

NFHS. 2016. *National Family and Health Survey (NFHS-4) 2015–16*. International Institute for Population Sciences (IIPS), Mumbai, India and International Classification of Functioning, Disability and Health (ICF).

NHA. 2018. *National Health Account for India: 2015–16*. Ministry of Health and Family Welfare, Government of India, New Delhi.

Reserve Bank of India. 2016. *RBI State Finance: A Study of State Budget*. Reserve Bank of India, Ministry of Finance, Government of India, New Delhi.

RHS. 2019. *Bulletin on Rural Health Statistics (RHS) in India*. Ministry of Health and Family Welfare. Government of India, New Delhi.

Savedoff, W. D. 2007. What Should a Country Spend on Health Care? *Health Affairs*, Vol. 26, No. 4.

Sen, A. 1999. *Development as Freedom*. Oxford University Press, Oxford.

UNICEF. 2019. *The State of the World's Children 2019: Children, Food and Nutrition, Growing Well in a Changing World Children, Food and Nutrition*, UNICEF, South Asia. https://www.unicef.org/media/60841/file/SOWC-2019-SA.pdf

Wagstaff, A., and van Doorslaer, E. 2003. Catastrophe and Impoverishment in Paying for Health Care: With Application to Vietnam 1992–1998. *Health Economics*, Vol. 12, No. 11, pp. 921–934.

WHO. 2019. *World Health Statistics 2019: Monitoring Health for the Sustainable Development Goals*. World Health Organisation, Geneva. https://apps.who.int/iris/bitstream/handle/10665/324835/9789241565707-eng.pdf

WHS. 2015–2020. *World Health* Statistics, *The Global Health Observatory*, World Health Organisation. Geneva. https://www.who.int/data/gho/publications/world-health-statistics

World Bank. 1993. *World Development Report: Investing in Health*. World Bank, Washington, DC.

3 Rejuvenating the public system
Efficiency in resource allocation[1]

Publicly provided healthcare continues to be relevant and expand in India. The system, however, is confronted with several challenges relating to inefficiency in resource utilisation and under-utilisation of services. The Ninth Five-Year Plan (GoI, 1997–2002) of India for the first time acknowledged that inefficiencies and problems exist in the healthcare system. This includes persistent gaps in personnel and infrastructure, especially at the primary healthcare level; sub-optimal functioning of existing infrastructure and poor referral services; not having appropriate personnel, diagnostic and therapeutic services and drugs in plethora of government, voluntary and private hospitals; massive interstate and interdistrict differences in performance reflected in health and demographic indices; poor availability and utilisation of services in most needy states and districts; sub-optimal intersectoral coordination; challenges of addressing emerging the dual burden of communicable and non-communicable diseases; escalating costs of healthcare; and ever widening gaps between what is possible and what the individual or the country can afford. Due to shortages of physical and human health infrastructure, along with poor availability of medicines and equipment in hospitals and healthcare centres, even the services that are assumed to be there in the public healthcare system were not available in practice. The high mismatch and shortage of drugs availability, non-availability of equipment and deteriorating buildings considerably limit the effectiveness of health staffs, rendering the system inefficient (Varatharajan, 1999). Such types of inaccessibility, inappropriateness and inefficiency result in under-utilisation of public healthcare services. Inefficient care generally leads to unnecessarily poor outcomes for the patients directly affected, measured either in terms of their health improvement, or in their broader satisfaction with the health system (Cylus et al., 2016). That is, inefficiency somewhere in the health system is likely to deny treatments and health improvement to patients who would otherwise have received treatment if resources had been better used. Such types of inefficiencies in economic terminology signifies wasted resources and mean a lot for a developing country like India where states have low fiscal space. The fiscal stress also forces the states to think innovatively for increasing the accountability and efficiency of resources use. Scholars have

DOI: 10.4324/9781032108438-4

pointed out that elimination of inefficiency from any system acts as a source of finance as it is equivalent to an increase in the resource availability (Berman and Sakai, 1989). Thus, improving the efficiency of the healthcare system is important.

The inefficiencies have been observed in all health systems of the world (WHO, 2000; Berwick and Hackbarth, 2012) relating to various dimensions like the failures of care delivery, failures of care coordination, overtreatment, administrative complexity, price failures, fraud and abuse, etc. (Cylus et al., 2016). The efficiency carries varied connotations. In economic terminology, efficiency means absence of waste, or using the resources as effectively as possible to satisfy people's needs and desires. It encompasses at least three components: allocative efficiency, technical efficiency and X-efficiency. Allocative efficiency is related with the reorganisation of the inputs (Samuelson and Nordhaus, 1992), technical efficiency is concerned with the technical relationship of the inputs with the outputs (Button and Weyman-Jones, 1992) and X-efficiency is often related to managerial aspects (Leibenstein, 1966). That is, allocative efficiency occurs when the resources are devoted to right activities while technical efficiency is achieved when a given health intervention or outcome is obtained through few resources (WHO, 1999). The misallocation of resources among the primary, secondary and tertiary sectors gives rise to allocative inefficiency, whereas an imbalance between installed capacity and recurrent resources to maintain it leads to technical inefficiency. Over-centralisation of financial decision making and underfunding of specific complementary inputs (such as drugs) can be cited as examples of X-inefficiency (Varatharajan, 1999).

As reported, the Ninth FYP envisions the expansion and improvement of health services to meet the increasing healthcare needs of the population. It felt the need to improve the health status of the population by optimising coverage and quality of care by identifying and rectifying the critical gaps in infrastructure, personnel, equipment, essential diagnostic and drugs. It envisions that the efforts will be directed to improve functional efficiency of the healthcare system through: a) creation of a functional, reliable health management information system and training and deployment of health personnel with requisite professional competence; b) multiprofessional education to promote teamwork; c) skill upgradation of all categories of health personnel, as a part of structured continuing education; d) improving operational efficiency through health services research; e) increasing awareness of the community through health education; f) increasing accountability and responsiveness to health needs of the people by increasing utilisation of the Panchayati Raj institutions in local planning and monitoring; and g) making use of available local and community resources so that operational efficiency and quality of services improve and the services are made more responsive to user's needs' (GoI, 1997–2002: 139). All of these dimensions are related to improving the efficiency of public system, though specific targets were not set. In 2005, the government of India launched the National Rural Health

Mission, which proposed several new provisions to improve the efficiency of the rural healthcare system, viz. identification of focused states (where mortality and morbidity indicators are worse) to allocate more resources in priority setting states and areas with an objective to reduce the variation in public health expenditure between high-focused and non–high-focused (mostly high-income) states categories. It came up with a plan to give priority to rural primary healthcare, especially to reduce the health outcome gaps between rural and urban. It made distinction of tied and untied funds in resource allocation. The allocation of untied funds to SC, PHC and CHC levels, especially to give them autonomy and meet the immediate/recurring requirements (medicine, water, equipment, etc.) of the centre, rerouting the allocation of central funds. The central allocated funds, which earlier passed through state budget/treasury route under the new provision of NRHM, now will bypass the state budget. These funds will be routed through state implementing agencies. The diversion in fund allocation from treasury route to society route was made to increase resource utilisation without any delay. However, after 2015, the fund again started transferring through treasury route, but the treasury would have to transfer money to the State Health Society within a minimum period of 15 days. Next is the engaging of local Panchayats and local agents in health policy design, creation and implementation. All these components focus on improving the performance and efficiency of the rural healthcare system. In 2013, the government of India also launched its Urban Health Mission to strengthen primary healthcare in urban India. Both of these together were subsumed and are now called the National Health Mission (NHM) that focus on strengthening and improving the efficiency of the PHC system of both rural and urban India. This chapter provides a discussion around these issues. There are two major inquiries in health policy circle literature: 'is it possible to improve population health by holding the current level of expenditure constant?'; and is it possible to improve the health-to-expenditure ratio by adjusting the allocation of additional resources?. These are discussed briefly in the chapter, along with a mention of functional efficiency, which can be termed as sources of inefficiencies.

Sources of inefficiency

In India, state governments are primarily responsible for healthcare provision. They therefore exercise major control over health-related functions, finance and administration, and other responsibilities. The efficiency therefore needs to be judged at the state level, especially whether a state has been able to develop an efficient healthcare system or any lack of one. One way of understanding the perspective of efficiency at the state level is to compare or match it with the so-called ideal healthcare system. By ideal system, here we mean a system that can fulfil the 'norm' prescribed by the national level policy guidelines. As we know, India has a three-tier structure of a healthcare system. The healthcare system, particularly at the primary care level, is prescribed on the basis of population norms. A system that fulfils this normative requirement can be visualised as an 'ideal' system which depends on size of the population of a state. The norms-based infrastructure in India consists of different layers of healthcare units: health sub-centres (SCs), primary health centres (PHCs), community health centres (CHCs), dispensaries (DSs), sub-divisional hospitals (SDHs) and district hospitals (DHs). The first three sets of healthcare units are primarily responsible for addressing the primary (preventive care, maternal and child care) healthcare needs of rural population, whereas remaining are located in the urban areas. Typically, one SC covers a population of 3000 in difficult/tribal or hilly areas and 5000 population in plain areas, and a requirement of one male and one female health worker is set for its proper functioning. On the other hand, one PHC would serve a population of 20,000 difficult/tribal and hilly areas, or 30,000 population in plain areas, and should consist of 4–6 indoor/observation beds. The PHCs are considered as a major cornerstone of rural health services, as it is the first port of a qualified doctor of the public sector in rural areas for the sick and those who directly report or referred from sub-centres for curative, preventive and promotive healthcare (GOI, 2006). Normally, one PHC acts as a referral unit for six sub-centres and refers outpatients and cases to CHC and higher order public hospitals located at sub-district and district levels. As per guidelines, there would be one CHC at 1,00,000–1,20,000 population with 30 beds and a sets of specialists and technical staffs consisting of physician, surgeon, obstetrician and gynaecologist, and a paediatrician. The design of primary healthcare in the rural area is such that a CHC is superimposed on a set of four PHCs and 24 SCs, indicating a set of 29 (1 + 4 + 24) units expected to cater to the healthcare needs of 1,00,000–1,20,000 rural population. Fulfilling the standards are the main driver for continuous improvements in quality. That is, the performance of individual centres and the collective system can be assessed against the set of standards. In order to provide an optimal level of quality healthcare, a set of standards is being recommended for these centres called Indian Public Health Standards (IPHS). The IPHS have been prepared keeping in view the resources available with respect to functional requirement of the centre with minimum standards such as building personnel, instruments and equipment, drugs and other facilities, etc. The overall objective of IPHS, which came into effect in 2006, is to provide healthcare that is quality oriented and sensitive to the needs of the community (IPHS, 2006). These standards would help monitor and improve the functioning of the centres. This section, in order to understand the functional efficiency of primary healthcare system, briefly describes the minimum normative prescription fulfilled by the states.

It is important to note that the normative framework in general involves public provisioning of healthcare services around three main parameters: buildings (physical infrastructure), personnel and materials (Varatharajan, 1999). The physical infrastructure is one of the key components of any health system, as it indicative of the existence of a unit, and the remaining two (personnel and materials) are built around this key component. Even if it is so, a proper balance among all of them is the necessary condition to achieve the desired level of efficiency of any system. This (physical) normative framework is structured in a way that can sufficiently meet the health/ morbidity requirement of the population. Any failure to establish such normative healthcare units can be termed as an imperfect system. A glance at the current status of normative public healthcare in the country reflects that around 1,58,417 SCs, 25,743 PHCs, 5624 CHCs, 1234 sub-divisional hospitals (SDHs) and 756 district hospitals (DH) were functioning in 2018–2019 (RHS, 2019). A quick view towards the normative numbers reflect a shortfall of 32,900 SCs (18%), 6430 PHCs (22%) and 2188 CHCs (30%) across the country (RHS, 2019). Ideally, there should have been a set of 28 SCs and PHCs in combination per one CHC to serve 100,000–120,000 population. In practice, most of the states fall short in fulfilling this combination. It ranges between one and ten in around seven states and between ten and 20 in 14 states (Table 3.1). More than half of the listed states in Table 3.1 could not fulfil the population based norm for SCs and PHCs, and more than two-third of stats could not fulfil normative requirement for establishing the CHCs.

Table 3.1 Normative functioning of primacy healthcare units across states of India

Number of SCs, PHCs per CHC in 2019 (in number)	1–10%	OR, TN, KL, RJ, HR, AS, GJ
	10–20%	HP, MH, UK, CH, UP, PN, MP, GA, WB, JK, AP, TL, KR, BR
Average rural population covered by SCs by range of population (2019)	< 3000	GA, KL
	3000–5000	HP, KR, GJ, UK, CH, TN, RJ, AP
	5000–7000	OR, MP, MH, PN, WB, AS, HR
	> 7000	JR, UP, BR
Average rural population covered by PHCs by range of population (2019)	10000–20000	HP, KL, KR, GA
	20000–30000	RJ, GJ, TN, CH, OR, UK
	30000–40000	AP, AS, TL, MH
	40000–50000	PN, HR, MP
	> 50000	BR, UP, WB, JK
Average rural population covered by CHC by range of population –(2019)	< 100000	KL, HP, GA, TN
	100000–200000	GJ, RJ, UK, CH, HR, JK, AS, MH, WB, MP, KR
	200000–500000	PN, TR, AP, UP
	> 500000	BR

Source: Rural Health Statistics (2019)

Note: AP – Andhra Pradesh, AS – Assam, BR – Bihar, CH – Chhattisgarh, DL – Delhi, GA – Goa, GJ – Gujarat, HR – Haryana, HP – Himachal Pradesh, JR – Jharkhand; KR – Karnataka, KL – Kerala, MP – Madhya Pradesh, MH – Maharashtra, OR – Odisha, PN – Punjab, RJ – Rajasthan, TN – Tamil Nadu, TL – Telangana, UP – Uttar Pradesh, WB – West Bengal

There is a high inadequacy of building of the centres – in the case of SCs, around 25% of the existing SCs do not have their own proper building for their regular functioning, and the range of inadequacy of own building in some cases goes up to 75% (Table 3.2). Varatharajan (1999) indicated that sub-centres are the first contact points for rural population and absence of basic structure even for those units that are described as 'functional' sends a wrong signal to the public regarding the character of public sector. The resulting lack of confidence sows the first seed of under-utilisation of services.

The next important component of better functioning of the healthcare system is the personnel at the facility. The SCs are the primary units of the healthcare system in India. As per norm, there should be one female health worker (ANM) and one male health worker (multipurpose health worker; MPHW) at a sub-centre. The shortfall of female health workers at these centres is currently low (around 3%), but around 62% of SCs do not have male health workers. This bias gives an impression that the SCs would provide care to female population, and that it, by design, excludes the second half (male) population for service access, as there is a low chance that male patients will report to female staff, particularly for family planning issues and in some cases for other types of care. The situation of health personnel at PHCs level is even more worrisome (RHS, 2019). Only around 5.9% of the PHCs found to be functioning with four-plus doctors, and only 31% of them have a female doctor. Around 10% of the PHCs function without a doctor and 38.4% and 24% of them, respectively, do not have a lab technician or a pharmacist. The personnel situation at the CHCs level is also not rosy. Around 82% of the CHCs do not have a combination of all four specialists consisting of surgeons, OB/GY, physicians and paediatricians, which should have been there as per the norms, and 59% of them do not have radiographers. The shortage of physicians is the major issue in most of the statistics (Table 3.2). There is a considerable variation across the states in the personnel situation. It is more grave in low-income states and in some of the high-income states (Table 3.2). The existing 1234 sub-divisional hospitals were found to be functioning with 13,750 doctors and 36,909 paramedical staffs as against the sanctioned position of 22,891 doctors and 52,526 paramedical staffs in March 2019. Similarly, the number of functioning district hospitals (DHs) was 756 hospitals in 2019, with 24,676 doctors and 85,194 paramedical staff as against the sanctioned position of 28,545 doctors and 90,969 paramedical staffs (RHS, 2019). On the one side, the burden of morbidity (communicable and non-communicable diseases) is increasing in the country, but at the same pace, the numbers of centres is not increasing, though there is significant change after the implementation of NRHM in 2005 (RHS, 2019).

The situation of the availability of equipment and other materials, including medicine, at most of the different layers of health centre is also grave; however, in some cases, proper data around these variables are not readily available. For supplying of medicine, there is hardly any norm set. However, under the recently launched Ayushman Bharat, the existing SCs are to be upgraded into health and wellness centres (HWCs). Of the total, about 7269

Table 3.2 Shortfall of human and other health infrastructure at primary care units in India

	Percentage of PHCs with or without doctor and other health personal-2019					Shortfall of health personnel at CHCs – 2019 (in percent)		Shortfall at SC – 2019 (in percent)	
	With 4+ doctors	Without doctor	Without lab tech	Without pharmacist	With female doctor	Of all four specialists (surgeons, OB/GY, physicians and paediatricians)	Of radiographers	Shortfall of health workers (male)	Percentage of SCs do not have own building
Andhra Pradesh	9.7					57.7	71.4	60.3	76.2
Assam			18.8	6.7	na	80.8	49.2	33.7	12.8
Bihar	29.7	45.2	17.3	13.6	10.5	86.3	99.3	87.5	43.3
Chhattisgarh			39.1	21.5	10.8	91.0	5.3	25.8	19.3
Gujarat		9.5	14.8	17.3	79.7	91.9	47.0	13.4	7.1
Haryana		22.3	49.7	35.2	29.0	96.7	53.0	37.7	35.9
Himachal Pradesh		18.6	63.8	25.8	28.6	98.6	72.4	68.5	24.0
Jharkhand		3.4	49.3	57.1	27.1	90.4	65.5	58.1	40.8
Karnataka		10.2	24.8	26.0	22.5	41.3	15.7	65.1	19.0
Kerala	0.1		47.5	0.0	67.8	96.1	100.0	36.8	20.8
Madhya Pradesh	1.8	25.4	59.4	38.2	12.2	91.6	30.7	61.2	26.6
Maharashtra	0.1	1.0	20.5	10.1	28.2	66.7	70.6	49.6	7.5
Odisha		25.4	68.3	40.6	104.8	84.4	82.5	51.3	28.3
Punjab		5.1	162.0	31.6	224.1	73.9	Surpl.	54.0	35.4
Rajasthan	1.1	9.1	20.8	76.0	5.7	80.1	39.9	97.4	21.2
Tamil Nadu	39.0		28.8	30.0	128.8	88.4	76.1	73.7	24.5
Uttarakhand	1.2	25.1	81.5	2.9	27.6	89.9	92.5	94.9	29.4
Uttar Pradesh	1.3		62.9	0.0	16.0	82.2	87.9	68.6	0.0
West Bengal	0.2	13.4	68.6	12.2	12.5	94.9	47.7	80.4	24.5
All India	5.9		38.4	23.9	31.0	81.8	59.0	62.3	24.7

Source: Rural Health Statistics (2019); more than 100% indicates the overstaffing or surplus

HWCs and SCs were found to have a regular supply of drugs for common ailments (RHS, 2019). Only about 9393 PHCs were found to be operational as 24/7 facilities in 2019 (RHS, 2019). The healthcare system of India not only faces a shortage of absolute number of centres/hospitals, but also a relative shortage of other inputs. There is no uniform pattern of shortfall of personnel and materials across facilities; some have serious shortfalls relative to the others. This could be attributed to the pattern of resource allocation towards the health sector across different service classifications.

If we look at the principle on which the health system was devised that 'nobody should be denied access the care for his inability to pay' and state would take the prime responsibility to treat them. This gives a narrative that effectively the objective of public healthcare system was to treat all type of ailments, but given the high mismatch between the existing facilities, how much the state could have delivered is summarised in Figure 3.1.

The public system seems to be effective at least to address a majority of morbidity (as inpatient) care in the 80. Around 60% of inpatient care demand is met by the public health system in 1986–1987. Even in late 80, the system was not so effectively delivering care for outpatient care ailment, as only around 22.5% ailments as outpatient received care from public system. However, there is a rise in outpatient services utilisation from public system after the implementation of NRHM/NHM with a significant rise in rural area. For instance, a major derive/initiative was undertaken in the NRHM for improving the institutional delivery of child, especially in the public system. We observed encouraging results towards securing high institutional delivery of child from public facility. It almost increased from 18% in 2004 to 69% in 2018–2019 (Figure 3.1). The system appeared to deliver more care to poorest segment of the society, as institutional delivery of child in public facility recorded one of the highest (74.4%) for the poorest. Similar impact are observed for urban area as well (Figure 3.1).

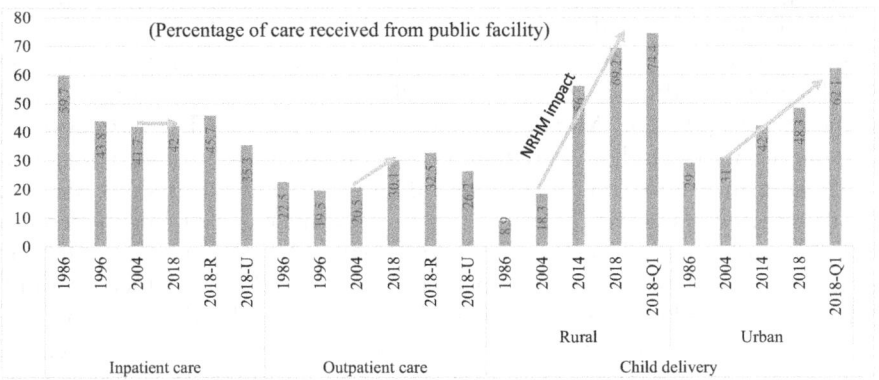

Figure 3.1 Public health system contribution in service delivery
Source: NFHS various rounds and NSS 75th round on Health 2018–2019

The health system seems to be performing well in some cases, while not in many other cases. For instance, more than 40% of the outpatient morbidity demand is treated by the single doctor or a small clinic, which is a major challenges. NFHS-4 data reported that more than half (55%) of households in India do not generally seek healthcare from the public sector, with a highest percentage in Uttar Pradesh (80%) and Bihar (78%), and lowest in Tripura (9%). The most commonly reported reason for not using government health facilities at the national level is the poor quality of care (48%), followed by 'no nearby government facility' (45%) and 'long waiting time at government facilities' (41%) as the most common reasons reported by the households that do not generally use government facilities. In addition to these reasons, around two-thirds (67%) of women reported at least one problem in accessing healthcare when they are sick. One-fourth of women cite money as a problem, 30% cite the distance to a health facility, 27% cite having to take transport as a problem, 37% of women report concerns that no female health provider is available, 45% of women report concern that no provider is available and 46% say that no drugs are available at facility. Most of these dimensions are the reflection of health system inefficiency which might have arisen due to underfunding of health sector or misallocation of existing resources towards the sector. The underfunding problems have already been reported in the previous chapter; the following section is devoted to report the allocation patterns and the need for restructuring of existing public funding, if any. This would be indicative towards the allocative efficiency of resources within the health system. Thereafter, a detailed analysis is provided of initiatives undertaken under the NRHM/NHM relating to improving the resource use efficiency.

Resource allocation pattern: services and sectoral classification

The allocation pattern of public funds speaks clearly about how the services are delivered in the country. Under the efficiency literature, it is well documented that the resource allocation may distort the health outcomes if the public health policies are not well targeted in order to improve specific targets (Hu and Mendoza, 2010; GoI, 2002–07). The allocation of resources, particularly towards high-tech equipment or advanced hospitals, may have little effect on public health if morbidity indicators show the need for increased resources for primary care. Any mismatch or low/inadequate allocation of public funds on medicine, material, supplies and equipment limit the health staff to perform better (NCMH, 2005). Allocated funds may yield little benefit if complementary services are lacking, e.g. roads or transportation services to hospitals and clinics and easy access to water and sanitation[2] (Wagstaff, 2002a, 2002b; Deolalikar, 2004). The allocation of funds towards water supply and sanitation (which is preventive in nature) generally have salubrious impact on both short-term and long-term healthy life in developing and poor countries and regions compared to the expenditure on medical, public health and family welfare (which are of both curative and preventive nature). Any concentration of health facilities in urban areas while facilities are missing from rural areas compels rural residents to travel longer distances than their urban counterparts to avail themselves of a health facility (Mahal and Fan, 2012). The rural residents many a time either postpone the care due to their low income (Shiva Kumar, 2005) or have to spend a higher share of their incomes on health and transportation. For this reason not only do the rural poor face the double burden of poverty and ill health, the financial burden of ill health can push even the non-poor into poverty (Hooda, 2017). The biased provision of health services can be one of the reasons of persistence of the rural-urban gap in health outcomes (like mortality, morbidity, undernourishment and burden of diseases are high in rural areas and twice as high among poorer segment of the society), which has even widened over time.[3] Thus, along with the size that is presented in the previous chapter, allocation patterns of public funds within the health sector also affects health outcomes (Breman and Shelton, 2001; Gumber, 1997; Ensor et.al., 2003). This section is therefore devoted to finding out the scope, if any, of change the composition and restructuring of public health spending.

Expenditures on medical, public health and family welfare are generally categorised as health expenditures in India, while expenditures on drinking water supply and sanitation receive less attention. The former is categorised as direct and the latter as indirect expenditure on health. These expenditure categories have some profound implications for service provision, as well as outcomes of the healthcare sector with advantages over the others. No doubt, direct health expenditure categories involve both curative as well as preventive components.[4] The expenditure on water supply, sanitation and nutrition sometimes even can have a more salubrious impact on the healthy life of the population, both the long term as well as in the short term, in cases of waterborne diseases and when mortalities due to undernourishment are high. The government expenditure on both direct and indirect health activities is reported to be around 1.55% of GDP in 2017–2018 BE (IPFS, 2018). The expenditure on direct health activities was 1.02% of GDP in 2015–2016 (NHPI, 2019).

The share of expenditure on direct health components at all Indian states level is recorded at over two-thirds of the total direct and indirect health expenditure of the states. The share of indirect health expenditure remained less than one-third. The share of expenditure on indirect health activities has declined over time on average, from 34.7% in 1995–2004 to 30.9% in 2015–2019. The National Rural Health Mission in 2005 for the first time identified the category of high-focused states (HFS; Bihar, Chhatisgarh, Jharkhand, Madhya Pradesh, Orissa, Rajasthan and Uttar Pradesh), based on high mortality and diseases burden, and others as non-HFS. The expenditure analysis by these categories shows that HFS spend a high amount on indirect health activities as compared to the non-HFS. The share of spending, however, in both the category of states is declining over time (Table 3.3). The

Table 3.3 Compositional distribution of health expenditure of states, 1995–2019

Compositional distribution (in %)		All states			HFS			Non-HFS		
		1995–2004	2005–2014	2015–2019	1995–2004	2005–2014	2015–2019	1995–2004	2005–2014	2015–2019
Direct and Indirect health spending	MPHFW – direct	65.3	67.3	69.1	64.0	66.5	66.3	69.1	70.5	72.4
	WSS – indirect	34.7	32.7	30.9	36.0	33.5	33.7	30.9	29.5	27.6
MPH and FW	MPH	84.5	86.4	85.5	80.9	84.0	82.6	85.8	87.1	86.3
	FW	15.5	13.6	14.5	19.1	16.0	17.4	14.2	12.9	13.7
MPH and FW	MPH – revenue	80.4	76.5	74.9	76.9	71.5	71.0	82.5	80.0	76.8
	MPH – capital	4.1	10.0	10.6	4.0	12.4	11.6	3.3	7.1	9.5
	FW – revenue	15.2	13.4	14.3	18.7	16.0	17.2	14.0	12.6	13.4
	FW – capital	0.3	0.2	0.2	0.4	0.0	0.2	0.2	0.3	0.3
MPHFW and WSS	Revenue	86.6	78.2	79.4	87.5	76.4	75.9	88.9	80.9	82.3
	Capital	13.4	21.8	20.6	12.5	23.6	24.1	11.1	19.1	17.7
WSS	Revenue	70.0	54.0	57.4	73.2	54.3	51.8	73.0	52.8	61.3
	Capital	30.0	46.0	42.6	26.8	45.7	48.2	27.0	47.2	38.7

Source: Estimated using data from Finance Accounts of the states and epwrfits; and https://main.mohfw.gov.in/sites/default/files/HEALTH%20SECTOR%20FINANCING%20BY%20CENTRE%20AND%20STATEs.pdf

Note: # – Total expenditure on health includes medical, public health, family welfare (HFW) and water supply, sanitation and nutrition (WSS)

low and declining trends of spending on water and sanitation facilities can result in low access to safe drinking water and sanitation facilities, which in turn results in high prevalence of waterborne disease, malaria, etc. (NCMH, 2005). It is quite likely that, in many states, as a result of low levels of education, a significant number of cases of disease and affliction may have been unreported or undetected, and/or not given importance to be reported until the last stages. The expenditure on preventive items should not only be sustained, but also be augmented.

Expenditures on direct health services, which comprises medical, public health and family welfare, is largely concentrated on medical and public health services and growing steadily over the period. This category is generally categorised as curative services in nature. As a corollary, the expenditure on family welfare, which largely comprised of preventive interventions and reproductive and child health, have been declining steadily in composition terms at all state levels, as well as in HFS and non-HFS states categories (Table 3.3). The share of family welfare in HFS, however, remained higher as compared to their non-HFS counterparts. It is imperative to note that that the expenditure on total direct health activities as a ratio of GSDP is declining over the period, except for a recent period (Hooda, 2015).

An important distinction of government health expenditure is the expenditure on revenue accounts (also known as current expenditure) and capital accounts. The current expenditure is recurring in nature consisting of wages and salaries of staffing and consumable of daily routine etc., while capital expenditure is considered as a sole determinant of creating physical infrastructure and buying equipment, etc. The state government spending on (direct) health is current in nature which leaves meagre resources for capital accounts to purchase drugs, medicines and equipment, and create infrastructure. From 1972–1985, the share of capital account at all state average was 12.0%. Its share, though, declined thereafter and remained stagnant at 4.86% for almost next 20 years from 1985–2005. Its share increased after the implementation of NRHM in 2005 and recorded around on average 10.35% from 2005–2020 for all Indian states (Chapter 2). The share of capital expenditure for high-focused states during these three phases was 12.23% between 1972–1985, 5.24% between 1985–2005 and 12.27% 2005–2020, and around 8.63%, 3.69% and 8.15%, respectively, for non-HFS. This indicates that HFS has prioritised their spending towards capital accounts after the NRHM intervention. The composition of health expenditure into revenue and capital accounts for different periods is provided in Table 3.3, which also reveals the same trends.

The capital expenditure on health in composition terms increased after the implementation of NRHM in 2005, but the share remained very low. The low share of capital expenditure is not problematic if state(s) already have achieved proscribed norms of health infrastructure and there is no shortfall of medical equipment in the existing health centres and hospitals. In reality, most Indian states are facing a shortfall in achieving the proscribed norms of health standards, as discussed previously. The low as well as declining share of capital expenditures further influence the recurring (revenue) expenditure to grow, as until and unless new health centres are created, new staffs will not be appointed. Such situations may affect the effectiveness of public expenditures to perform.

The budget classifies government expenditure into plan and non-plan components. By definition, plan expenditure is considered as an important component for the welfare of society. It arises out of schemes freshly introduced in an ongoing Five-Year Plan (FYP) period. In the same period, non-plan expenditure arises out of schemes carried forward from previous FYP periods. Non-plan expenditures generally support the old schemes of the governments, and plan expenditures are the new schemes because new schemes add to the economy's productive capacity as the old schemes did in the past. The plan expenditure reflects the government's investment in enhancing the economy's productive capacity. Expenditures on plan components, in compositional terms, increased from 38% in 2004–2005 to 53% in 2016–2017. This is a healthy indication to add in the productive capacity of the state in health sector. The increment in plan components remained more noticeable in middle-income states compared to the low-income and high-income states (for details, see Hooda, 2015). This may mean that middle-income states have launched more new health schemes compared to the low-income and high-income states, and have added in productive capacities. The plan and non-plan classification provided a robust analysis of the government's initiatives towards new health schemes; such distinctions in the budget, however, have been stopped in the recent past, from 2016–2017 onwards.

In practice, it may be difficult to segregate government health expenditures into an alternative classification like expenditures on preventive or curative functions. Similarly, it is extremely difficult to analyse the expenses directed towards primary, secondary, tertiary or quaternary care, from a strictly budget-based analysis. The National Health Account (NHA 2018), however, provided a detailed segregation of the total current health expenditure of both the government and private sectors taken together. Around 51.7% of the current health expenditure is reported to be curative in nature, which attributed towards both inpatient (34.4%) and outpatient (17.3%) services, followed by prescribed medicines (27.5%) and a marginal share on preventive care (6.9%). The rest of the current health expenditure is reported on patient transportation, laboratory and imaging services, therapeutic appliances, governance and health system administration, etc. If one includes the prescribed medicines, over-the-counter drugs and those provided during an inpatient, outpatient or any other event involving a contact with healthcare provider, then the share of total pharmaceutical expenditure accounted for around 35.4% of the total current health expenditure (NHA, 2018).

The classification of current health expenditure (for both public and private sectors) as primary, secondary and tertiary care note that primary care constituted around 45.1%, secondary care 35.2% and tertiary care 15.2%, while governance and supervision constitutes 3.1% of the total current health expenditure. The share of expenditure of these services in private setting noticed to be around 43% on primary, 40% on secondary and 16.2% on tertiary care services. When it comes to the classification of current health expenditure of the government sector, it turned out to be around 51.5% on primary care, 22% on secondary care, 13% on tertiary care, 10.7% on governance and supervision, and 2.8% on others services (NHA, 2018). It is important to note that the 12th Plan document of the then-Planning Commission of Government of India earmarked that under the relative proportions of primary, secondary and tertiary care spending, the state should increase and spend 70% of the total health budget on primary care. The preceding analysis reveals that the earmarking of 70% of the health budget on primary care is still nowhere close. The analysis of budget documents for some of the states for two points of time – that is, the year before starting the 12th plan (i.e., 2007–2008) and end year of 12th plan (i.e., 2011–2012) – reveals that the compositional share of primary care remained almost the same (55–56%) at both the points of time for the all-states average. The share of primary care in HFS increased slightly, while it declined marginally for non-HFS (Table 3.4). There have been ups and downs in the share of primary care in each of the states; only five states observed the increasing share of primary care. The share of tertiary care in states like Andhra Pradesh, Karnataka and Gujarat recorded increasingly high proportions; these are the states where insurance-driven models were experienced amongst the others. There is no valid empirical justification for 70% of primary care being the ideal composition (Rao, n.d.); however, if one looks at the Kerala model – which is considered as one of the best healthcare delivery models in the country and perhaps in the world – the share of primary care was recorded 75% in 2011–2012 (Table 3.4). Other states can divert attention towards that.

The regional dimensions of government health expenditure reveals that it is highly concentrated toward urban areas (Table 3.5). An analysis of budget documents before the launch of NRHM reflects that out of the total health spending, the share of urban health spending was almost three-fourths and the remaining one-fourth was rural health spending (for details, see Hooda, 2015). The share of rural in compositional terms was about 22.3% in 1995–1996 and 24.5% in 2004–2005, which slightly increased to 25.5% in 2015–2016. The share of urban spending was 36.2% in 2015–2016. If one includes the other expenditures like medical education, training, research and general expenditure, which is urban in nature),[5] it further will go up and its share will be more than double the existing share.[6] The share of rural spending recorded a high rate (about 35.7%) in low-income states compare to middle-income (about 21.4%) and high-income (15.8%) states. The classification of total direct and indirect expenditure into rural or urban shows that expenditures on rural components was high in low-income states (43%), followed by 39% and 27% in middle-income and high-income states, respectively (Hooda,

Table 3.4 Government health expenditure on primary, secondary and tertiary care, 2007–2008 to 2011–2012

| | Compositional distribution by the respective year total (%) | | | | | | | | Rs. in crore | |
| | Primary care | | Secondary care | | Tertiary, including medical education | | Others | | Total | |
	2007–2008	2011–2012	2007–2008	2011–2012	2007–2008	2011–2012	2007–2008	2011–2012	2007–2008	2011–2012
Orissa	36	44	9	9	20	19	34	28	750	1643
West Bengal	40	44	48	42	10	14	2	0	1677	4112
Maharashtra		66		4		18		12		5892
Gujarat	57	54	11	12	27	31	5	3	1617	3898
Bihar	85	68	3	7	11	23	1	3	1675	2921
Chhattisgarh	61	58	10	8	13	13	16	22	572	1390
Haryana		65		1		20		14		1466
Himachal Prad	70	61	28	19	2	19	0	1	321	820
Madhya Pradesh	62	51	10	13	18	26	11	10	1762	3501
Punjab	54	59	18	16	17	15	12	10	839	1941
Jharkhand	68	61	12	10	18	18	2	12	573	1365
Rajasthan	50	47	6	10	28	23	17	20	1858	3753
Uttrakhand	59	62	24	15	12	16	5	7	364	903
Uttar Pradesh	56	60	20	18	23	22	1	1	4151	6698
Andhra Pradesh	53	46	12	9	24	38	11	7	2859	5502
Karnataka	47	42	18	18	35	40	0	0	1972	3384
Kerala		75		14		9		1		1019
Tamil Nadu	58	54	4	4	26	25	11	17	2303	5262
HFS	60	56	12	12	20	22	8	10	22115	43233
Non-HFS	52	54	17	13	24	25	7	8	65338	160181
All states	56	55	15	13	22	24	7	9	87453	203414

Source: Based on Sujata Rao (n.d.)

Table 3.5 Regional distribution of health expenditure, 1995–2016

Regional distribution	Low-income states				Middle-income states				High-income states			
	1995–1996	2004–2005	2009–2010	2015–2016	1995–1996	2004–2005	2009–2010	2015–2016	1995–1996	2004–2005	2009–2010	2015–2016
Rural	38.7	42.8	38.5	36.7	29.8	38.8	20.6	21.3	27	27.5	18.4	19.1
Urban	26.9	29.4	30.0	31.9	38.1	32.6	38.3	38.0	29.1	27.2	39.3	37.2
Others	34.4	27.8	31.5	31.4	32.1	28.6	41.1	40.6	43.9	45.3	42.2	43.7

Source: Finance Account of the State Governments provided by Controller Auditor General (CAG), Finance Department, various states Government; Original Budget Paper, various state, Original Budget Paper, Department of Finance, State Governments; MoHFW, n.d.

2015). The share of rural health (both direct and indirect) in GSDP constituted less than 1% and nearly 1%, respectively, in urban areas in 2004–2005 (Hooda, 2015). However, the share of rural as well as urban health expenditure as percentage of GSDP shows declining trends from 1987–1988 to 2004–2005, with a more pronounced declined in rural health spending. This reveals that India is having an urban curative centric healthcare system which was inherited from colonial rule at the time of independence.

The further classification of government health expenditures in staffing (salary) and non-staffing (non-salary) categories generally called economic classifications are other important dimensions. The staffing expenses constitute the largest proportion – over 90% – of the total spending. This leaves little fund to purchase machinery, equipment, drugs, material and supplies – the non-staffing category. A high proportion of expenditure on wages and salaries – and, as a corollary, a low proportion on drugs and material supplies — is evocative of poor service delivery in terms of quality. However, it can also be argued that in principle, the first claim of the priorities of expenditure on merit goods like health should be on appropriate staffing. This may be followed by expenditure on drugs and material supplies to make the service delivery more effective. The non-staffing components, however, cannot be ignored. Historically, low levels of non-staffing in the country have probably resulted in high out-of-pocket (OOP) expenditures, particularly on the purchase of medicine and testing, of which medication purchasing constitutes around 70% within the total OOP expenditure (Hooda, 2017). A reasonable level of public spending on the purchase and distribution of medicine would have eminent importance especially to reduce the burden of medication-related OOP in the country. The state's spending towards procuring and providing free medicine is essential; states like Tamil Nadu and Kerala have started procuring and distributing medicine to the needy. Rajasthan also joined the same effort later on, and the central government recently made some efforts with the establishment of the Jan Aushadhi Kendra programme across the country.

The sectoral, service and regional classifications of health expenditures show a biased spending towards some care, services and areas as compared to their counter groups. Now one question emerges whether India needs to restructure the existing structure and pattern of healthcare spending. One argument is that the healthcare system inputs such as expenditure or other resources may be directed towards creating some outputs that are not priorities for society. For example, providing very high-cost end-of-life cancer treatments may create benefits for the individuals involved, but society may judge that the limited money available to the health system may be better spent on other interventions that create (in aggregate) larger health gains. Second, if a health system does not secure the minimum cost of medicines and other inputs, less output either in terms of quantity of patients treated or quality of care provided will be possible for a given level of expenditure. Studies have also mentioned that if a patient's medical tests are unnecessarily ordered or duplicated, there is a waste of resources and other individuals may be forced to forego needed care (Cylus et al., 2016). Such processes generate inefficiency in the system. In the Indian context, we would argue that any restructuring in the inputs should be based on the distinctive need of both rural-urban, staffing–non-staffing, preventive-curative and other components separately. Sometime, the per capita cost of serving a densely populated area may be lower, due to technological indivisibility and economics of scale, than that for a widely dispersed population. On the contrary, a densely arranged population may have greater needs either due to higher reporting of incidents or due to enhanced vulnerability from proximity to afflicted individuals. On the rural side, the low availability of private health facilities, high burden of mortality, morbidity and disease with high proportion of population enforces us to argue that every state needs to provide comprehensive public health facilities to meet the demands of rural residents at least to create more Indian Public Health Standard (IPHS) health centres which are very few (only 11%) at present (RHS, 2019). In India, health outcomes at aggregate level are lower than neighbouring developing countries and could not achieve the Millennium Development Goals targets. The gaps in rural-urban health outcomes are still high. The country also faces a shortage of physical infrastructure and human resources for health. The overall health spending in the country is lower than the required level of resources. Therefore, restructuring in health expenditure should not be done by changing the nature of existing resources allocated to health, but rather should be done through additional spending in the health sector. Rural health gets priority under NRHM, which is discussed in the following section.

Resource allocation under NHRM/NHM: efficiency of resource use

The government of India made a landmark reform in the healthcare sector to provide accessible, affordable, equitable and quality healthcare services with the launch of the National Rural Health Mission in April 2005. In order to provide accessible, affordable and quality healthcare to rural and vulnerable populations, the NRHM classified the high-mortality, largely low-income, states as empowered action group (EAG) states. These are generally known as high-focused states (HFS) and others as non–high-focused states (non-HFS) in the major state category.[7]

The mission made a commitment to increase the public health spending to '2–3% of GDP' by the end of the Eleventh Five Year-Plan (GOI, 2005). The expenditure on NRHM was an umbrella programme subsuming various centrally sponsored schemes in health and family welfare, including the Reproductive and Child Health II (RCH-II), National Disease Control Programmes for malaria, tuberculosis, kala azar, filaria, blindness and iodine deficiency, Integrated Disease Surveillance Programme, etc. This was a centrally funded programme; however, the state governments are asked to increasing their funding (along with the centre) in health. The devolution of central funds to states was based on conditionality. The states need to increase their own spending at a specified rate in tandem with increased central funding. Less than expected increase in state spending reflects their inadequate absorptive capacity to utilise central funds properly. A few new provisions were also made, such as that the central allocated funds which were earlier passed through the state budget/treasury route will bypass the state budget and will be routed through state implementing agencies. The diversions in fund allocation from treasury route to society route was made to increase the resource utilisation without any delay. The tied and untied distinction was also made in overall fund allocation. However, with the implementation of 14th finance commission recommendations in 2015–2016, the states are given more fiscal autonomy in the name of cooperative federalism, most of the tied-untied distinctions were abolished and treasury route was adopted again with some modification.

The analysis of health expenditure trends across HFS and non-HFS shows a declining trend as a ratio of GSDP in both categories states (Figure 3.2). However, expenditure in per capita terms shows increasing trends in both these categories of states (Figure 3.2). The conflict between increases in per capita spending but decreasing as a share of GSDP reveals that the responsiveness of change in health expenditure relative to GSDP is lower than the responsiveness to population. Per capita fund requirements to provide the basic health facility is higher in HFS, but the responsiveness of health expenditure to population is low (Figure 3.2). The funds allocation exclusively on NRHM components is not only increasing as percentage of GSDP, but expenditure of HFS also recorded higher as compared to the non-HFS (Figure 3.2). This reflects that NRHM funds are allocated on priority and need bases in the specified states.

The NRHM is a central sponsored programme; therefore, the central government is committed to transferring more funds in the state health sector. The release of central funds, however, many times has been noticed to be less than the commitment of spending made in the budget. The release of funds

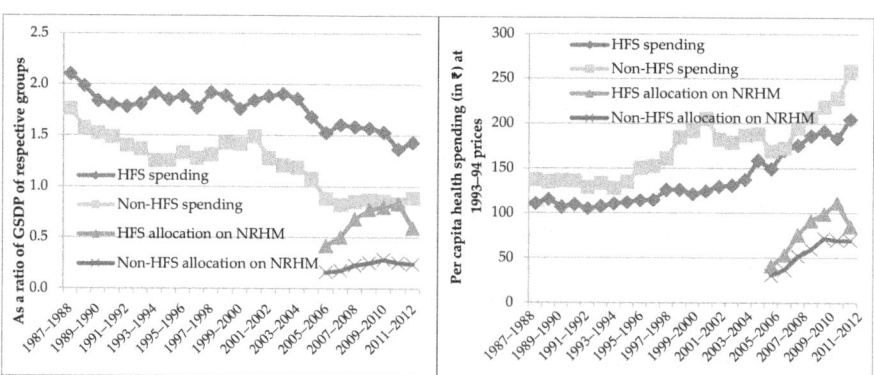

Figure 3.2 Trends in health expenditure as percentage of GSDP and in per capita terms: pre- and post-NRHM analysis

Source: Reserve Bank of India (various years); Government of India (n.d.)

Note: The NRHM items include expenditure on RCH flexipool, NRHM flexipool, infrastructure maintenance, IIPI (pulse polio) and National Disease Control Programmes (NDCP)

found to be less by 18% and 15% funds than the commitments made by central government in HFS and non-HFS, respectively (Table 3.6). Except for Rajasthan, the release of funds always remained lower than the commitment of spending in many other states. Another dimension of central transfer was that along with the commitment of more central devolution to states, the states were asked to increase their own spending at a specified rate in tandem

Table 3.6 Status of funds utilisation and budgetary priority of states to health (percentages)

State	Fund released vs. fund utilised: NRHM spending		Budgetary commitment vs. actual spending: state's spending in health	
	Amount released by GOI as a ratio of commitment under NRHM: 2005–2006 to 2012–2013	Absorptive capacity: unspent amount with states as a ratio of total fund released by GOI under NRHM: 2005–2006 to 2012–2013	Revised estimates as a ratio of budget estimates: 2011–2012	Account (actual spending) as a ratio of budget estimates: 2010–2011
Andhra Pradesh	81.3	29.1	101.8	96.6
Assam#	76.5	7.1	104.6	76.9
Bihar#	72.6	–19.1	110.7	82.6
Gujarat	86.0	–11.0	104.7	101.2
Haryana	90.1	–13.8	117.4	109.4
Himachal Pradesh#	96.5	–23.8	99.0	127.0
Karnataka	83.1	–8.8	103.6	102.4
Kerala	83.9	17.1	98.8	93.5
Madhya Pradesh#	84.4	–1.4	107.6	109.9
Maharashtra	83.6	–15.0	106.1	107.4
Orissa#	90.8	21.9	94.2	87.5
Punjab	96.2	47.6	97.1	89.8
Rajasthan#	103.4	4.7	106.1	88.3
Tamil Nadu	86.6	10.2	101.0	105.4
Uttar Pradesh#	77.3	19.4	103.4	95.9
West Bengal	84.0	56.1	94.6	101.7
High-focused states (all #)	82.0	6.4	104.6	93.5
Non–high-focused states	84.8	12.5	102.7	101.7

Source: Reserve Bank of India (various years); Government of India (n.d.)

Note: $:Expenditure on medical, public health, family welfare, water supply and sanitation

with increased central funding. The evidence suggests that many state governments failed to absorb the funds allocated by the central government. Around 6.4% and 12.5% of the central funds remained unspent in HFS and non-HFS states, respectively (Table 3.6), which indicates inadequate absorptive capacity of the state governments to utilise the allocated central funds. The absorptive capacity remained high in HFS as compared to the non-HFS. The funds utilisation status remained low in West Bengal and Punjab, where around 56% and 48% central allocated funds were not utilised. This may mean that state governments could not scale up the programme directed by the central government. The lack of inadequate availability of human resources and weak capacity to plan and execute plans have probably limit the state government to absorb the central fund adequately.

It is important to note that government budget is a most important policy instrument of every government. This contains spending commitments made by the government in the budget towards social (including health), economic and general services. In the budget presentation, mostly provisional budget estimates of the expenditure are presented for the next financial year. There may be differences in budget estimates, revised estimates and what government actually allocates (actual expenditure) for a particular sector in the coming year. The ratio of actual expenditure to budget estimates reflects the priority and politics behind fund allocation to a sector. How priority has been accorded to the health sector is assessed by studying the budget document of state governments. The value of this ratio for the health sector ranges between 127% and 77% in different states. This means overspending, as well as gap in actual (account) spending and budget estimates (BE). The actual spending found less than BE in almost eight states out of the total listed states in Table 3.6, an indication of low priority to health sector by the particular states. This ratio is accounted around 93.5% in HFS, which is less than the average ratio of non-HFS. The low level of fiscal capacity or priority of HFS might have come in the way in fulfilling the expenditure obligations/commitments for the health sector.

Despite having health as a responsibility of state governments, the central government in India does intervene directly in establishing major hospitals to assist medical education and research and also intervene through Central Plan and Centrally Sponsored Schemes – which are implemented through state budgets.[8] Until 2002–2003, most of the central schemes were routed through the states' budgets and the funds were being transferred as grants to the states as consolidated funds – but because of nationwide externalities of some of the health services, the central government has initiated important interventions under the National Common Minimum Programme[9] (NCMP), the most important of them being the National AIDS Control Organisation (NACO) and the National Rural Health Mission (NRHM, 2005). Now most of the central funds (particularly the NRHM funds) routed through the states' implementing agencies[10] – particularly though the involvement of Panchayati Raj institutions,[11] i.e. district Panchayats and village Panchayats. The changing routes of central transfer might have invited some implications for the Indian healthcare sector, as central transfer to state now has two features: a) central funds that pass through state budgets in terms of CSS/CPS; and b) central transfers that bypass the state budget. It is important to mention here that the central transfer to states through CSS/CPS is an important policy initiative of the central government to support various health programmes running in the state. This helps in meeting the recurring and non-recurring requirements of these programmes, especially those related to communicable and non-communicable diseases such as trachoma, blindness control programmes, family welfare programmes, and others. An in-depth analysis suggests that the expenditure in this category declined from 0.16% of GDP in 1990–1991 to 0.08% GDP in 2004–2005 (Figure 3.3). The decline in central transfer means some of the central sponsored health programmes discontinued. The declining share of CSS/CPS before the implementation of NRHM certainly has reduced the budgetary resources provided for dealing with several existing major communicable and non-communicable disease programmes such as trachoma, blindness control, family welfare, etc. This is very serious worry on the sustainability of some of the existing health programmes. The long-term sustainability of any of these central sponsored health programmes, to a large extent, depends on continuous funding support from the central government. The declining behaviour or uncertainties in resource flows from centre to state would certainly affect the implementation process and effectiveness of these programmes at the state level and more particularly the needy (poorer) states. The implication is that now state governments have to bear most of the burden of health expenditures to finance these programmes from their own resources.

The other component of central spending is the central transfer to NRHM that bypasses the state budget and implements through decentralised agencies. The central transfer on this component shows an increasing trend as a share of GDP from 2005–2006 to 2008–2009 (Figure 3.3). The increase in central funds that are routed through decentralised agencies can be a healthy indication for better delivery of health services in rural areas.

With the implementation of NRHM, some of the central funds, which were earlier passed through states' budgets (through Centrally Plan and Sponsored schemes; CPS/CSS), started bypassing the state budgets. This changing route of central transfer has put limitations on central sponsored health programmes running through CPS/CSS. The share of central transfer in CPS/CSS has come down significantly as percentage of GDP. This declining share of central transfer from CPS/CSS has resulted in discontinuation of some of the health programmes running in the villages, specifically the plus polio and national disease control programmes. This has also made the financial relationship in a federal country like India more complex and health expenditure data more complex to understand. The central spending which bypassed the state budget under NRHM shows increasing trends as percentage of GDP from 2005–2006 to 2011–2012. The bypassing nature of central transfer can

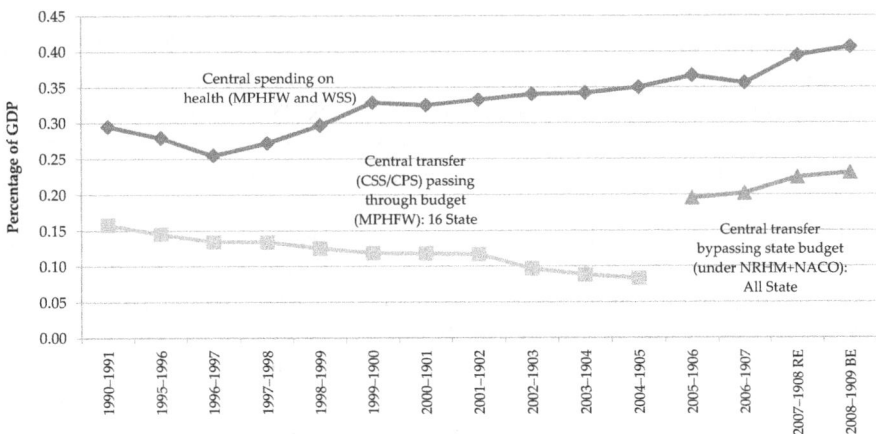

Figure 3.3 Changing patterns of central transfer to states in health: pre- and post-
NRHM analysis

Source: Finance Account of State Governments; Indian Public Finance Statistics; NRHM Expenditure Statement

probably lead to unintended consequences to mobilise the funds from states' own exchequers, as they may contend that NRHM is a financial responsibility of centre government. Second, the central funds that pass through the state implementing agencies became difficult to monitor – specifically, whether these funds have been implemented effectively at the ground level.

In order to assess the sustainability of central sponsored (CSS/CPS) health programmes, the NRHM components are studied here. The NRHM consists of some of the new schemes and repackages many of the existing health schemes which are now bypassing the state budget. The National Disease Control Programmes (NDCP), which was earlier with the Department of Health, has now been made part of the NRHM. Similarly, the earlier schemes of the Department of Family Welfare – such as reproductive and child health programme (RCH), immunisation, contraception, information education and communication (IEC), training and research, area projects and other family welfare services – are all included in the NRHM. The new initiatives under the NRHM are mostly financed through what is called the 'mission flexible pool' which provides for activities like selection and training of a new cadre of community health workers called Accredited Social Health Activist (ASHA), upgradation of health facilities (community health centre and public health centres) to first referral unites (FRU) and facilities meeting the new Indian Public Health Standards (IPHS), constitution of patient welfare committees called Rogi Kalyan Samiti (RKS) and district hospital management committees, mobile medical units, untied funds for sub-centres, preparation of district action plans, and so forth. There have been some changes in the centrally sponsored schemes which are now falling under the NRHM umbrella. The earlier RCH programme (RCH1) was funded as a fixed set of activities. Under the NRHM, the earlier form of the RCH programme is being phased out. In RCH2, most activities are funded through an RCH flexible pool[12] which supports decentralised planning and flexible programming by the states (NRHM, 2005). This shows that NRHM have included many of schemes which were covered under the CSS/CPS.

The study of expenditure on different components of NRHM throw some light on the sustainability of earlier programmes sponsored through CSS/CPS. The NRHM mission flexible pool, which provides much of 'new' funds to the states, constituted a higher amount and shows increasing trends as percentage of GDP over the period, except the two more recent years. Its share in compositional term has also increased from 13.2% in 2005–2006 to 35.2% in 2012–2013 (Table 3.7). The RCH flexible pool, which provides the greater flexibility to states spending on RCH-related activities, constitutes a higher amount and shows increasing trends as percentage of GDP. In compositional terms, its share increased from 17.6% in 2005–2006 to 26.4% in 2012–2013. The expenditure on maintenance of infrastructure, however, put on the priority at the time of launch of NRHM. This component had higher amount as percentage of GDP in 2005–2006, but started declining thereafter. In compositional terms, its share stood around half of the NRHM funds (about 46.9%) in 2005–2006, but declined to 33.3 percent in the year 2012–2013 (Table 3.7). One of the possibilities of declining in the expenditure of this component is that central government has allocated funds on a conditional basis that state governments need to increase their own spending at a specified rate in tandem with the increased central funding. The inadequate absorptive capacity of state governments probably has come in the way that expenditure on these components has not been increased. With regards to the programmes relating to NDCP, the expenditure from these programmes, in composition terms, declined significantly from 14.4% in 2005–2006 to 4.5% in 2012–2013. Similar trends are reflected in the case of plus polio programmes. This raises the question of sustainability of these programmes running in the states. Therefore, it can be argued that overall increment in expenditure on NRHM components is a healthy indication for the healthcare sector. But the changing pattern of health expenditure, through different routes, leaves some questions on sustainability of some of the programmes. It has also made the health expenditure more complex to understand. It can also be argued on one hand that increased funds which pass through state implementing agencies are expected to improve the delivery system of health services in the rural areas, but on the other hand are making centre-state finance relations more complex to understand.

Similar to the trends in NRHM components which shows increasing trends on RCH and mission flexipool at aggregate level, the same trends emerge for high-focused and non–high-focused states (Table 3.8), while the share of infrastructure in declining in both the category of states. The

Table 3.7 Trends and composition of fund allocation on NRHM components (percentages)

NRHM programmes	2005–2006	2006–2007	2007–2008	2008–2009	2009–2010	2010–2011	2011–2012	2012–2013
RCH flexipool	17.6 (0.039)	23.3 (0.060)	24.8 (0.083)	30.5 (0.115)	27.5 (0.110)	26.0 (0.103)	32.5 (0.106)	26.4 (0.018)
NRHM flexipool	13.2 (0.029)	24.3 (0.063)	30.1 (0.101)	29.0 (0.109)	33.1 (0.132)	35.0 (0.138)	33.8 (0.110)	35.2 (0.024)
Infrastructure maintenance	46.9 (0.104)	31.4 (0.081)	30.2 (0.101)	27.3 (0.103)	28.4 (0.114)	29.9 (0.118)	29.1 (0.095)	33.1 (0.022)
IPPI (pulse polio)	8.0 (0.018)	8.4 (0.022)	4.9 (0.016)	5.2 (0.020)	4.1 (0.016)	2.6 (0.010)	2.3 (0.007)	0.9 (0.001)
National Disease Control Programme (NDCP)	14.4 (0.032)	12.5 (0.032)	10.0 (0.033)	7.9 (0.030)	6.9 (0.028)	6.5 (0.026)	2.2 (0.007)	4.5 (0.003)
Total NRHM Fund (in Crore)	7548.9 (0.223)	10171.1 (0.257)	15356.8 (0.335)	19969.8 (0.377)	24440.1 (0.400)	28641.1 (0.394)	27191.3 (0.326)	6401.0 (0.068)

Source: NRHM Expenditure statement

Note: These expenditure categories include total fund allocated by central and state governments and includes all Indian states (high-focused – North East and other than North East; and non–high-focused states). Figures in parentheses are as percentage of GDP (at factor cost, current prices 2004–2005 series) and figures not in parentheses are the composition of total health expenditure.

Table 3.8 Trends and composition of fund allocation on NHM components for HFS and non-HFS (percentages)

		High-focused states						Non-high-focused states					
		2005–2006 to 2011–2012	2012–2013	2013–2014	2014–2015	2015–2016	2016–2017*	2005–2006 to 2011–2012	2012–2013	2013–2014	2014–2015	2015–2016	2016–2017*
A.	NRHM-RCH flexible pool	59.36	60.45	68.11	69.76	69.29	74.56	56.24	62.68	63.30	69.14	62.19	60.50
1.	RCH flexible pool	29.04	31.60	35.51	34.18	32.00	35.89	19.78	26.00	26.95	29.15	28.67	31.82
2.	Mission flexible pool	23.29	23.89	27.69	31.45	33.52	35.26	32.70	33.12	33.31	37.15	30.42	26.87
B.	Infrastructure maintenance	32.93	36.73	29.09	26.44	26.27	20.48	36.30	32.34	32.61	25.90	32.04	32.92
C.	Flexible pool for communicable disease control programmes	6.40	2.04	2.09	2.74	3.23	3.64	5.40	3.50	2.55	3.32	3.78	4.88
D.	Flexible pool for non-communicable disease programmes	1.31	0.78	0.71	1.06	1.21	1.33	2.06	1.49	1.54	1.64	2.00	1.71
Total	(A + B + C + D)	100	100	99.98	99.24	97.52	96.90	100	100	99.92	96.83	95.01	93.96
E.	National Urban Health Mission flexible pool	0.00	0.00	0.02	0.76	2.48	3.10	0.00	0.00	0.08	3.17	4.99	6.04
G.T	Grand Total (A + B + C + D + E)	100	100	100	100	100	100	100	100	100	100	100	100
	Share of central release in NHM total expenditure	88.43	74.65	74.98	77.18	66.21	77.88	88.57	71.90	76.64	73.94	68.02	64.78

Source: National Health Mission, State/UT-wise details of Central Release, State share credited and Expenditure from the F.Y. 2005–2006 to 2016–2017, MOHFW, Govt. of India. https://nhm.gov.in/images/pdf/FMG/FMG_RTI/Central_Release_State_Share_Credited_and_Expenditure_undr_NHM.pdf

share of mission flexipool for non-HFS is declining over time, while it is increasing in case of HFS. The share of NUMH is also increasing with marginal share. It is interesting to note that out of the total expenditure on NHM components (centre plus states), the share of centre release shows declining trends, indicating centre is shifting its responsibility on the states.

Rerouting the transfer of funds

With the implementation of NRHM/NHM, the mode of funds transfers from central to state governments started bypassing the treasury route and funds were directly transferred to implementing agencies. However, the High-level Expert Group 2010 of Government of India suggested reform for efficient management of public expenditures and raised concerns about accountability of fund transfers outside the state treasuries. It is suggested that all central scheme funds should be released to implementing agencies through state treasuries. Based on the recommendations, the central government started releasing NHM funds to implementing agencies through state treasuries from April 2014. The state-level implementing agencies further release the funds to district level, to block level and to the lower-level implementing agencies. This change in the architecture of fund flows affects the process of budget execution significantly, in case if any delay in releasing funds in any part, like from centre to treasury and from treasury to state health society (SHA) and then SHA to other sub-implementing units. Reporting for 2015–2016 reveals about the substantial delay in release of funds from state treasuries to bank accounts of State Health Societies in most states (Figure 3.4). There is gap in fund transfer to SHA of more than three months. In Bihar and

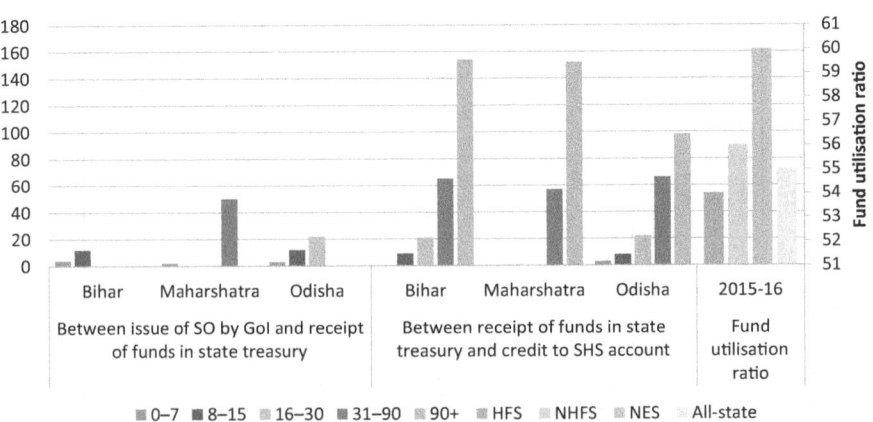

Figure 3.4 Number of days taken to credit central share in SHS account: 2015–2016

Source: Prepared using data from Choudhury et al. (2017)

Maharashtra, about 80–85% of all funds received were credited to the bank account of State Health Societies (SHS) with a time lag of more than two months (Choudhury et al., 2017). Many a time, a high volume of transferred funds reaches SHA during December, while there was less delay on part of SHA as it immediately (within in few days) transfers the received funds to the next level of sub-implementing units. The high delay in fund transfer to SHA resulted in low level of fund utilisation in most of the states. The fund utilisation turned out to be around 55% at all state levels, and it ranges between 54% in HFS to 56% in NHFS and 60% in Northeast states (Figure 3.4)

Conclusion

The composition of health expenditure shows that health spending is dominated by urban and curative cares, whereas the spending in rural areas and on preventive cares is very low. The overall (both rural and urban) health expenditure shows declining trends as a share of GDP. These declining trends, however, are more pronounced in rural areas in most of the Indian states. Within in the rural healthcare spending, the expenditures towards salary components is high, whereas spending on essential medicine, drugs and equipment is very low. The capital expenditure, which is the sole determinant of physical infrastructure, is recorded as very low in all the Indian states. The share of capital expenditure in total state budget expenditures and in GSDP has even come down during the study period. Such trends of capital expenditure are likely to force or push back against the recurring expenditure to grow.

The government of India has set the ambitious goal of increasing the government health spending up to 2–3% of GDP by the end of the Eleventh Five-Year Plan. This was a strong commitment towards the health sector; the spending at the end of plan is recorded 1.2% of GDP, less than the commitments made. Another feature of NRHM was to provide possible help to needy states, filling the gap in health outcome and facility between lagging and more advanced states. These states are categorised into high-focused and non–high-focused states, respectively. The findings indicate that the NRHM has given adequate priority to needy states. The health expenditures in these states show increasing trends compare to the non–high-focused states.

Under the mission, the central government asked the state governments to increase their own spending at a specified rate in tandem with the increased central funding. The state government did not show the pace to increase its spending at the required level. Therefore, the transfer of central funds to the states, which was based on some conditionality, could not be utilised by the state governments adequately. The inadequate absorptive capacity of state governments to utilise the funds properly further resulted in slowing down the NRHM implementation. It can be argued that a lack of inadequate availability of human resources and weak capacity to plan and execute plans probably limit the state government to absorb the central funds adequately.

The delay in resource allocation is a serious problem, which needs greater attention.

Notes

1 This chapter draws some inferences and data from my previously published work originally published in S. K. Hooda. 2015. Government Spending on Health in India: Some Hopes and Fears of Policy Changes. *Journal of Health Management*, Vol. 17, No. 4, pp. 458–486 Copyright 2015 © Indian Institute of Health Management Research. All rights reserved. Reproduced with the permission of the copyright holders and the publishers, SAGE Publications India Pvt. Ltd, New Delhi.

2 However, there can be a variety of reasons of weak impact or no impact of public spending on health outcomes, including corruption and patronage, and there may be a case that a unit's worth of public spending does not necessarily buy a unit's worth of service (Pritchett and Summers, 1996).

3 Peters et al. (2002: 1–2) reported that the rural-urban gap in health outcomes is not only persistent, but widening.

4 The distinction between curative and preventive expenditure depends critically upon the basis for reference. For instance, expenditure on treating any tuberculosis-afflicted person may be considered as curative from the point of view of the individual, but given the contagiousness of the disease, from the society's point of view, this may be categorized as preventive expenditure.

5 It is quite likely that the expenditure on medical education, training and research, public health and general expenditure are most urban in nature.

6 It is not quite easy to argue who are the beneficiaries of this high spending in urban areas. That is, it cannot be easily deciphered that all the beneficiaries from this expenditure are mostly urban residents; there is a high probability that people from rural areas go to avail themselves of care at urban health facilities.

7 The mission covers the entire country, but 18 states are chosen as high focus states. These include all special category states (which include North-eastern, Sikkim, Himachal Pradesh, Uttarakhand and Jammu and Kashmir) and the low-income general category states (i.e., Uttar Pradesh, Bihar, Chattisgarh, Jharkhand, Orissa, Madhya Pradesh and Rajasthan).

8 Most of the CSS directed at augmenting health services are (almost) 100% financed by the centre and routed through the state budget. There are some central schemes where the central funding components are 88%, 75% and 50%.

9 Until the Eleventh Five-Year Plan, the funding for the scheme came entirely from the central budget. This has been made a shared cost programme, with central and state governments contributing 85% and 15%, respectively.

10 But part of NRHM funds also flow through the state treasuries and are reflected in the state health budget (Berman and Ahuja, 2008). According to their observation, about 31% of NRHM allocations during 2005–2008 were to flow through treasury. Specifically, they mentioned that over 60% of all central government health allocation is now routed through NRHM – out of which, about 69% bypasses state budgets.

11 Funds are transferred from the centre to the district health missions through the State Health and Family Welfare Society. The direct transfer of funds to the Zilla Parishad are done through the State Health and Family Welfare Society for implementing the NRHM. The District Health Mission is then implemented by the Zilla Parishads (district Panchayats). It will control, guide and manage all public health institutions in the district, sub- health centres (SHC), primary health centres (PHC) and community health centres (CHC). Village Panchayats will select, appoint and supervise the Accredited Social Health Activist (ASHA)

to act as an interface between community and public health system. The design also allows for the allocation of untied funds at SC, PHC and CHC levels. The healthcare system and the estimated expenditure requirements are expected to be built from the village upwards.

12 The flexible pool also incorporates 'pooled' funds of external funding agencies such as the World Bank and Department of International Development (DFID) (Berman and Ahuja, 2008).

References

Berman, P., and Ahuja, R. 2008. Government Health Spending in India. *Economic and Political Weekly*, Vol. 46.

Berman, P., and Sakai, S. 1989. The Costs of Public Primary Health Care Services in Rural Indonesia. In P. Berman et al. *Bulletin of the World Health Organization*, Vol. 67, No. 6, pp. 685–694. https://apps.who.int/iris/handle/10665/47469

Berwick, D., and Hackbarth, A. 2012. *National Research Council (US); Institute of Medicine (US)*. Editors S. H. Woolf and L. Aron. National Academies Press, Washington, DC, 2013.

Breman, A., and Shelton, C. 2001. *Structure Adjustment and Health: A Literature Review of the Debate, Its Role-players and Presented Empirical Evidence*. Working Paper WG6:6, June. Commission on Macroeconomics and Health (CMH). http://library.cphs.chula.ac.th/Ebooks/HealthCareFinancing/WorkingPaper_WG6/WG6_6.pdf

Button, K. J., and Weyman-Jones, T. G. 1992. Ownership Structure, Institutional Organization and Measured X-Efficiency. *American Economic Review*, Vol. 82, No. 2, pp. 439–445.

Choudhury, M., Mohanty, R. K., and Garg, A. 2017. *Utilisation, Fund Flows and Public Financial Management under the National Health Mission: A Study of Selected States*. National Institute of Public Finance and Policy (NIPFP), New Delhi. https://www.nipfp.org.in/media/medialibrary/2017/11/WHO_PFM_Report_Sep_2017.pdf

Cylus, J., Papanicolas, I., and Smith, P. 2016. *Health System Efficiency: How to Make Measurement Matter for Policy and Management: European Observatory on Health Systems and Policies*. Health Policy Series Number 46. Copenhagen (Denmark).

Deolalikar, A. 2004. *Attaining the Millennium Development Goals in India: Role of Public Policy and Services Delivery*. World Bank, Washington, DC.

Ensor, T., et al. 2003. Public Expenditure Review of the Health and Population Sector Program in Bangladesh. In Abdo S. Yazbeck and David H. Peters (Eds.), *Health Policy Research in South Asia*. World Bank, Washington, DC. https://openknowledge.worldbank.org/bitstream/handle/10986/15071/272100PAPER0Health0policy0research.pdf?sequence=1&isAllowed=y

GOI. 1997–02. *Ninth Five-Year Plan Document 2002–07, Planning Commission*. Government of India, New Delhi.

GOI. 2019. *National Health Profile of India*. Ministry of Health & Family Welfare, Government of India, New Delhi.

Government of India. n.d. *NRHM Expenditure Statement*. Ministry of Health and Family Welfare, Government of India, New Delhi.

Government of India. various year. *Government Budget, Demand for Grants of Various States*. Ministry of Finance, New Delhi.

Government of India. 2002–07. *Tenth Plan Document (2002–07)*. Planning Commission, Government of India, New Delhi.

Government of India. 2005. *Mission Documents of the National Rural Health Mission (NRHM)*. Government of India, New Delhi. http://mohfw.nic.in/nrhm.html

Gumber, A. 1997. Burden of Diseases and Cost of Ill Health in India: Setting Priorities for Health Interventions during the Ninth Plan. *Margin. National Council of Applied Economic Research*, Vol. 29, No. 2.

Hooda, S. K. 2015. Government Spending on Health in India: Some Hopes and Fears of Policy Changes. *Journal of Health Management*, Sage, Vol. 17, No. 4.

Hooda, S. K. 2017, April 22. How Effective Are Health Policy Interventions? Health Payments and Household Well-being. *Economic and Political Weekly*, Vol. 52, No. 16, pp. 54–65.

Hu, B., and Mendoza, R. U. 2010, April. Public Spending, Governance and Child Health Outcomes: Revisiting the Links. *Journal of Human Development and Capabilities, UNICEF, Policy and Practice*, Vol. 14, No. 2, pp. 285–311.

IPFS. 2018. *Indian Public Finance Statistics (IPFS)*. Ministry of Finance, Government of India, New Delhi.

IPHS. 2006, March. *Indian Public Health Standards (IPHS) for Primary Health Centres Guidelines*. Government of India, New Delhi.

Leibenstein, H. 1966. What Can We Expect From a Theory of Development? *Kyklos*, Vol. 19, No. 1, pp. 1–22. https://doi.org/10.1111/j.1467-6435.1966.tb02490.x

Mahal, A., and Fan, V. Y. 2012. Expanding Health Coverage for Indians: An Assessment of the Policy Challenge. In *India Policy Forum, 2011–12*. http://testnew.ncaer.org/image/userfiles/file/IPF-Volumes/Volume%208/2_Ajay%20Mahal.pdf

MoHFW. n.d. *Health Sector Financing by Centre and States/UTs in India*. Ministry of Health and family Welfare (MoHFW). Government of India, New Delhi. https://main.mohfw.gov.in/sites/default/files/883514734NHA.pdf https://main.mohfw.gov.in/sites/default/files/HEALTH%20SECTOR%20FINANCING%20BY%20CENTRE%20AND%20STATEs.pdf

NCMH. 2005. *Report of the National Commission on Macroeconomics and Health, National Commission on Macroeconomics and Health (NCMH)*. Ministry of Health & Family Welfare, Government of India, New Delhi.

NFHS. 2016. *National Family and Health Survey (NFHS-4) 2015–16*. International Institute for Population Sciences (IIPS), Mumbai, India and International Classification of Functioning, Disability and Health (ICF).

NHA. 2018. *National Health Accounts Estimates for India*. Ministry of Health & Family Welfare, Government of India, New Delhi, November 2019.

Peters, D., Yazbeck, A., Sharma, R., Ramana, G., Pritchett, L., and Wagstaff, A. 2002. *Better Health Systems for India's Poor*. Human Development Network. World Bank, Washington, DC.

Pritchett, L., and Summers, L. H. 1996. Wealthier is Healthier. *Journal of Human Resources*, Vol. 31, No. 4, pp. 841–868.

Rao. n.d. Inter-State Comparisons on Health Outcomes in Major States and A Framework For Resource Devolution For Health, Background Paper 14th Finance Commission, available at Centre for Economic and Social Studies Nizamiah Observatory Campus, Hyderabad, Andhra Pradesh, India https://fincomindia.nic.in/writereaddata/html_en_files/oldcommission_html/fincom14/others/39.pdf

Reserve Bank of India. various issues. *RBI State Finance: A Study of State Budget*. Reserve Bank of India (RBI), Ministry of Finance, Government of India, New Delhi.

RHS. 2019. *Bulletin on Rural Health Statistics (RHS) in India*. Ministry of Health and Family Welfare. Government of India, New Delhi.

Samuelson, P., and Nordhaus, W. 1992. *ECONOMICS*, 9th Edition. The McGraw-Hill, Irwin College.

Shiva Kumar, A. K. 2005. Budgeting for Health Some Considerations. *Economic and Political Weekly*, Vol. 40, No. 14, pp. 1319–1396.

Varatharajan, D. 1999. *Improving the Efficiency of Public Health Care Units in Tamil Nadu, India*. Research Paper No. 165, December, 1999. Takemi Program in International Health, Harvard School of Public Health, Boston, MA.

Wagstaff, A. 2002a. Inequality Aversion, Health Inequalities, and Health Achievement. *Journal of Health Economics*, Vol. 21, No. 4, pp. 627–641.

Wagstaff, A. 2002b. Poverty and Health Sector Inequalities. *Bulletin of the World Health Organization*, Vol. 80, No. 2, pp. 97–105.

WHO. 1999. *World Health Report*. World Health Organization, Geneva.

WHO. 2000. *The World Health Report 2000: Health Systems Improving Performance*. World Health Organisation, Geneva. https://www.who.int/whr/2000/en/whr00_en.pdf

Part 2

Institutional reforms

Decentralisation in service delivery

The idea of institutional reforms is increasingly being applied to accelerate the process of economic development, as well as for shaping the sector-specific outcome from an efficiency point of view that influences the outcomes directly or indirectly via improving the efficacy of resource utilisation. Institution ideas initially arise in critical response to inadequacy of neoclassical theory in dealing with uneven performance of economies across space and time, and its limited potential to explain the persistence of inefficient institutions and the role of ideology in choice determination of individuals. Neoclassical economics completely ignores the 'power' dimension in policy making. It does not deal with the incentives and behaviour of political actors, or the influence of the political process on targets for growth, stability or the division of public investment among sectors. It is being increasingly realised that these factors play a crucial role in explaining persistent unevenness across space and time. Their framework offers no scope to integrate politics into economics and does not help to capture the real time phenomenon of economic outcome as influenced by political institutions. Institutions are taken for granted for observing the social rules, conventions and other elements of the structural framework of social interaction in the mainstream economics. These inadequacies led to a shifted focus on the role of political and individual ideologies, institutions and incentives in explaining economic and sector specific performance.

In a more fundamental work on institutions and their possible channels that influence economic performance, North (1990) pointed out that institutions are everywhere, and ignoring them would lead to incompleteness of conclusions and policy implications. Many scholars thereafter identify that institutions (the political system, the federal structure, the bureaucracy, the fiscal system, the welfare state, the institutions of industrial policy, and so on) have significant impact on different outcomes and economic performance of a country or region. The chapters in this section provide an in-depth understanding and analysis of the role of political institutions (that strengthen people participation and representation in politics) and federal institutions (the devolution of decentralised power to local governments and local agents

DOI: 10.4324/9781032108438-5

and people) specifically to find out whether they successfully addresses the problems of underfunding and inefficiency in resource utilisation of health sector.

The Chapter 4 brings an argument that the appalling situation of low levels of public spending in healthcare is not likely to change, unless low-cost, high-quality and equitable healthcare becomes a political demand and an electoral issue that would come only from higher participation of people in politics. It hypothesizes that greater participation of people in the electoral process allows political authorities to align their decisions with the interests and priorities of the public. One can even expect an increase in welfare spending if more excluded groups (like women and minorities) are incorporated into the political process through constitutionally mandated consensual rules. It specifically examine whether an increase in participation and greater representation of diversified groups in politics leads to concomitant rise in welfare expenditures like health.

The effectiveness of increases in government spending on healthcare is influenced by the level of good governance achieved by the country, which refers to the institutional structure. Among the many forms of institutions, an institution of federalism (decentralisation) has been advocated as a powerful means of improving the provision of public goods such as healthcare services and outcomes of the healthcare sector. It is argued that devolving power to local governments would improve service delivery, equity, accountability, effectiveness, efficiency and thereby utilisation of health services and health outcomes. The Chapter 5 postulates that a high amount of public spending on healthcare services sometimes will not contribute substantially, if the existing facilities or funds are not implemented and managed through proper channels or through effective government interventions like community participation or decentralisation. This is because the decentralised mechanism improves accountability, effectiveness and efficiency of service delivery by bringing decision makers closer to the people and by enhancing the participation of the community in the decision making and implementation processes. Their close relations with the local people enables them to know the local problems and needs, and they are therefore in better position to establish the right priorities than a central or regional government far away.

In order to fully evaluate the gains from decentralisation, the conceptual clarity on what constitutes decentralisation, how it can be empirically captured and what its constituent elements are discussed in the chapter in detail. The measures of decentralisation are then used to examine their impact on improving the efficacy of allocated public funds that can have significant impact on health sector outcomes.

Within the health sector, recommendations are made several times to involve the community and decentralisation to achieve specific outcomes. For instance, the National Rural Health Mission in 2005 seeks to improve access to healthcare facilities, enable community ownership of services, strengthen public health systems, enhance the equity and accountability of the providers, and most importantly, strengthen and deepen the levels of decentralisation by increasing the resources available to the Panchayats. While the responsibility of implementation of this programme rests with the state governments, the NRHM seeks to empower the Panchayats to manage, control and be accountable for health services. The Panchayats are critical to the planning, implementation and monitoring of the NRHM in the village. Village-level committees called village health and sanitation committees (consisting of educated villagers, school principals, women, minority communities, etc.) are entrusted with the planning and implementation of health programmes in the village to achieve equity and efficiency in healthcare through decentralising the services. This committee envisions local people taking leadership in health management of the health system and its related matters, and provided them with an amount of Rs. 10,000 to help poor women during health emergencies, pregnancy and spread of diseases). This committee therefore is a significant mechanism for engendering inclusiveness in health planning. Under the mission, the interface between the community and public health system at the village level is entrusted through a female accredited social health activist (ASHA) for spreading awareness about the importance of basic facilities and health programmes in the village and made accountable to the Gram Sabha (a formal Panchayat meeting consisting of villagers, Panchayat representatives and health functionaries). The Mission also introduced a cash incentive programme called Janani Suraksha Yojana (JSY) to promote institutional delivery, along with some other committees called Rogi Kalyan Samiti (RKS) and Sakshar Mahila Samooh (SMS), etc. for planning and implementation of health programmes that involve communities. All of these initiatives explain a sustained process of decentralisation that involve community, local agents and local governments for effective delivery of health services in rural India. We believe that the gain from these initiatives depend on how these initiatives have been implemented at ground level and helped in improving the health service delivery system in rural area. These initiatives involve various dimensions of community and local agents participation, and therefore, evaluating their impacts is not straightforward. In order to fully understand the benefit from various dimensions of decentralisation, a field survey is conducted at households, panchayat and health functionaries level especially to identify the impact of the degree of community participation and engagement, and the extent of decentralisation in the health sector, on health service delivery, particularly in improving the access to maternal and child healthcare utilisation and improving overall health system functioning. In Chapter 6 entitled 'Decentralisation, access and service delivery'.

Reference

North, D. C. 1990. *Institutions, Institutional Change and Economic Performance.* Cambridge University Press, Cambridge.

4 Politicising the reprioritisation of health expenditures[1]

One of the major concerns across the world has been allocation of a sizeable amount of public funds to healthcare to achieve better healthcare outcomes. Some studies have suggested that every country should spend at least 5% of its GDP on healthcare (Savedoff, 2007). The quantified goals of spending, however, are not based on much solid analysis, while based on international comparisons and immense unmet needs; one could argue that government should spend more on healthcare than it has been in the past. However, when one looks at the pattern of budgetary spending on healthcare internationally, it is reported to be highly unequal. The developed countries tend to invest/spend a sizeable amount of public funds on healthcare as compared to developing ones (Chapter 2). A low level of public spending is a reflection of government failure in providing a reasonable level of health facility.

It is unfortunate to observe that the healthcare sector of a group of developing countries even suffers from an absolute underfunding problem, along with a disproportionally high disease burden. A WHO report states that they together claim close to 90% of all maternal deaths, and it is perhaps the consequence of underfunding of their health sector (WHO, 2008). If one goes by this narrative, one would argue that income (level of development) has a direct influence on healthcare expenditures. A closer look at the pattern of healthcare spending of developed and developing countries, however, suggests that income alone cannot be the sole criteria of higher spending. This is because the expenditure pattern is reported to be highly unequal, even in countries and regions with similar levels of economic development like the OECD (Organisation for Economic Cooperation and Development) and within developing countries. When one looks at countries around India, the low-income countries like Nepal and Bangladesh, whose per capita GDP is less than per capita GDP of India, spend more public funds on health than India. Being a developing country, Sri Lanka also allocates more public funds on health than India (Chapter 2), indicating in addition to economic prosperity, other factors influence the size/growth of expenditure that a country would allocate for health.

In the Abuja Declaration (2000), it is narrated that the resource allocation towards health can be influenced by a government's desire to allocate funds for health which generally depends on fiscal resources available with

DOI: 10.4324/9781032108438-6

the government in a financial year (Abuja Declaration, 2000). This is because, in the budget making process, the Ministry of Finance of a country generally identifies priority and non-priority areas. Some sectors are being prioritised over the others, depending on the available fiscal resources with the government (Lu et al., 2010) and the amount of money needed to address the growing health needs of young-older age population and rural-urban residents and addressing burden of (communicable and non-communicable) diseases (Hitiris and Posnett, 1992). One can expect higher allocation of resources and budgets toward welfare services like healthcare from states having high fiscal capacity, as more spending towards any sector requires more fiscal space (WHO, 2010; Durairaj and Evans, 2010). Thus, low resource availability or any fiscal stringency can come in the way of fulfilling the obligations and commitments towards the expenditure on healthcare. In the case of India, where healthcare is a state subject, it is observed that some of the high fiscal capacity states tend to allocate less per capita public funds on healthcare (Chapter 2) even if they are higher in need (Chapter 3). While, some low fiscal capacity states observed allocating higher amount on healthcare. Thus, one would agree with the WHO conclusion that size and growth of healthcare expenditures between and within developing countries are vulnerable not to economic (level of income or fiscal capacity) reasons, but rather to political context (WHO, 2008).

There have been several attempts to identify the degree to which discrepancies in healthcare expenditure is explained by income (level of development), fiscal capacity and other economic factors. A brief review can be found in Hooda (2016). Most of such studies have tried to reach consensus on whether health has been accorded highest priority amongst the goals of social and economic development of a country. How politics and political factors can influence the size and growth of health expenditure of a country have received a little place in empirical estimation. This chapter aims to find out whether spending on health has a political context in Indian states. This specifically tries to identify whether low levels of spending on healthcare can be reprioritised through politics. The following section briefly discusses how political approaches are being (or can be) used for reprioritisation of health expenditure.

Conceptualising the political approach to expenditure reprioritisation

A body of literature suggests that government ideology, political and electoral factors – to a certain degree – explain the difference in expenditures on public health systems (De la Maisonneuve et al., 2016; Bellido et al., 2019). The democratic countries and those with higher degrees of political liberty do tend to allocate a higher share of government expenditure and GDP towards health, even after controlling for confounding factors (Tandon et al., 2014). This notion is based on the premises that the elected representatives and governments are more sensitive and responsive towards satisfying the peoples' interests so as to win the next election (Baum and Lake, 2003). However, by considering largest democratic (India) and non-democratic (China) countries of the world, some studies have reported that public healthcare conditions in democratic country India is recorded worse than in non-democratic China (Ma and Sood, 2008; Dummer and Cook, 2008). An in-depth analysis from a study suggests that development ideology and systematic pressure from the lower classes have a greater impact on government investment in public health than the regime type, even after controlling the economic growth (Joshi and Yu, 2014). The political competition was also found to be very important for health expenditure to grow, as it enforces the elected incumbent government to spend more on public healthcare (Datta, 2020), however, an earlier study did not find any impact of political competition on the development expenditure (Chhibber and Nooruddin, 2004).

In the case of India, a report from an ex-official member of erstwhile Planning Commission (PC, which used to be a most powerful body for setting up various developmental agendas and priorities for the country before the National Institution for Transforming India [NITI Aayog]) states that political representatives in practice often do not seek resources for health (Kumar, 2015). Other sectors such as industry, agriculture, trade, and infrastructure take up the priority on the demands list. The sporadic demand in the healthcare sector is mostly limited to the tertiary care hospitals for the respective political constituencies (Kumar, 2015). The official reported that the appalling situation of low levels of public spending in healthcare is not likely to change, unless low-cost, high-quality and equitable healthcare become a political demand and an electoral issue. This can come from higher participation of people in political process. Studies have also suggested that with an increase in political participation, government's expenditure on welfare activities generally increases (Vatter and Ruefli, 2003).

Theoretically, the power resource theory in political science describes that social classes are the main agents of societal change and that their balance of power determines policy outcomes. It states that the size of a welfare state can be explained in terms of power resources of social classes (Esping-Andersen, 1990; Vatter and Ruefli, 2003). An effective political system in general 'empowers' the citizens by widening the access to political processes such as the introduction of various forms of proportional representation. One can even expect an increase in welfare spending like health if more excluded groups (like women and minorities) are incorporated into the political process through constitutionally mandated consensual rules (Gronbjerg, 1977). Earlier empirical evidence suggests that countries that are progressive in the standing of women in political and economic forums seem to possess a strong relationship to governments that spend more on healthcare as a portion of GDP. Household-level studies have also suggested that pediatric health, as well as public health, improves when women are empowered within the family (Thomas, 1990; Duflo, 2005). More public water sources are made available when village Panchayats are reserved for women (Duflo, 2005), and female leaders in village councils tend to provide more public goods of equal quality at a lower price and implemented more pro-women policies (Beaman et al., 2012). Higher representation of women in the local council in Sweden and Norway resulted in increasing the spending on child-care and education, respectively (Svaleryd, 2009; Halse, 2009). A study from 24 Indian villages found that equal political representation of women increases the opinion congruence between elites and masses (Lindgren et al., 2009). Cross-countries presentation show that a higher percentage of women in national parliament leads to higher government spending on health as a share of GDP. That is, government health spending is positively associated to female representation in parliament/assembly.

This conversation reveals that political factors can shape public policy debates (Crepaz, 1998; Vatter and Ruefli, 2003). Within the political factors, the democratic election process creates an environment conducive to decision makers (political party) having appropriate and up-to-date information about the preferences and problems of the local people (Oates, 1977). It is an effective channel for people to express their priorities and negotiate their wants, and a motivating environment for decision makers to effectively address people's needs (Akin et al., 2001; Faguet, 2004). People, through political participation, tend to influence and shape policies in their favour, such as those related to welfare services including healthcare (Besley and Coate, 1997; Besley et al., 2005). Greater participation in the electoral process allows political authorities to align their decisions with the interests and priorities of the general public. The median voter hypothesis reflects that low-income democratic countries (where the majority of voters are likely to be poor), governments should place a greater emphasis on spending in sectors like healthcare.

No doubt, low resource availability or any fiscal stringency can come in the way of fulfilling the obligations and commitments towards expenditures on welfare activities. However, it would be interesting to examine whether high participation and representation of diverse groups in politics can enforce the state to allocate more funds towards the healthcare sector out of their budget even if they have low fiscal space; and if it can influence decision makers to spend more on healthcare, even if their level of income/development is low. This will help us to understand whether political factors influence the government's priority towards health out of their budget and GDP. This can reflect upon the political economy of reprioritisation of budgetary allocation towards the healthcare sector – that is, whether with an increase in participation and greater representation of diversified groups in politics can cause concomitant rise in welfare expenditures like healthcare which can be observed in the context of Indian states.

Based on the preceding theoretical and empirical narratives, this chapter hypothesises that one can expect an increase in welfare spending if more excluded groups (like women and minorities) are incorporated into the political process through constitutionally mandated consensual rules. This is simply because their greater participation in the electoral process allows political authorities to align their decisions with the interests and priorities of the general public. An effective political system in general 'empowers' the citizens by widening the access to political processes such as the introduction of various forms of proportional representation. Thus, with an increase in political participation, government's expenditure on welfare activities expected to increase (Vatter and Ruefli, 2003).

To put this phenomena to empirical testing, a comprehensive approach that includes several political indictors is adopted that captures political participation and representation (PPR) of diversified groups in politics in Indian states. It includes total voter turnout and representation of diverse population groups in assembly and Panchayat politics. Using information on such political indicators, an index of PPR is constructed by employing principal component analysis (for PCA estimation refer Kundu, 1984). The indicators are: a) percentage of total voter turnout in assembly election of a state; b) total number of women who voted in assembly election as percentage of men who voted in assembly election; c) percentage of women contestants in assembly elections; d) percentage of women contestants elected in assembly election of a state; and e) women and reserved class Panchayat representatives as a share of total Panchayat representatives in a state. The comprehensive nature of this index provides an understanding of citizens' participation and representation, as well as the level of democracy in a particular state and expectation to influence the government spending on health. Table 4.1 presents the progress of PPR across states and time. The level of

Table 4.1 Trends and variation in the level of political participation and representation across Indian states

State	Election years data used for PPR calculation	PPR value		
		1987–1988	*2000–2001*	*2011–2012*
Andhra Pradesh	1985, 89, 94, 99, 04, 09	3.11	4.83	5.38
Assam	1985, 91, 96, 01, 06, 11	3.33	3.39	5.14
Bihar	1985, 90, 95, 00, 05, 10	2.42	3.28	5.49
Gujarat	1985, 90, 95, 98, 02, 07, 12	4.33	3.24	4.37
Haryana	1987, 91, 96, 00, 05, 09	3.37	3.58	3.65
Himachal Pradesh	1985, 90, 93, 98, 03, 07, 12	3.96	4.92	4.51
Karnataka	1989, 94, 99, 04, 08, 12	3.58	3.51	3.82
Kerala	1987, 91, 96, 01, 06, 11	4.08	4.40	4.86
Madhya Pradesh	1985, 90, 93, 98, 03, 08	3.00	4.11	5.09
Maharashtra	1985, 90, 95, 99, 04, 09	3.21	3.52	3.69
Orissa	1985, 90, 95, 00, 04, 09	2.76	4.28	4.55
Punjab	1985, 92, 97, 02, 07, 12	3.29	4.25	5.24
Rajasthan	1985, 90, 93, 98, 03, 08, 12	3.23	3.78	5.20
Tamil Nadu	1989, 91, 96, 01, 06, 11	4.82	3.41	4.50
Uttar Pradesh	1989, 91, 93, 96, 02, 07, 12	2.98	2.80	4.60
West Bengal	1987, 91, 96, 01, 06, 11	3.28	3.66	5.33

Source: State Election Report of different states for various years, available at http://eci.nic.in/eci_main1/ElectionStatistics.aspx

political participation and representation varies across states. It shows an increase trend over time with a wide variation across the states.

Incorporating confounding factors

There is no uniform consensus on what factors generally influence the size and growth of health expenditures. Much of the discussion, since the first seminal work of Newhouse (1977), is centred on whether income of a country or region is the major determinant of health expenditures, and if yes, whether income elasticity of health expenditures is less or greater than 1. Based on the size of the income elasticity coefficient, studies have suggested the associated policy implications for financing and distribution of healthcare resources. Healthcare is reported as a necessary good (if responsiveness is insensitive to income change, i.e. elasticity <1) in some studies (Gerdtham et al., 1992; Di Matteo and Di Matteo, 1998; Bhat and Jain, 2004; Sen, 2005; Baltagi and Moscone, 2010; Xu et al., 2011), while healthcare was reported as a luxury good (if responsiveness is sensitive to income change, i.e. elasticity >1) in other studies (Newhouse, 1977; Hitiris and Posnett, 1992; Wilson, 1999). In some low-middle–income countries, income turned insignificant in influencing the public spending on health (Lu et al., 2010). The advocates of 'health as a luxury good' argued that health is a kind of commodity that is best left to market forces, whereas advocates of 'health as a necessary good' often support the idea of greater government intervention in the healthcare sector (Culyer, 1988; Di Matteo, 2003; Baltagi and Moscone, 2010).

The fiscal disabilities of states arising from unequal capacities in raising revenues is another important factor that can influence a government's priority to allocate for health. This is simply because more spending in health requires more fiscal space (WHO, 2010; Durairaj and Evans, 2010). Amongst the other demand-side and supply-side factors, other covariates that have been incorporated in many cross-country and cross-region studies have included population age structure of those aged under 15 years and above 60–65 years (Leu, 1986; Hitiris and Posnett, 1992), epidemiological proxies like HIV prevalence, infant and maternal mortality rate and life expectancy (Lu et al., 2010; Murthy and Okunade, 2009; Dregen and Reimers, 2005), technological progress and variation in medical practices like surgical procedures and numbers of specific medical equipment (Baker and Wheeler, 2000; Weil, 1995), health system characteristics like service provision (Gerdtham et al., 1998), health financing sources like taxes and social insurance (Leu, 1986; Hitiris and Posnett, 1992; Gaag and Stimac, 2008; Wagstaff and Bank, 2009) and external funds (Gaag and Stimac, 2008), and provider payment mechanism (Gerdtham and Jönsson, 2000; Murthy and Okunade, 2009). These are important in explaining the level of and growth in health expenditures. The selection of variables (and techniques) is generally guided by data limitations. For instance, health system characteristics such as healthcare financing indicators, provider payment mechanisms and service provision have recently been recognised as important variables (Xu et al., 2011), but they could not be tested extensively in literature due to data limitations.

Choice of variables

Studies have used cross-sectional bivariate (Newhouse, 1977), cross-sectional multivariate (Leu, 1986; Gerdtham et al., 1992), static and dynamic panel techniques (Gerdtham et al., 1992, 1998; Hitiris and Posnett, 1992; Barros, 1998; Roberts, 1999; Farag et al., 2009; Xu et al., 2011), unit roots and cointegration analysis (Gerdtham and Löthgren, 2002; Okunade and Karakus, 2001; Hartwig, 2008; Baltagi and Moscone, 2010), while a few have applied two-way causation and Granger-causality tests (Erdil and Yetkiner, 2009). Considering the fact that estimators are highly sensitive to the data, variables and method that one employs, this chapter uses a single country – India – as a case and obtains a set of rationally selected variables and techniques for estimation to avoid some of the aforementioned problems. One advantage of taking states as sample units is that it would simply avoid the limitation of data aggregation – a methodological problem – when considering countries with different settings and varying levels of economic development in a single estimation. This takes care of the simple econometric assumption that data should be drawn from the same population, particularly to compare the sample units and to get robust estimates. The Indian case is especially important because of its federal structure in nature where states are governed under the same constitution, but have freedom to draft their own policies on subjects classified as state subjects under the constitution. Healthcare is placed under the state subject in India. It is each state's responsibility to devise and implement comprehensive health policies – acknowledging the political and economic environment in the states – in order to meet the health needs of its population. Apart from socio-cultural, economic and political diversities, Indian states have several factors in common, as well. Given the obligatory constitutional framework and social, economic and political diversity, estimation by considering state as sample unit is important to understand how different covariate influence the expenditure on health.

The study has taken state government expenditure on healthcare (*he*), an important component of healthcare financing, as dependent variable. It includes expenditure on medical services, public health, family welfare, water supply and sanitation. The log value of real per capita (at 1993–1994 prices) health expenditure *(lnhe)* is used in the estimation. Data are compiled from finance accounts of individual states and 'RBI-State Finance: A Study of State Budget, Government of India'.

The index of PPR, discussed previously, is the main explanatory variable. This is a comprehensive index which captures voter turnout and representation of diversified groups, including women, in assembly and Panchayat elections. This gives an understanding of citizens' participation and representation, as well as the level of democracy in a particular state. Based on the theoretical and empirical notion, this index is expected to influence government spending on health. The index is constructed using data from the state election reports of different states for all state elections years (Table 4.1). Note that state assembly elections in India generally take place every five years. The index value, therefore, is kept constant for consecutive years in the panel data setting of a particular state. The log value of PPR (*lnPPR*) is used in the analysis. A significant and positive coefficient value reflects that a high participation of diversified groups in electoral process influences the growth of government spending on health. We have also tried to find out whether high degrees of political participation and representation do tend to influence the government to allocate a higher share on health from total budget and GDP, even after controlling for confounding factors.

The fiscal capacity (*fc*) reflects the revenue generating capacity of the government. A high revenue-generating capacity ensures greater autonomy for government to meet the growing expenditure obligations and requirements for the provisioning of different welfare services, including healthcare. The total government expenditure as a share of GDP is used as fiscal capacity variable in Xu et al. (2011), reflecting the fiscal space for a given GDP level. The report of the Finance Commission of India (GOI, 2013) states that states' own revenue resources or revenue-generating capacity (either taken in per capita terms or as a share of GDP or share in total expenditure of the state) is the best measure of fiscal capacity of the state rather than the earlier measures. This chapter uses per capita total own (tax plus non-tax) revenue of a state as a measure of fiscal capacity. This reflects the availability of resources with the state governments to meet their expenditure obligations, thus providing greater autonomy to spend according to their priorities. It is presumed that a state would allocate large amounts on healthcare if more resources are available with them, whereas a state with low resource capacity will find it difficult to fulfil the expenditure obligations and commitments to a particular sector. This presumption is based on the notion that more spending in healthcare requires more fiscal space (WHO, 2010; Durairaj and Evans, 2010). This variable is used as log of per capita state own revenue *(lnfc)* in the analysis. The data is taken from Economic and Political Weekly Research Foundation (epwrf) Online Services on India Time Series.

Many studies have considered income (per capita GDP) as the primary covariate to determine health expenditure. It is based on the premise that as the per capita income increases, the pressure on state machinery to provide better and varied health services increases. This may either be due to an increase in incidence of the so-called lifestyle diseases such as diabetes, cancer and cardiovascular diseases, or the government as a 'welfare state' may spend more to provide comprehensive healthcare facilities across the regions. The government, in the face of its increased ability, may spend more on health to meet the increased demand for services. How far this phenomenon is true for Indian state is tested empirically – specifically, whether health expenditure grows with an increase in state income. The real per capita GDP of states (at 1993–1994 prices) is taken as a measure of state income, and its log value *(lngdp)* is used in the analysis. GDP data are taken from National Account Statistics, Ministry of Statistics and Programme Implementation, Government of India. The size of the coefficient of this variable tells whether income elasticity of health expenditure is greater than or lower than 1.

Within the demographic characteristics, population age structure is expected to influence health expenditure. Therefore, age was more often used as a covariate of health expenditure in earlier estimations. Generally, the shares of the young (under 15 years of age) and/or old (above 60, 65 or 75 years of age) people in the total population are the most commonly used indicators. The notion behind the use of these indicators is that these two age groups use more healthcare services. For instance, in countries where population ageing is fast approaching, health systems face high pressure to cope with increasing needs of the population (Xu et al., 2011). This phenomenon, however, may be true for countries (especially high-income ones) where either the elderly population is high or population ageing is fast approaching. The same may not be true for a developing country like India, where ageing is not a dominant issue or a deciding factor for increasing government spending. Therefore, one would not expect the government to redirect or increase its spending on health with an increase in elderly population. We believe that India's demographic structure poses a different challenge to its health system compared to other developed and developing nations. One can envision that the changing epidemiological profile of India – especially the rising burden of non-communicable diseases (NCDs), along with a high load of communicable diseases – presents a formidable challenge to the country's healthcare system. According to WHO (2011), NCDs were responsible for 53% of deaths in India in 2008. Evidence suggests that the highest proportion of NCD deaths occur in the productive years of life (i.e. under the age of 60). Alongside the double burden of diseases, in 2019, the infant mortality rate (IMR) of India was around 28.3 per 1000 live births, whereas that of Sri Lanka was 6.1 and under-5 mortality rate was 34.3 and 7.1 per 1000 live birth. The life expectancy at birth of an average Indian (about 66) is at least 13 years lower than that in high-income countries and even lower than of Sri Lanka (about 79 years) (WHO, 2015). According to the latest UNICEF report 2019, almost half of Indian children suffer from malnutrition, which is worse than the situation in some countries in sub-Saharan Africa (UNICEF, 2019). The latest National Health and Family Health Survey of India reported that more than 50% of women suffer from anaemia (NFHS, 2016). There is still a huge gap in rural-urban health outcomes. Further, an increase in the incidence of the so-called lifestyle diseases also poses various challenges. This reflects that the total population count, across age groups, poses great challenge to the country's healthcare system. In such a situation, it becomes important for India to improve its overall healthcare system in order to provide comprehensive healthcare facilities to the general population. This is even more important because there is shortfall in the provisioning of basic health services across states (RHS, 2019). Therefore, instead of considering the age structure of a particular population, overall population density in a region/state will be more useful, as each age group requires different types of healthcare facilities. We have presumed that state feels immense pressure to provide healthcare services of the requisite level to its entire population. Therefore, overall population density (pd) is taken as a covariate of health expenditure, and its log value ($lnpd$) is used in the analysis. The data is compiled from Census of India, Government of India.

The mortality, morbidity or epidemiological profile of a country/state generally reflects the diseases and health problems that need to be addressed through an efficient health system. Various proxies of such need factors like HIV prevalence (Lu et al., 2010), TB incidence (Xu et al., 2011) and maternal mortality rate (Murthy and Okunade, 2009) have been used as covariates of health expenditure. In the present study, infant mortality rate (IMR) is taken as a proxy of need factors. We believe that infant mortality is a superior and more reliable measure than other health indicators like life expectancy. While infant mortality figures are based on actual data, life expectancy figures are based on extrapolations from child mortality data. The IMR also reflects the health status of both the mother and the child in a country or state. We have presumed that the government is more sensitive to IMR than other mortality and morbidity indicators. The log value of IMR ($lnIMR$) is used in the analysis. The data are explored from Sample Registration System, Office of the Registrar General, Government of India.

However, it is important to note that there is no theoretical understanding on whether the coefficient signs for demographic and mortality indicators are positive or negative. In simple terms, one can argue that a less healthy population will, on average, require more resources and thus result in greater demand for healthcare and an increase in per capita health expenditure. On the contrary, states may have ensured better outcomes through high spending, reflecting two-way causation problem in the model. Therefore, we do not strongly support the signs of the coefficients of these indicators.

We have also tried to take states' priority to health as another explanatory variable. Whether the healthcare sector has been given priority by a state under adverse macroeconomic conditions is estimated in Chapter 2. As reported previously, any adverse conditions might have affected the overall public finances, but also affected the overall public spending in general and on the healthcare sector in particular of many states. A state able to manage high spending on healthcare in adverse conditions is referred to as 'high priority' accorded by the respective state; otherwise, it is referred to as 'low priority'. Using this connotation, we have derived state priority indicators in dichotomous (dummy) form. It takes value 1 if expenditure on health is positive during adverse condition or fiscal stringency period, and 0 otherwise. The purpose to include this variable is to find out how states have accorded priority to health. The state's priority (sp) is used as dummy variable (1 = high priority, 0 = otherwise) in the analysis.

The National Rural Health Mission (NRHM, 2005) classifies states having high fertility and mortality rates as high-focused states (HFS), and others as non-HFS. The state classification dummy is introduce to understand 'whether states with the same level of economic development follow the same trends when increasing health spending'. The value 1 is assigned to high-focused states (Assam, Bihar, Madhya Pradesh, Orissa, Rajasthan and Uttar Pradesh, except Himachal Pradesh) and 0 otherwise.

Estimation procedure

The estimation is done by considering 16 major states representing 90% of the population of India for the period from 1987–1988 to 2011–2012. The overall sample consists of a balanced panel of 400 observations covering 25 time series and 16 cross-section units. The panel data allows us to control and test for cross and time-invariant effects and to conduct appropriate analysis in the presence of those invariant effects (Baltagi, 2013; Greene, 2008). The specification of estimated panel equation is as follows:

$$lnhe_{st} = \beta_0 + \beta_1 lnsgdp_{st} + \beta_2 lnPPR_{st} + \beta_3 lnfc_{st} + \beta_4 lnIMR_{st} + \beta_5 lnpd_{st} + \beta_6 spd_{st} + \beta_7 scd_{st} + v_s + \varepsilon_{st} \ldots \tag{1}$$

Where, *lnhe* is log of real per capita public expenditure on health, *lnPPR* is log of political participation/representation index, *lnsgdp* is log of real per capita State's GDP representing state's income, *lnfc* is log of real per capita state's own revenue representing fiscal capacity of a state, *lnIMR* is log of infant mortality rate, *lnpd* is population density in a state, *sdp* is dummy variable reflecting state's priority to health sector, *sdp* is dummy of state classification into high-focused and non–high-focused states, *vs* is state-specific residual, *εst* is standard residual with the usual assumption of zero mean, uncorrelated with v and other explanatory variables, and homoscedasticity, *s* is state (16 states), and t is time from 1987–1988 to 2011–2012 (25 years).

Equation 1 can be estimated employing OLS estimators by simply stacking the data over *s* and *t* into one long regression with NT observations. The usual OLS output treats each of the *t* years as independent pieces of information, but there is minimal information, given the positive error correction. This leads to an overstatement of estimator precision, which can be very large. Therefore, one needs to use panel-corrected standard errors whenever OLS is applied in a panel setting. It is important to note that the OLS estimators will be inconsistent if the true model is a fixed effects model (Cameron and Trivedi, 2005). In such a situation, it becomes important to choose either a fixed effects (FE) model or a random effects (RE) model. The RE specification helps us to gauge the impact of different covariates as they change across states, while the FE model measures the impact of a change in any of these variables within a state. The Hausman specification test is applied to choose between FE and RE models. The Hausman test

(Ho: difference in coefficients not systematic) estimates show significant differences in the coefficients estimated by the consistent FE estimators and efficient RE estimators; therefore the FE model is more appropriate (see Hooda, 2016). That is, exogeneity of the regressors with respect to the time-invariant error terms was rejected, leading us to consider the FE model. In addition, simple descriptive statistics (presented in Table 4.2) show relatively high within-variance in many of the independent variables, suggesting a low statistical efficiency of RE model.

In order to ensure robust results and minimise the potentially confounding effects of unobserved state-specific attributes, the FE model is employed. Note that the OLS estimates are inconsistent, though results are reported to see the changes in the size of coefficient.

Furthermore, even after controlling for time-invariant country-fixed effects, the residual may contain time-varying factors that may be correlated with explanatory variables, which may lead to biased estimates for the coefficients. The FE model assumes that independent variables are strictly exogenous. Resultantly, its estimates will be inconsistent with models having endogenous variables and/or lagged dependent variables as regressors. In our case, 'state priority' dummy is derived from the dependent variable and is therefore endogenous in nature. Moreover, government's budgetary allocations for the healthcare sector (the dependent variable) generally depend on the amount allocated during the previous year. That is, current year fund allocation depends on what the government allocated in the previous year's budget. Thus, the introduction of lagged dependent variable in the analysis assumes importance. The models with a lagged dependent variable, which is correlated with the fixed effects, produce biased estimates. In order to provide efficient estimates, a dynamic panel set by Arellano-Bond is estimated using a Generalised Method of Moments (GMM) approach. The Arellano-Bond estimator corrects for the endogeneity in the lagged dependent variable and provides consistent parameter estimates, even in the presence of endogenous independent variables (Cameron and Trivedi, 2005). It also allows for individual fixed effects, heteroscedasticity and autocorrelation within individuals.

The first step of the GMM procedure is to remove individual effects by introducing instrumental variable(s) of endogenous regressors. Finding valid external instruments, however, is not easy. One of the main advantages of the GMM approach is that it draws instruments from within the data set, as lagged value of the instrumented or dependent variable. The normality assumption tests the exogeneity of instruments using the Sargan test. The GMM procedure therefore gains efficiency compared to OLS by exploiting additional moment restrictions. The estimated dynamic panel equation estimated using GMM is as follows:

$$\text{lnhest} = \alpha + \beta_0 \text{lnhe}_{st-1} + \beta_1 lnsgdp_{st} + \beta_2 lnPPI_{st} + \beta_3 lnfc_{st} + \\ \beta_4 lnIMR_{st} + \beta_5 lnpd_{st} + \beta_6 spd_{st} + \beta_7 scd_{st} + v_s + \varepsilon_{st} \ldots \quad (2)$$

lnhest-1 is the lagged dependent variable. Other variables have already been defined in Equation 1. In the dynamic model, the Sargan test (H0: over identifying restrictions are valid) shows that the population moment conditions specified in the model are correct. Estimates show that the H0 is not rejected, because Prob-value turned out to be (Prob > 0.05) in all estimations. The Arellano-Bond (H0: no autocorrelation) test for zero autocorrelation in first-differenced errors shows that the Arellano-Bond serial correlation test with 1st lag significant and 2nd lag insignificant tells us that the model is correctly specified at lag one (for details, see Hooda, 2016).

Preliminary findings

Table 4.2 summarises cross-state and time series variation in variables used in the analysis. The percentage difference between minimum and maximum values of dependent variables shows high time series (within) variation (97%) compared to cross-sectional (between) variation (85%). The percentage difference between the minimum and maximum values is reported to be high in time series compared to the cross-sectional variation in per capita income, fiscal capacity and political factors. On the contrary, cross-sectional variation is found to be greater in infant mortality rates and population density as compared to their time series differences in the maximum and minimum values.

The dependent variable (per capita health expenditure) and all covariates (political factor, income, fiscal capacity, population density, infant mortality rates) shows an upward trend in most of the states (Table 4.3), but there remains a considerably high variation across states. States like Tamil Nadu, Kerala, Himachal Pradesh and Punjab allocate a sizeable amount of public funds on healthcare, and consequently, their healthcare outcomes (like IMR) are better compared to other states. Assam and Haryana, despite spending a good amount of money on health, could not manage better outcomes. Some of the low-income states (Bihar, Orissa and Madhya Pradesh) spend low amounts on healthcare, and their healthcare outcomes are also poor. West Bengal and Maharashtra ranked low in per capita health spending, but secured good outcomes. It seems that the variation in health expenditure is not because of the preferences of individual states or because of prevailing mortality burden in the state. Some high-income states allocate low funds to the healthcare sector despite high prevalence of mortality burdens. Whether the differences in health expenditure are attributed to a state's income or state's interest (political factors) in promoting the sector, fiscal disability arising from unequal revenue-raising capacity or due to varying cost of providing health services, regional diversity, socio-economic conditions and demographic characteristics of a particular state is empirically examined in the next section.

Table 4.2 Summary statistics of selected variables across space and time

Variable		Mean	Std. dev.	Min.	Max.	Percentage diff.	Obs.
PCHE (in Rs.)	Overall	192	124	66	887	−92.6	400
	Between		112	89	580	−84.7	16
	Within		59	15	498	−97.0	25
PPR (index value)	Overall	3.88	0.70	2.42	5.49	−55.9	400
	Between		0.42	3.16	4.48	−29.5	16
	Within		0.56	2.56	6.21	−58.8	25
PCSGDP (in Rs.)	Overall	12875	7006	3034	38571	−92.1	400
	Between		4402	4905	19424	−74.7	16
	Within		5556	2926	32022	−90.9	25
PCFC (in Rs)	Overall	1175	706	221	3514	−93.7	400
	Between		530	343	2028	−83.1	16
	Within		484	220	3075	−92.8	25
IMR (in years)	Overall	63	23	10	127	−92.1	400
	Between		19	15	93	−83.9	16
	Within		13	26	105	−75.2	25
PD (sq km)	Overall	399	227	87	1014	−91.4	400
	Between		227	107	877	−87.8	16
	Within		54	231	577	−60.0	25
Percentage of total voter turnout	Overall	65.5	9.3	23.8	84.3	−71.8	400
	Between		7.0	52.4	77.4	−32.3	16
	Within		6.4	29.0	83.4	−65.2	25
Percentage of women voted to men voted	Overall	84.9	10.1	57.2	108.0	−47.0	400
	Between		9.3	70.2	103.0	−31.8	16
	Within		4.7	64.8	105.7	−38.7	25
Percentage of women contested	Overall	4.9	2.2	0.0	10.0	−100.0	400
	Between		0.8	3.9	6.5	−40.0	16
	Within		2.1	1.6	9.9	−83.8	25
Percentage of contested women elected	Overall	6.2	3.0	1.1	14.0	−92.1	400
	Between		1.7	3.1	10.0	−69.0	16
	Within		2.5	0.0	15.8	−100.0	25
Percentage of elected women and minority groups in PRIs		30.3	5.5	22.4	40.1	−44.1	16/400

Source: Author's estimates

Table 4.3 Trends in selected variables across states

States	Real PCHE (Rs.)		Real PCSGDP (Rs.)		Real PCFC (Rs.)		Pop. Density (per sq. km)		IMR (per 1000 live births)	
	1987–1988	2011–2012	1987–1988	2011–2012	1987–1988	2011–2012	1987–1988	2011–2012	1987–1988	2011–2012
Andhra Pradesh	134	230	6948	25357	815	2463	225	310	79	43
Assam	156	301	6185	17892	360	1552	278	393	102	55
Bihar	66	146	4254	9536	326	515	463	787	101	44
Gujarat	185	257	7952	28601	964	2632	199	308	97	41
Haryana	157	452	10159	35549	1368	2939	343	581	87	44
Himachal Pradesh	413	704	7087	29488	720	2847	87	124	82	38
Karnataka	145	247	6875	23380	839	2495	222	312	75	35
Kerala	140	315	6482	31044	754	2774	723	893	28	12
Madhya Pradesh	133	232	6254	17530	603	1828	137	222	120	59
Maharashtra	140	225	9475	38571	1105	2976	237	369	66	25
Orissa	106	181	4840	19050	345	1549	191	271	126	57
Punjab	149	338	12190	32981	1124	3196	376	587	62	30
Rajasthan	198	277	5285	15519	552	1386	119	200	102	52
Tamil Nadu	163	339	7440	34296	740	3514	414	521	76	22
Uttar Pradesh	82	167	5304	13060	405	1223	439	723	127	57
West Bengal	81	162	6328	17494	411	898	709	1014	71	32
States' avg.	**153**	**286**	**7066**	**24334**	**714**	**2174**	**323**	**476**	**88**	**40**

Source: Author's estimates

Impact of political and other factors on health expenditures

Table 4.4 presents a relationship between health expenditure, political factors, income, fiscal capacity and other variables. Per capita health expenditures appear to be positively correlated with levels of political participation and representation index, fiscal capacity of the states and with per capita income. The trends in IMR are negatively correlated with health expenditure, indicating that states which spend low amounts on health have the least healthy population. The demographic (population density) characteristic also shows negative association with health expenditure.

A robustness check of the results is done using advanced techniques. For instance, the OLS coefficient estimates of PPR were 'high' compared to other advanced robust techniques. The results obtained from this technique may be biased because some of the explanatory variables included in the model are not exclusively exogenous; they could result in correlation with the error term, and thus provide inconsistent estimates. Consequently, OLS presents biased estimates. In panel setting, even if one uses panel-corrected standard errors while applying OLS, the estimates will still be inconsistent if the true model is a fixed-effects model. As reported in the methodological section, the FE and GMM models are more suitable for our study. Therefore, we do not place much emphasis on results obtained from OLS estimation technique, though results are presented and discussed here.

The bivariate empirical investigation suggests that greater participation and representation of diverse groups in the electoral process leads to a significant rise in government spending on health (Table 4.5). The analysis from a bivariate analysis suggests that size of the coefficient for political factors turned out to be higher (1.46) than the income elasticity coefficient (0.58) and fiscal capacity variable coefficient (0.48) in the OLS estimation. The fixed effect and dynamic panel (GMM) estimates also reveal that size of coefficient of PPR higher than the income and fiscal capacity variables

Table 4.4 Correlation between selected variables

	lnpche	*lnpcsgdp*	*lnpcfc*	*lnPPR*	*lnimr*	*lnpd*	*spd*	*scd*
Lnpche	1	0.547	0.624	0.631	−0.262	−0.447	0.200	−0.047
lnpcsgdp	0.5465	1	0.4563	0.5485	−0.4723	0.0465	0.297	−0.1847
lnpcfc	0.6236	0.4563	1	0.9251	−0.486	−0.0333	0.2688	−0.5704
lnPPR	0.6312	0.5485	0.9251	1	−0.5432	0.0669	0.3495	−0.5159
lnimr	−0.2616	−0.4723	−0.486	−0.5432	1	−0.4971	−0.2903	0.5128
lnpd	−0.4467	0.0465	−0.0333	0.0669	−0.4971	1	0.1697	−0.4057
spd	0.1997	0.297	0.2688	0.3495	−0.2903	0.1697	1	−0.3232
scd	−0.0473	−0.1847	−0.5704	−0.5159	0.5128	−0.4057	−0.3232	1

Source: Author's estimates; variables description have been provided in methodological section

Table 4.5 Impact of economic and political factors on health expenditure: bivariate analysis

Eq. estim.	Independent variable	Pooled: OLS	Panel: FE	Dynamic panel: GMM
PPR on HE (eq-i)	PPR	1.46*** (0.112)	1.065*** (0.068)	0.33*** (0.063)
	Constant	3.17*** (0.151)	3.69*** (0.092)	0.508*** (0.130)
	L1			0.82*** (0.0329)
Income on HE (eq-ii)	lnpcgsdp	0.586*** (0.036)	0.521*** (0.021)	0.210*** (0.024)
	Constant	−0.347 (0.337)	0.262 (0.214)	−0.425 (0.150)
	L1			0.703*** (0.035)
Fiscal capacity on HE (eq-iii)	lnpcfc	0.480*** (0.030)	0.502*** (0.023)	0.183*** (0.024)
	Constant	1.817 (0.209)	1.670 (0.180)	0.109 (0.127)
	L1			0.736*** (0.035)

Source and note: Author's Estimates; ***, **, * are 1%, 5%, and 10% significance level; N = 400 (n = 16, t = 25); Adj-R2, Housman specification and Sargan test values are not reported.

in the bivariate analysis without controlling other confounding factors (Table 4.5).

It is interesting to note that the empirical estimates fall in value when one moves from a bivariate regression to multivariate regression. The coefficient values also fall when on move towards a more advanced robust technique, say from pooled (OLS) to panel (FE) and then to dynamic panel (GMM) estimation (Table 4.6). This indicates a decline in the magnitude of coefficient with the inclusion of other observed determinants and estimation techniques. For instance, the coefficient value of PPR was 0.57 in OLS estimations, when controlled for income, fiscal capacity and other confounding factors. The coefficients value of income (0.31) and fiscal capacity (0.14) remained even lower than PPR coefficient (0.57) in OLS estimation. The coefficient value of PPR also noticed to be higher than fiscal capacity variable in FE and GMM estimate, when control for all confounding factors. However, the coefficient values of PPR in FE (0.19) and GMM (0.097) estimation were slightly lower than the coefficient of income (FE 0.32 and GMM 0.16), but remained statistically significant with a positive sign (Table 4.6).

Table 4.7 provides an interesting insight about the impact of PPR. It reveals that if, on average, political participation/representation of diverse population groups is high in any state/year, then spending on healthcare is likely to be high even if state's fiscal capacity is low. This is reflected from the interaction variable of fiscal capacity and PPR dummy. A popular notion is that government's desire to increase healthcare spending is highly dependent on the availability of financial resources with the states, failing which the probability of fulfilling expenditure obligations towards the sector may be low; however, interaction terms suggest that even if fiscal capacity is low,

Table 4.6 Politicising health expenditure: pooled and panel regression estimates

	Pooled: OLS	Panel: FE	Dynamic panel: GMM
lnPPR	0.571*** (0.089)	0.191** (0.076)	0.097* (0.073)
lnsgdp	0.312*** (0.074)	0.317*** (0.068)	0.156** (0.059)
lnfc	0.141** (0.063)	0.152** (0.052)	0.045 (0.046)
lnimr	−0.237*** (0.041)	0.334*** (0.076)	−0.022 (0.064)
lnpd	−0.425*** (0.0299)	0.632*** (0.143)	−0.11** (0.046)
scd	0.190*** (0.0378)		−0.016 (0.057)
spd	0.0516* (0.028)	0.0208 (0.018)	0.057** (0.018)
Adj-R2 and L1	R2 = 0.7314	R2 = 0.5443	lnhe.L1 = 0.679*** (0.037)
M1: z (p > z)			−3.403 (0.0007)
M2: z (p > z)			1.1504 (0.2500)
Sargan: chi2 (P > chi2)			304.2 (0.068)

Source and Note: same as Table 4.5; lnhe.L1 is one lag value of dependent variable (lnhe)

Table 4.7 Prioritising budget and GDP for health through politics: an interaction regression analysis

		Pooled: OLS	Panel: FE	Dynamic panel: GMM
Prioritising budget for health through PPR (eq-i)	lnpcfc	0.198*** (0.045)	0.303*** (0.038)	0.124*** (0.034)
	Interaction fc*ppr	0.128*** (0.016)	0.066*** (0.010)	0.023** (0.010)
	Constant	2.573*** (0.215)	2.431*** (0.209)	0.424** (0.181)
	L1			0.712*** (0.036)
Prioritising GDP for health through PPR (eq-ii)	lnpcgsdp	0.336*** (0.052)	0.389*** (0.034)	0.187*** (0.037)
	Interaction gdp*ppr	0.081*** (0.013)	0.036*** (0.007)	0.006 (0.008)
	Constant	0.973** (0.383)	1.047*** (0.265)	−0.267 (0.242)
	L1			0.698*** (0.035)

Source and note: see Table 4.5; interaction variables are lnpcfc*ppr dummy and lnpcgsdp*ppr dummy in eq-i and eq-ii. For interaction variables, a dummy of PPR is created with value 1 for years/states more than average value of PPR index and 0 otherwise, using its value an interaction term is created with fiscal capacity (lnpcfc) and income (lnpcgsdp) variables.

high participation of population in politics can influence the government to spend more on healthcare. Similarly, if, on average, political participation and representation of diverse population groups is high in any state or year, then spending on healthcare is likely to be high, even if the state's income is low. This is reflected from the interaction variable of income and PPR dummy. This analysis reveals that political participation assumes greater significance in influencing the government to allocate more funds from the budget and GDP for the healthcare sector.

This analysis suggests that with an increase in political participation and representation, one can assume a concomitant rise in welfare spending like health across states of India. In other words, greater participation in the electoral process allows political authorities to align their decisions with the interests and priorities of the general public. Thus, one can argue that political factors do matter in determining public spending on healthcare. That is, one can expect an increase in welfare spending if, overall, more excluded groups are incorporated into the political process through constitutionally mandated consensual rules. This estimation suggests that participation of diversified groups in electing a political representative makes the elected government sensitive to satisfying their interests – especially to win the next election (Przeworski et al., 2000). This is important in public policy discourse, particularly for ensuring state interventionism in welfare activities like provision of health services. Some other studies that have tried to examine the impact of other dimensions of political factors have reported a positive impact of variable 'political competition' on public healthcare expenditure in Indian states (Datta, 2020; Kosec et al., 2018, Chaudhry and Mazhar, 2018; Ghosh, 2010; Besley and Burgess, 2002). These studies suggest that government formed after a competitive assembly election tends to spend more on public healthcare.

As regards to the impact of level of development measured through income, the coefficient values of the impact of per capita income decline in magnitude and precision with the inclusion of other possible determinants of per capita health expenditure and robust technique. However, the income elasticity estimates, across different estimators, remained significant in influencing the growth in health expenditure. The income elasticity of health expenditure ranges between 0.15 and 0.59 across these estimations (Table 4.5, Table 4.6 and Table 4.7), which is less than 1. In contrast to the findings of equal to or greater than 1 (largely in case of advanced countries), income elasticity in the Indian context turned out to be less than 1. These empirical results suggest that health is not a luxury good; rather, it is a necessary good in India. The low value of income elasticity estimates allow us to argue that the public health sector has not been given high priority amongst the goals for social and economic development of the country.

It is true that the government's desire to increase health spending mainly depends on the availability of financial resources. The fiscal capacity of a particular state turns significant in influencing public health expenditure. The coefficient value of fiscal capacity variable ranges from 0.04–0.48 in different bivariate and multivariate estimations presented in Table 4.5, Table 4.6 and Table 4.7. In Table 4.5 and Table 4.7, the coefficients of fiscal capacity variable were significant in FE estimation, while positive but insignificant in GMM estimation in Table 4.6. Overall, it can be argued that with higher fiscal capacity (an indication of high resource availability and autonomy with the state governments), government spending on health will be higher. Low resource availability or fiscal stringency can get in the way of fulfilling the expenditure obligations and commitments for providing better healthcare services in the country. This is in line with the argument that high resource allocation towards any sector requires more fiscal space with the government. In order to meet the expenditure obligation for any particular sector, states will have to focus on generating revenue from their own sources, either through widening the tax base or by improving the administrative and technical efficiencies for resource collection. An increased fiscal capacity not only provides autonomy to allocate resources to different sectors, but also reduces fiscal dependency on central transfers.

The estimates from dynamic panel show that the coefficient value of lagged dependent variable turned out to be significant in both bivariate and multivariate estimations presented in Table 4.5, Table 4.6 and Table 4.7. The coefficient value of a lagged dependent variable was also observed as higher than any other covariate in the analysis in dynamic panel estimations. This means that – in addition to other factors – policy decisions taken in the past (for instance, previous year budget allocations for various health schemes) define, to a considerable degree, the future path of policy development and the level of state interventionism in the health sector.

The coefficient estimates of demographic factors like population density and infant mortality rate are negative and significant in OLS estimation, while they turned positive and significant in FE estimation. The former, however, turned negatively insignificant in the dynamic panel estimation, while the latter was negatively significant. Coefficient estimates of these variables have remained inconclusive in the analysis.

The coefficient value of government priority variable turned positive and significant, indicating that the health sector has been given significant priority in states that have managed to sustain growth trend, even in times of fiscal stringency and/or under adverse macroeconomic conditions as compared to their counterparts.

One important finding of the study is that the coefficient estimates of most of the important covariates show an upward bias in magnitude and precision due to the absence of unobserved control determinants of per capita health expenditure and an advanced robust estimation technique.

The findings of this study, however, do not rule out the possible confounding effects of simultaneity bias in the estimation. One can evaluate the sensitivity of empirical estimates through the inclusion of more/other confounding factors and instruments, techniques, etc. This study has added new dimensions such as establishing the importance of political factors and fiscal capacity in public policy discourse, which are very significant. No doubt, we have also reassessed the elasticity estimates with robust samples and techniques. The results of elasticity estimates are more or less consistent with the other study estimates on developing countries/regions.

Conclusion

The estimates suggest that with the widening of access to political participation and representation of diverse population groups, one can see a concomitant rise in government spending on health, indicating that state intervention in welfare activities increases with political participation. More interestingly, if, on average, political participation/representation of diverse population groups is high in any state, then spending on health is also likely to be high – even if state's income is low. In that sense, political participation assumes greater significance in influencing the government to allocate more funds to the health-care sector amongst the other economic development factors of the state. The government's desire to increase healthcare spending is highly dependent on the availability of financial resources with the states, failing which the probability of fulfilling expenditure obligations towards the sector may be low.

In contrast to the estimates of previous studies that income elasticity of health expenditure is greater than 1, this study suggests that income elasticity is less than 1. No doubt, higher income contributes to higher public spending on health, but having a coefficient value of less than 1 indicates that health is a necessary good. The low-income elasticity estimates indicate that the public healthcare sector has not been given high priority amongst the goals for social and economic development in the country.

We noticed that the coefficient estimates of most of the important covariates are biased upward in magnitude and precision due to the absence of control for unobserved determinants and of an advance robust estimation technique. Thus, inclusion or exclusion of more or other confounding factors and instruments/techniques, etc., may influence the results. This study concludes that no approach/study/technique in itself represents the whole truth, but each study is a grain-sized contribution to the estimation process. However, given the diverse nature of explanatory variables and techniques used, this study has added new dimensions: establishing how political participation and fiscal capacity variables matter in influencing public policy, particularly government expenditure on welfare activities like health services. Our results on elasticity estimates are more or less consistent with those of many previous studies.

Note

1   This chapter draws from certain inferences and data previously published in S. K. Hooda. 2016. Determinants of Public Expenditure on Health in India: A Panel Data Analysis at Sub-National Level. *Journal of Quantitative Economics*, Vol. 14, No. 2, pp. 257–282, Springer Nature, https://doi.org/10.1007/s40953-016-0033-8.

References

Abuja Declaration. 2000. *The Abuja Declaration: Ten Years On.* www.who.int/healthsystems/publications/abuja_report_aug_2011.pdf?ua=1

Akin, J. P., Hutchinson, P., and Strumpf, K. 2001. *Decentralized and Government Provision of Public Goods: The Public Health Sector in Uganda.* Working paper WP-01–35. MEASURE Evaluation: Carolina Population Center, University of North Carolina and Chapel Hill. www.cpc.unc.edu/measure/publications/pdf/wp-01-35.pdf

Baker, L. C., and Wheeler, S. K. 2000. Managed Care and Technology Diffusion the Case of MRI. *Health Affairs*, Vol. 17, pp. 195–207.

Baltagi, B. H. 2013. *Econometric Analysis of Panel Data*, 5th Edition. John Wiley & Sons Ltd., West Sussex, England.

Baltagi, B. H., and Moscone, F. 2010. Health Care Expenditure and Income in the OECD Reconsidered: Evidence from Panel Data. *Economic Modelling*, Vol. 27, No. 4, pp. 804–811.

Barros, P. 1998. The Black Box of Health Care Expenditure Growth Determinants. *Health Economics*, Vol. 7, pp. 533–544.

Baum, M. A., and Lake, D. A. 2003. The Political Economy of Growth: Democracy and Human Capital. *American Journal of Political Science*, Vol. 47, No. 2, pp. 333–347. www.jstor.org/stable/3186142

Beaman, L., et al. 2012. Female Leadership Raises Aspirations and Educational Attainment for Girls: A Policy Experiment in India. *Science*, Vol. 335, No. 6068, pp. 582–586. www.ncbi.nlm.nih.gov/pmc/articles/PMC3394179/#

Bellido, H., et al. 2019. Do Political Factors Influence Public Health Expenditures? Evidence Pre- and Post-great Recession. *The European Journal of Health Economics*, Vol. 20, pp. 455–474.

Besley, T., and Burgess, R. 2002. The Political Economy of Government Responsiveness: Theory and Evidence from India. *Quantitative Journal of Economics*, Vol. 117, No. 4, pp. 1415–1451. http://doi.org/10.1162/ 003355302320935061

Besley, T., and Coate, S. 1997. An Economic Model of Representative Democracy. *Quarterly Journal of Economics*, Vol. 112, No. 1, pp. 85–114.

Besley, T., Pande, R., and Rao, V. 2005. Participatory Democracy in Action: Survey Evidence from India. *Journal of the European Economics Association*, Vol. 3, No. 2–3, pp. 648–657.

Bhat, R., and Jain, N. 2004. *Analysis of Public Expenditure on Health Using State Level Data.* Indian Institute of Management, Ahmadabad, Gujarat, June.

Cameron, C. A., and Trivedi, P. K. 2005. *Microeconometrics: Methods and Applications.* Cambridge University Press, Cambridge.

Chaudhry, A., and Mazhar, U. 2018. *Political Competition and Economic Performance: Empirical Evidence from Pakistan.* Economics Discussion Papers, No 2018-27, Kiel Institute for the World Economy. http://www.economicsejournal.org/economics/discussionpapers/2018-27

Chhibber, P., and Nooruddin, I. 2004. Do Party Systems Count? The Number of Parties and Government Performance in the Indian States. *Comparative Political Studies*, Vol. 37, No. 2, pp. 152–187.

Crepaz, M. M. L. 1998, October. Inclusion versus Exclusion: Political Institutions and Welfare Expenditures. *Comparative Politics*, Vol. 31, No. 1, pp. 61–80.

Culyer, A. J. 1988. *Health Care Expenditures in Canada: Myth and Reality, Past and Future.* Canadian Tax Foundation, Toronto, Ont.

Datta, S. 2020. Political Competition and Public Healthcare Expenditure: Evidence from Indian States. *Social Science & Medicine*, Vol. 224. https://doi.org/10.1016/j.socscimed.2019.112429

De la Maisonneuve, C., Moreno-Serra, R., Murtin, F., and Martins, O. J. 2016. *The Drivers of Public Health Spending: Integrating Policies and Institutions*. OECD Economics Department Working Papers, 1283, OECD Publishing, Paris. https://doi.org/10.1787/5jm2f76rnhkj-en

Di Matteo, L. 2003. The Income Elasticity of Health Care Spending: A Comparison of Parametric and Nonparametric Approaches. *The European Journal of Health Economics*, Vol. 4, pp. 20–29.

Di Matteo, L., and Di Matteo, R. 1998. Evidence on the Determinants of Canadian Provincial Government Health Expenditures: 1965–1991. *Journal of Health Economics*, Vol. 17, No. 2, pp. 211–228.

Dregen, C., and Reimers, H. E. 2005. Health Care Expenditures in OECD Countries: A Panel Unit Root and Cointegration Analysis. *International Journal of Applied Econometrics and Quantitative Studies*, Vol. 2, pp. 5–20. IZA Discussion Paper n. 1469.

Duflo, E. 2005. *Gender Equality in Development*. Bureau for Research in Economic Analysis of Development, Policy Paper No. 011. http://ipl.econ.duke.edu/bread/papers/policy/p011.pdf

Dummer, T. J. B., and Cook, I. G. 2008. Health in China and India: A Cross-country Comparison in a Context of Rapid Globalization. *Social Science & Medicine*, Vol. 67, No. 4, pp. 590–605.

Durairaj, V., and Evans, D. B. 2010. *Fiscal Space for Health in Resource-poor Countries*. World Health Report-2010. Background Paper No. 41. www.who.int/healthsystems/topics/financing/healthreport/41FiscalSpace.pdf

Erdil, E., and Yetkiner, I. H. 2009. The Granger-causality Between Health Care Expenditure and Output: A Panel Data Approach. *Applied Economics*. Taylor & Francis, Vol. 41, No. 4, pp. 511–518.

Esping-Andersen, G. 1990. *The Three Words of Welfare Capitalism*. Princeton University Press, Princeton.

Faguet, J. P. 2004. Does Decentralization Increase Responsiveness to Local Needs? Evidence from Bolivia. *Journal of Public Economics*, Vol. 88, pp. 867–894.

Farag, M., et al. 2009. Does Funding from Donors Displace Government Spending for Health in Developing Countries? *Health Affairs*, Vol. 28, No. 4, p. 1045.

Gaag, J. van der, and Stimac, V. 2008. *Towards a New Paradigm for Health Sector Development*. Amsterdam Institute for International Development, Amsterdam.

Gerdtham, U. G., and Jönsson, B. 2000. International Comparisons of Health Expenditure: Theory, Data and Econometric Analysis. In A. J. Culyer and J. P. Newhouse (Eds.), *Handbook of Health Economics*. Elsevier, Amsterdam, pp. 11–53.

Gerdtham, U. G., and Löthgren, M. 2002. New Panel Results on Cointegration of International Health Expenditure and GDP. *Applied Economics*, Vol. 34, No. 13, pp. 1679–1686.

Gerdtham, U. G., et al. 1998. The Determinants of Health Expenditure in the OECD Countries: A Pooled Data Analysis. In P. Zweifel (Ed.), *Health, The Medical Profession, and Regulation*. Kluwer Academic Publishers, Boston, pp. 113–134.

Gerdtham, U. G., Sogaard, J., et al. 1992. An Econometric Analysis of Health Care Expenditure: A Cross-section Study of the OECD Countries. *Journal of Health Economics*, Vol. 11, No. 1, pp. 63–84.

Ghosh, S. 2010. Does Political Competition Matter for Economic Performance? Evidence from Sub-national Data. *Political Studies*, Vol. 58, No. 5, pp. 1030–1048. http://doi.org/10.1111/j. 1467-9248.2010.00823.x

Government of India. 2013. *14th Finance Commission of India, Background Paper on Estimating True Fiscal Capacity of States and Devising a Suitable Rule for Granting Debt Relief based on Optimal Growth Requirement.* Government of India (GOI). http://fincomindia.nic.in/writereaddata%5Chtml_en_files%5Cfincom14/others/32.pdf

Greene, W. H. 2008. *Econometric Analysis*, 5th Edition, Pearson Education, Published by Dorling Kindersley Pvt. Ltd., New Delhi.

Gronbjerg, K. 1977. *Mass Society and the Extension of Welfare, 1960–1970.* University of Chicago Press, Chicago.

Halse, A. 2009. *A Woman's Touch: The Impact of Gender on Political Priorities.* Thesis, Centre of Equality, Social Organization, and Performance (ESOP), University of Oslo. www.esop.uio.no/research/masterthesis/Halse.xml

Hartwig, J. 2008. What Drives Health Care Expenditure? Baumol's Model of Unbalanced Growth Revisited. *Journal of Health Economics*, Vol. 27, No. 3, pp. 603–623.

Hitiris, T., and Posnett, J. 1992. The Determinants and Effects of Health Expenditure in Developed Countries. *Journal of Health Economics*, Vol. 11, pp. 173–181.

Hooda, S. K. 2016. Determinants of Public Expenditure on Health in India: A Panel Data Analysis at Sub-National Level. *Journal of Quantitative Economics*, Springer Publication, Vol. 14, No. 2, pp. 257–282.

Joshi, D. K., and Yu, B. 2014. Political Determinants of Public Health Investment in China and India. *Asian Politics & Policy*, Vol. 6, No. 1, pp. 59–82. https://doi.org/10.1111/aspp.12087

Kosec, K., Haider, H., Spielman, D. J., and Zaidi, F. 2018. Political Competition and Rural Welfare: Evidence from Pakistan. *Oxford Economic Papers*, Vol. 70, No. 4, pp. 1036–1061.

Kumar, R. 2015. Lack of Social or Political Demand for Good Health Care in India: Impact on Unfolding Universal Health Coverage. *Journal of Family Medicine and Primary Care*, Vol. 4, No. 1, pp. 1–2. http://doi.org/10.4103/2249-4863.152234

Kundu, A. 1984. *Measurement of Urban Processes: A Study in Regionalisation.* Popular Prakashan, Bombay.

Leu, R. R. 1986. *Public and Private Health Services: Complementarities and Conflicts, Chapter the Public-private Mix and International Health Care Cost.* Basil Blackwell, Oxford.

Lindgren, K.-O., et al. 2009, November. Who Knows Best What the People Want: Women or Men?: A Study of Political Representation in India. *Comparative Political Studies*, Vol. 42, No. 1. https://doi.org/10.1177/0010414008324992

Lu, C., et al. 2010. Public Financing of Health in Developing Countries: A Cross-national Systematic Analysis. *The Lancet*, Vol. 375, No. 9723, pp. 1375–1387.

Ma, S., and Sood, N. 2008. *A Comparison of the Health Systems in China and India.* www.rand.org/pubs/occasional_papers/OP212.html

Matteo, L. D. 2003. The Income Elasticity of Health Care Spending. *The European Journal of Health Economics*, Vol. 4, No. 1, pp. 20–29. https://doi.org/10.1007/s10198-002-0141-6

Matteo, L. D., and Matteo, R. D. 1998. The Fiscal Sustainability of Alberta's Public Health Care System. *SSRN Electronic Journal*, Vol. 2, No. 2. https://doi.org/10.2139/ssrn.3046639

Murthy, V., and Okunade, A. 2009. The Core Determinants of Health Expenditure in the African Context: Some Econometric Evidence for Policy. *Health Policy*, Vol. 91, No. 1, pp. 57–62.

Newhouse, J. P. 1977. Medical-care Expenditure: A Cross-national Survey. *The Journal of Human Resources*, Vol. 12, No. 1, pp. 115–125.

NFHS. 2016. *National Health and Family Welfare (NFHS-4): 2015–16*. Ministry of Health and Family Welfare, Government of India (GOI).

NRHM. 2005. *Mission Documents of the National Rural Health Mission (NRHM)*. Government of India (GOI). http://mohfw.nic.in/nrhm.html

Oates, W. 1977. *The Political Economy of Fiscal Federalism*. Lexington Books, Lexington, Massachussets (MA), D.C.

Okunade, A. A., and Karakus, M. C. 2001. Unit Root and Cointegration Tests: Time-series Versus Panel Estimates for International Health Expenditure Models. *Applied Economics*, Vol. 33, No. 9, pp. 1131–1137.

Przeworski, A., Alvarez, M. E., Cheibub, J. A., and Limongi, F. 2000. *Democracy and Development: Political Institutions and Well-being in the World, 1950-1990*. Cambridge University Press, New York.

RHS. 2019. Bulletin on *Rural Health Statistics* (RHS) *2019*. Ministry of Health and Family Welfare, Government of India, New Delhi.

Roberts, J. 1999. Sensitivity of Elasticity Estimates for OECD Health Care Spending: Analysis of a Dynamic Heterogeneous Data Field. *Health Economics*, Vol. 8, No. 5, pp. 459–472.

Savedoff, W. D. 2007. What Should a Country Spend on Health Care? *Health Affairs*, Vol. 26, No. 4.

Sen, A. 2005, June. Is Health Care a Luxury? New Evidence from OECD Data. *International Journal of Health Care Finance and Economics*, Vol. 5, No. 2, pp. 147–164.

State Election Report. various years. *Statistical Report on the Legislative Assembly Election, Individual State Election Reports, Election Commission of India*. Government of India, New Delhi, http://eci.nic.in/eci_main1/ElectionStatistics.aspx

Svaleryd, H. 2009. Women's Representation and Public Spending. *European Journal of Political Economy*, Vol. 25, No. 2, pp. 186–198. https://econpapers.repec.org/article/eeepoleco/v_3a25_3ay_3a2009_3ai_3a2_3ap_3a186-198.htm

Tandon, A., et al. 2014. Reprioritizing Government Spending on Health: Pushing an Elephant Up the Stairs? *WHO South-East Asia Journal of Public Health*, Vol. 3, No. 3, pp. 206–212. www.who-seajph.org/article.asp?issn=2224-3151;year=2014 ;volume=3;issue=3;spage=206;epage=212;aulast=Tandon

Thomas, D. 1990. Intra-Household Resource Allocation: An Inferential Approach. *The Journal of Human Resources*, Vol. 25, No. 4, pp. 635–664. www.jstor.org/stable/145670

Vatter, A., and Ruefli, C. 2003. Do Political Factor Matter for Health Expenditure: A Comparative Study of Swiss Cantons. *Journal of Public Policy*, Vol. 23, No. 3, pp. 301–323.

Wagstaff, A., and Bank, W. 2009. *Social Health Insurance Vs. Tax-financed Health Systems: Evidence from the OECD*, World Bank, East Asia & Pacific. https://doi.org/10.1596/1813-9450-4821

Weil, T. P. 1995. Comparisons of Medical Technology in Canadian, German, and US Hospitals. *Hospital & Health Services Administration*, Vol. 40, pp. 524–533.

WHO. 2008. *The World Health Report 2008 – Primary Health Care* (Now More Than Ever). www.who.int/whr/2008/en/

WHO. 2010. *Health System Financing: The Path to Universal Coverage, World Health Report*. World Health Organisation (WHO), Geneva.

WHO. 2011. *Non Communicable Diseases Country Profile 2011*. www.who.int/ nmh/publications/ncd_profiles2011/en/, accessed on 15/04/2013.

WHO. 2013 and 2015. *World Health Statistics, 2013 & 2015*. World Health Organization, Geneva.

Wilson, R. M. 1999. Medical Care Expenditures and GDP Growth in OECD Nations. *American Association of Behavioral and Social Sciences Journal*, Vol. 2, pp. 159–171.

World Bank. 2009. *World Development Report-2009*. World Bank, Washington, DC.

Xu, K., Saksena, P., and Holly, A. 2011. *The Determinants of Health Expenditure: A Country-Level Panel Data Analysis*. Result for Development Institute, World Health Organization, Working Paper, December 2011. https://www.who.int/ health_financing/documents/report_en_11_deter-he.pdf

5 Decentralisation in health

Rationale, measurements and effectiveness[1]

Well-documented phenomena are that public investment in health influences health outcomes positively (Barenberg et al., 2016; Arthur and Oaikhenan, 2017; Rahman et al., 2018), reduces health gaps/inequalities (Barenberg et al., 2016), addresses many preventable and untimely deaths (GBD, 2018) and helps in achieving universal health coverage. If health system advances and investments made do not keep the pace with population health needs, one can expect slow progress in securing better health outcomes (GBD, 2018). Any restriction on spending would have devastating impact on child mortality (Breman and Shelton, 2001; Maruthappu, 2015), especially for low-income groups in developing countries (Gupta et al., 2001; Gwatkn, 1999 & 2000) more than the high-income countries (Tandon, 2005). Despite such encouraging results, health systems of many developing countries are facing underfunding problems, alongside inefficiencies in utilisation of the scanty amounts of funding allocated towards the sector. The inefficiency in fund utilisation is a general phenomenon in the context of policies addressing unemployment, poverty, inequality and management of public health services which require a set of institutional reforms (Cassel, 1995). Citing a relationship between life expectancy at birth with the resources that countries devote to health, Berman and Bitran (2011) presented a high variability in the relationship between performance and spending, demonstrating the weak link between these two. It indicated that variables like quality of policies and institutions play a greater role for health system performance. The study by Chaudhury et al. (2006), while citing a case of absenteeism of health staffs from health facility of 35–40%, indicated that the weak institutions for supplying public goods like healthcare are a significant barrier to economic development in many countries. The much recent discussion of economic development therefore revolves around the role of institutions that strengthen governance.

The idea of institutional economic reforms is increasingly being applied to understanding and accelerating the process of economic development, as well as for shaping the sector-specific outcome from an efficiency point of view that influences the outcomes directly or indirectly via improving the efficacy of resource utilisation. Earlier, the idea of institutions arose in

DOI: 10.4324/9781032108438-7

critical response to the neoclassical theory – in particular, the inadequacy of the neoclassical theory in dealing with uneven performance of economies across space and time, and its limited potential to explain persistence of inefficient institutions and role of ideology in choice determination of individuals (North, 1997). Neoclassical economics does not deal with the incentives and behaviour of political actors, or the influence of political processes on target for growth, stability or the division of public investment among sectors (Eggertsson, 1997).

It is increasingly being realised that these factors play critical roles in explaining persistent unevenness across space and time. Literature indicates that neoclassical economics completely ignores the 'power' dimension in policy making (Schmid, 1978). The framework has also been criticised for construction of its own 'idealised' world, one that it does not encompass the reality and efficacy of transaction costs (Williamson, 1990). The framework offers no scope to integrate politics into economics and does not help to capture the real-time phenomenon of economic outcomes as influenced by political institutions. Institutions are taken for granted in mainstream economics for observing the social rules, conventions and other elements of the structural framework of social interaction (Bardhan, 1989). These inadequacies led to a shifted focus on the role of political and individual ideologies, institutions and incentives in explaining economic performance.

In a more fundamental work on institutions and their possible channels that influence economic performance, North (1990) pointed out that institutions are everywhere, and ignoring them would lead to incompleteness of conclusions and policy implications. While analysing the geography and institutions in the making of modern world income distribution, Acemoglu et al. (2002: 1231) argued that among the areas colonised by European powers during the past 500 years, those that were relatively rich in 1500 are now relatively poor. This reversal in relative incomes appears to reflect the effect of institutions. Among the determinant factors (like institutions, geography and trade) of income level around the world, Rodrik et al. (2004) showed that quality of institutions – in particular, the role of property rights and the rule of law – matter more (positively) in determining the income. In an example, Przeworski (2005) observed that the countries which were ruled by dictatorships grow slowly, whereas growth is recorded faster in democratic countries. To understand why some economies have good economic performance while others do not, many scholars identify that institutions – the political system, the bureaucracy, the fiscal system, the welfare state, the institutions of industrial policy, and so on – have significant impact on different outcomes and economic performance of a country or region. Chang (2007) and Kaufmann et al. (2002) showed high and positive correlation between quality of governance and per capita income across many developed and developing countries. Hall and Jones (1999) found huge differences in output per worker across countries in the world. They argue that the difference in output is caused by differences in the so-called social infrastructure (that which is formed by the institutional structure of the economy) rather than difference in capital and human capital.

While explaining the performance of economies over space and time, scholars have emphasised the role of institutions in economic development. They suggest some measures for improvement in institutions of developing countries as a way of promoting their economic development. One important dimension that emerges is that not only are many of the 'global standard' institutions inappropriate for developing countries, but the institutional reforms that are directly derived from the experiences of the developed countries do not work for them. It is argued that the institutions can vary across space and time. They cannot be imported. They are endogenous (North, 1990, 1997). Their form and their functioning depend on the conditions under which they emerge and endure. The characteristics and effects of particular institutions depend on the conditions under which they function. Same institutions can – and do – serve different and/or multiple functions in -different countries or regions, and perform differently.

The literature in health economics argues that institutions and governance are central in determining the efficacy of public spending. The countries with good governance levels secured better health outcomes (Makuta and O'Hare, 2015), even with lower or the same levels of spending (Farag et al., 2013). A study by Rajkumar and Swaroop (2008) found that a 1-percentage-point increase in the share of public health spending in GDP lowers the under-5 mortality rate by 0.32% in countries with good governance (measured by corruption index) and 0.20% in countries with average governance, but has no impact in countries with weak governance. The impact of spending in improving the maternal mortality, underweight children under age 5 and tuberculosis mortality increased significantly with increase in levels of good governance (measured by the Country Policy and Institutional Assessment [CPIA] index).[2] The impact of increase in government health expenditure on MDGs outcomes was none/minimal in countries with low CPIA governance level (Wagstaff and Claeson, 2004). The impact (size of coefficient) of the increase in government spending on health thus depends on the level of good governance achieved by the country that refers to the intuitional structure.

Decentralised institutions

In recent times, among the many forms of institutions that affect the economic performance of a country, the institution of federalism (decentralisation) has been advocated as a powerful means of improving the provision of public goods such as healthcare services and outcomes of the healthcare sector. It is argued that devolving power to local governments would improve service delivery, equity, accountability, effectiveness and efficiency, and thereby utilisation of health services and health outcomes. A high amount of public spending on healthcare services sometimes will not contribute substantially, if the existing facilities or funds are not implemented and managed through proper channels or through effective government interventions like community participation or decentralisation (Hanmer et al., 2003). The decentralised mechanism improves accountability, effectiveness and efficiency of service delivery (Litvack et al., 1998; Bossert and Beauvais, 2002) by bringing decision makers closer to the people and by enhancing the participation of communities in the decision making and implementation processes. Their close relation with the local people enables them to know the local problems and needs, and they are therefore in a better position to establish the right priorities than a central or regional government far away (Peabody et al., 1999). The theory of public economics argues that local governments have more and better information regarding their constituents, and they may be better able to enforce and coordinate policies and programmes at the local level (Oates, 1994; Prud'homme, 1995). Being at a close proximity to those in charge also enables citizens to better monitor the responsible parties' performance and hold them accountable.

The health reformists argue that decentralisation can enhance the participation of local communities in decisions regarding health policy objectives, goals, strategies, planning, financing, implementation and monitoring, which are important to improve healthcare outcomes (Lieberman, 2002). It also promotes intersectoral coordination, increases accountability, reduces duplication and improves implementation of health programmes. This, in turn, affects the quality and coverage of health services delivery – and thereby health outcomes – especially in reducing the mortality rates in many countries to varying degrees (Robalino et al., 2001). The marginal benefits from decentralisation were greater in some low and middle-income countries (Khaleghian, 2003; Ebel and Yilmaz, 2002) like India (Mahal et al., 2000; Asfaw et al., 2004), Argentinean provinces (Habibi et al., 2001) and China (Yee, 2001); however, no or negative benefits were seen in some others (Treisman, 2000; Montoya and Vaughan, 1990). Studies have argued that outcomes of the impact of decentralisation are affected by how the decentralised policies are designed, measured (Ebel and Yilmaz, 2002) and implemented –the absence of which may pose risks and present challenges that may lead to deterioration in the provision of health services, and consequently to poor health outcomes (Lieberman, 2002). For instance, Nigeria has a system of decentralised delivery of primary healthcare servicesI, but has several problems relating to ambiguity in sharing of responsibilities between the three tiers of local governments (Johan and Jacob, 2016). The absence of trust between authorities of the health governance system and local communities caused a delay in preventing the spread of Ebola (Mishra, 2015). A significant number of functionaries were transferred to local governments in Indonesia in 2001, but with limited power relating to appointment and dismissal of personnel (Hoffman and Kaiser, 2002).

Some scholars, however, believe the inherent assumptions behind the pro-decentralisation stance are simply weak or absent in developing countries. Hence, the benefits of decentralisation may not be realised. One counterargument is that decentralisation does not automatically bring about productive efficiencies. Bardhan (2002) contends that information asymmetries between the central authority and sub-national governments might cause serious problems with regard to the kind of services delivered to the public. Because of these information asymmetries, coordination problems may also arise (Azfar et al., 1999). In the public health context, sub-national governments do not necessarily have the right people for the job, nor do they know how to best implement programmes. Improper implemented decentralisation may pose significant risks and challenges that may lead to a deterioration in the provision of healthcare services and consequently to poor healthcare outcomes (Lieberman, 2002). Another argument against decentralisation is about diseconomies of scale. That some healthcare programmes may not be better performed at local levels because either they require a national perspective or may not be cost effective. The effectiveness of decentralisation depends on the existence of strong planning and executive capacity at local levels, which brings a heavy and new management burden on local governments (Litvack and Seddon, 1999). Some experiences of developing countries reveal that local governments suffer from a shortage of qualified personnel and managers to shoulder the new responsibilities. This undermines the competence of local bodies to plan and execute the new tasks (Collins and Green, 1994). The problem can further be complicated if there is lack of clearly defined accountability and responsibility between and within different actors at the central, regional and local levels (Arun and Ribot, 1999).

The confrontation and unwillingness or half-hearted tendency from a central or regional body to delegate power and authority to local bodies may also undermine the effect of decentralisation on delivery of efficient, responsive and qualitative healthcare services at lower levels (Gilson and Mills, 1995; Pokharel, 2000). Decentralisation may also aggravate inequalities in service access between rich and poor areas. Local authorities in rich areas can mobilise substantial resources to attract qualified personnel and to deliver high-quality and efficient services compared to poor areas. This may exacerbate the inequalities between poor and rich areas and communities. Sometime, local bodies may not necessarily reflect the interests and developmental priorities of the communities they represent. It is possible that local elites and dominant individuals may hijack the decentralised power and authority to pursue their own interests and may not promote efficiency and equity (Collins, 1989; Mills et al., 1990). The problem can be more severe if the expected participation of the community does not materialised. Evidence from some countries suggests that poorly designed and hastily implemented decentralisation have serious consequences for healthcare service delivery (Collins and Green, 1994; Gilson et al., 1994; Kolehmaine-Aitken and Newbrander, 1997). These have resulted, in some cases, in backlash against the reforms and started initiatives for 'recentralization' (Bossert and Beauvais, 2002: 14).

Bossert and Beauvais (2002) provide an analytical framework to describe and compare the type and degree of decentralisation in Ghana, Uganda,

Zambia and the Philippines, and developed a new approach (Decision Space Approach) to understand the effective process of decentralisation in a particular country, but we believe that institutions can vary across space and time – and therefore, comparing the effective processes of decentralisation across countries by putting them into the same framework is problematic and will distort the results. As argued earlier, institutions are endogenous. Their form and their functioning depend on the conditions under which they emerge and endure. That is, the characteristics and effects of particular institutions depend on the conditions under which they function. Similar institutions can – and do – serve different or multiple functions in different countries or regions. We believe that for any effective policy suggestion on the process of decentralisation, one needs to compare only those regions which fall under one legal provision.

The literature provides a possible explanation that decentralisation can improve healthcare sector performance. However, in order to fully evaluate the gains from decentralisation, conceptual clarity on what constitutes decentralisation, how it can be empirically captured and what its constituent elements are need to be incorporated in a measure of decentralisation. The theoretical construct argues that the measurement of decentralisation is highly context specific (North, 1997). The manner, instruments and mechanisms through which decentralisation gets grounded in any region or country has to be kept in mind in order to identify the parameters that can be used to capture the spatial and regional variations in the quantum of decentralisation. The impacts of decentralisation are highly sensitive to the way the decentralisation variables are measured (Ebel and Yilmaz, 2002).

The community driven development of World Bank define that decentralisation is a wide concept, which includes political, administrative, and fiscal decentralisation, and coordination among them is highly important. This involves devolution of powers and authorities to local governments. While examining the impact of decentralisation on health outcomes the existing studies used a narrow definition of decentralisation like either the political (Mahal et al., 2000), or fiscal decentralisation at Panchayat (Asfaw et al., 2004) and state level (Robalino et al., 2001) or both (Yee, 2001). These measures seem to be weak[3] simply because they covered limited dimensions of decentralisation.[4] The gamut of issues that involve comprehensive dimensions of the devolution of different powers (like, fiscal, functional, administrative and political powers) to local bodies have not been captured while measuring its effectiveness on health sector.

How a more comprehensive measure of decentralisation improves the efficacy of allocated public funds that can have significant impact on health sector outcomes remained unresolved specifically in Indian context. The pursuit of improving the performance of public health system from expenditure point of view in a country like India is imperative, because, public funding, particularly in rural area, is one of the single most important sources of health system funding. It is therefore necessary to ensure that the allocated funds to health sector are deployed effectively and that such expenditure is in line with the local preferences. In conditions when tax and non-tax revenue sources are under stress, the effectiveness of every rupee that is spent becomes even more important. The high morbidity, undernourishment, burden of disease and ageing population on one side and escalating healthcare costs from private sources on the other side add pressure to find out the tools of improving the performance of the public healthcare system. This motivates us to look at different dimensions of decentralisation and construct appropriate measures of the decentralised form of governance in Indian states that are governed under the same constitution, but one can expect the variation in its implementation in different states and thereby differential impact on efficacy of allocated resources and health outcomes. This chapter provides a conceptual framework and methodology for the robust measures of the extent of decentralisation across major states of India and compares how these states have performed to achieve a desired level of decentralisation. The estimated dimensions of decentralisation are then associated with selected health outcome parameters (like the IMR) while measuring the efficacy of healthcare spending.

Decentralisation initiatives within the healthcare sector

Community participation and decentralisation concepts have already been discussed as a part of health policy making in India since the Bhore Committee 1946 through the Second National Health Policy 2002. During this period, India constituted several other committees on health and took several measures to reform the healthcare delivery system. However, India failed to design and classify how to involve decentralisation and community participation in improving the healthcare service delivery system in the country. The government of India launched its National Rural Health Mission in 2005. The mission was designed to provide effective healthcare to rural people in general and women and children belonging to weaker sections of society in particular. This is because of low levels of institutional delivery and birth attended by skilled health personnel and inadequate level of post-natal care received by the mother and child with a higher rate amongst the poorest and most deprived sections of the society. The mission also concerned areas that are detrimental to health, like poor sanitation, lack of nutrition, lack of availability of clean drinking water, etc. Along with a commitment of increase in public spending on health to 2–3% of GDP, the mission designed the implementation of several initiatives through a highly decentralised policy framework (NRHM, 2005). It is believed that significant amounts of public funds will not contribute substantially if the existing facilities are not managed through proper channels or through effective government interventions, community participation or decentralisation in governance. Overall, the NRHM seeks to improve access to healthcare facilities, enable community ownership of services, strengthen public health systems, enhance the equity and accountability of the providers and most importantly, strengthen and deepen the levels of decentralisation by increasing the resources available to the Panchayats (Nagarajan, 2017).

While the responsibility of implementation of this programme rests with the state governments, NRHM seeks to empower the Panchayats to manage, control and be accountable for health services. Block-level Panchayat Samitis will coordinate the work of Panchayats within their jurisdictions and serve as links to district-level hospitals. The Zilla Parishad will lead these, which will control, guide and manage all public health institutions in the district. The Panchayats are critical to the planning, implementation and monitoring of the NRHM in the village. Thus, the success and efficacy of NRHM depends on Panchayat-level community ownership steered through village-level health committees, and through a strong public sector healthcare system, as well as on the well-functioning Panchayats (Nagarajan, 2017). The village-level committee called Village Health and Sanitation Committee (VHSC)[5] was entrusted with the planning and implementation of health programmes in the village to achieve equity and efficiency in healthcare use through decentralising the services. This committee envisioned that local people would take leadership in management of the healthcare system (a part of community participation) and its related matters. This committee therefore is a significant mechanism for engendering inclusiveness in health planning. Further, to make NRHM objectives more functional and effective, the concept of ASHA workers (women from the village) was also introduced to provide and spread awareness about the importance of basic facility and health programmes in the village. Earlier ANM and Anganwadi works were critical to spreading awareness about healthcare and related matters due to their scarcity. The involvement of large number of ASHA workers is crucial for women's community participation in the healthcare service delivery system, especially to spread awareness among households which were earlier used to depending on informal sources such as social networks for information access about the key health-related problems. The detail on all these dimensions is provided in Chapter 6. Here, we have discussed decentralisation reforms that are initiated as a part of democratic political process.

Dimensions of decentralisation: the measurements

The government of India has taken several initiatives to promote decentralisation policy as a part of the democratic decentralised political process, as well as within the health sector. Before measuring the impact of decentralisation, thus, it became important to understand what constitutes decentralisation, what its constituent elements are and how it can be empirically captured in both contexts like decentralisation initiatives as: a) democratic decentralised political process; and b) within the healthcare sector. The decentralisation initiatives that have been taken as a health sector reforms process (especially under NRHM) are discussed in detail in Chapter 6.

India has been placing the strength of decentralisation in its development policy agendas since the time of independence. Direct democracy, however, was strongly mandated during the early 1990s through the 73rd and 74th

Constitution Amendment Acts (CAA). These Acts enabled the state legislatures to transfer – if they chose to do so – adequate powers and responsibilities to local bodies to enable them to prepare and implement schemes for economic development and social justice. The 73rd Constitution Amendment Act provided a viable way of transferring political,[6] fiscal and administrative powers to rural local bodies. This also made a provision of some mandated actions, like constitution of the State Election Commission (SEC),[7] the State Finance Commission (SFC),[8] the District Planning Committees (DPCs)[9] and Gram Sabhas[10] to ensure an effective way and process of decentralisation in India. The responsibility on 29 functions,[11] under the Eleventh Schedule, is also sought to be entrusted to local Panchayats in planning and implementation of works of local significance. This Act, in a way, provides a formal instrument of a *minimum* level of rural decentralised governance in India by enabling state legislative bodies to transfer functional, financial and functionaries (administrative) powers to local governments along with delegation of political powers to ensure participation of people in grass-roots politics and policy.

Giving discretionary powers to the states to devolve power to PRIs can greatly dilute the decentralisation process in a state, as state(s) may not devolve important functions to the PRIs, and so the functionaries and funds also do not get correspondingly devolved to them. Therefore, the extent of adequate devolution of personnel control (functionary), funds and function powers may vary across states, which will impact the magnitude of the decentralisation process in that particular state and, in turn, affect outcomes of the healthcare sector. The extent of decentralisation would be high in states that have devolved adequate and balanced 3Fs powers to PRIs; in the reverse case, it would be low. We have presumed that the state that devolves inadequate powers and authorities to local governments in effect treats its local bodies as agents of the state government and no participatory approach is followed. This would certainly affect the extent of decentralisation in governance in the state and reduce local participation in grass-roots plans and policies in sectors like healthcare. Thus, devolution of decentralisation powers to local bodies is central to local governance measurements and for improved outcomes of the health sector.

India has initiated decentralisation as a political process that entrusts power to local government and within the health sector that involve local agents (community and elected representatives) in health policy making, monitoring and implementation. This section, based on the decentralisation initiatives undertaken under the 73rd CAA, first isolate the core dimensions to capture the comprehensive measure of decentralisation. These dimensions are then converted into measurable parameters, along with elaboration of a methodology to combine these parameters. Specifically, to capture the diversity in devolution of powers, we have constructed a comprehensive measure of decentralisation at state level using information on 18 indicators of funds, functions and functionaries (3Fs) powers which have been devolved to local Panchayats under the 73rd CAA on matters and activities related to health (Table 5.1). This index does not only capture the extent of

Table 5.1 Indicators and methods for calculating decentralisation indices at the state level

Political Participation Index (PPI)

Constitution of State Election Commission (SEC)	If, Yes = 5, No = 0
Holding Elections to PRIs every Five Years	If Yes = 5; No = 0
Share of women and reserved class Panchayats representatives	If ≤25 = 1; if >25 and ≤29 = 2; if >29 and ≤33=3; if >33 and ≤37 = 4; if >37 = 5
Percentage of total voters' turnout in assembly election	If < 45% = 1; 45–65% = 3; > 65% = 5
Total women who voted in assembly elections as percentage of men who voted in assembly election	If < 75% = 1; 75–85% = 3; > 85% = 5
Percentage of women contestants in assembly election	<2% = 1; 2–3% = 3; >3% = 5
Percentage of women elected in assembly election	<4% = 1; 4–6% = 3; > 6% = 5
Political Participation Index (PPI) #	**Arithmetic mean of all above items is computed and it is normalised to be between 0 and 100 by using the formula: PPIi = (PPIi × 100)/5**

Sub-Index of Functions Devolution

De facto transfer of six health and health-related functions to Panchayats	[(Number of functions transferred/6) × 5]
De facto transfer of remaining 23 functions to Panchayats	[(Number transferred/23) × 5]
Has activity mapping been conducted on six health functions? ##	[(Number of functions for which activity mapping is done/6) × 5]
Has activity mapping been conducted for the remaining 23 functions?	[(Number of functions for which activity mapping is done/23) × 5]

a. Functions devolution sub-indices

Sub-Index of Finances Devolution

Authorisation to the village Panchayats as per the PRIs Act to collect appropriate taxes, duties, tolls and non-taxes fees	[(Number of taxes items assigned/38) × 5] [(Number of non-taxes items assigned/29) × 5]
PRIs own revenue as percentage of expenditure of PRIs	Less than 5% = 1; 5–10% = 2; 11–15% = 3; 16–20% = 4; More than or equal to 21% = 5

PRIs own revenue as percentage of state's own revenue	Less than 1% = 1; 1–2% = 2; 2–3% = 3; 3–4% = 4; more than 4% = 5
Per capita (as per rural population) real expenditure (at 1993–1994 prices) by PRIs on core services (like health, education, water supply, street light, roads, etc.)	Less than Rs. 50 = 1; 51–100 = 2; 101–150 = 3; 151–200 = 4; more than 200 = 5
Constitution of State Finance Commission (SFC)	If no SFC constituted = 0; Only 1st SFC report received = 2; 2nd SFC report received = 3; 3rd SFC report received = 5; (used highest score)
Timely Actions on the latest SFC's major recommendations	> Two years = 1; <2 years>one year = 2; < 1 year > six months = 3; < Six months = 5
Percentage of funds devolved to PRIs that are 'untied' to any scheme	<5% are untied = 1; 5–25% untied = 2; 25–50% untied = 3; 50–75% untied = 4; >75% untied = 5
Release of funds to PRIs: compliance of the state government in sending the TFC grant without delay (data from NCAER)	>60 Days = 1, 45–60 = 2, 30–45 = 3, 15–30 = 4, <15 Days = 5
Is the allocation of SFC funds to the PRIs based on an apportionment formula?	If allocation is based on development or equitable criteria and include more than three items = 5, if three items = 4; if two items = 3; if one item = 2; if ad-hoc grant = 1
b. Finances devolution sub-indices	Arithmetic mean of all finance items
Sub-Index of Functionaries Devolution	
Whether staff transferred, for instance, whether: (i) only general staff transferred; (ii) functionaries of departments transferred but without any control over them by elected representatives; (iii) functionaries of departments transferred with some degree of control invested in the elected representatives (such as sanction of leave); (iv) functionaries transferred and under substantial control of the elected representatives	If item (iv) = 5; if item (iii) = 4; if item (ii) = 3; if item (i) = 1; if no information average of below three items
How many functionaries have been transferred?	[(Number of functionaries transferred/29) × 5]

(Continued)

Table 5.1 (Continued)

General support to Panchayats at present: government has specified expert institutions and entities to support PRIs for preparation of annual plans and for capacity building (data from NCAER)	Yes = 5 No = 1
What is the amount of money provided for the training of PRI's elected functionaries in the state budget? (Rs per year per elected functionary) (data from NCAER)	Less than or equal to Rs. 1000 = 1; More than Rs. 1000 = 5
Has the state's department of Panchayati Raj brought out its annual report for the last fiscal year?	Yes = 5, No = 0
c. Functionaries devolution sub-indices	**Arithmetic mean of all functionaries items**
Devolution Index to Health (DIH)###	**Arithmetic mean of a, b and c.; The DI value, further, is normalised to be between 0 and 100 by the formula: DIi = (DIi × 100)/5**

Source: Central Finance Commission and State Finance Commission (individual states), Status of Panchayati Raj Report 2007 & NCAER. 2007. An Index of Devolution for Assessing Environment for Panchayati Raj Institutions in the States. Draft Report, National Council of Applied Economic Research (NCAER), New Delhi, March

Note: # – For PPI, the assembly election data for the period 1992–2005 is considered for individual states. ## – Under the Schedule 11 of the 73rd Constitutional Amendment, the 29 functions were transferred to PRIs; the activity mapping indicates whether systematic efforts at clarifying the roles and responsibility of PRIs on the transferred functions is carried out or not. ### – The detail of selected indicators is provided in Appendices 5.1, 5.2 and 5.3.

fiscal decentralisation (funds), but also gives adequate or appropriate weight to the structure and content of devolution, as manifested in the agency to which the power is transferred (functionary) and the purpose for which the power is transferred (function). This comprehensive nature of the index makes it distinct and robust as compared to the earlier measures which have captured only two or three indicators of decentralisation (see, for example, Mahal et al., 2000; Asfaw et al., 2004) while examining its impact on health outcomes. This index is constructed for major states of India using scaling score method (Table 5.1). This index is called Devolution Index for Health (DIH) here. This index is used to see the effectiveness of government health spending in states where local institutions are functionally, financially and administratively viable, and vice-versa. The limitations of data information on different dimensions of decentralisation allows us to measure it at some points of time, while indices of fiscal and political decentralisation are constructed for longer periods due to availability of time series data.

Amongst the other forms of decentralisation, decentralising the budget (fiscal decentralisation, which provides responsibilities to local bodies relating to revenue raising, expenditure allocations and other finances) is the most important form of decentralisation, which enables local governments to meet the needs of people and better provisioning of local services, such as the healthcare. However, its effectiveness also requires calibration with other dimensions, particularly with political and administrative decentralisation. Political participation brings decision making closer to the people, and thereby increases democratisation. Without political decentralisation, participatory decision making seems to be impossible. The political participation helps in deciding the preferences of local residents. A more active political participation of the population, particularly of the women, is expected to align the decisions of local authorities to the interests and priorities of the population (Asfaw et al., 2004). Since political decentralisation strengthens the effectiveness of fiscal decentralisation, an index of political participation and representation that give more weight to women representatives in assembly- and Panchayat-level politics is also used while measuring the impact of decentralisation on health outcomes. This index provides a better understanding of citizens' participation, as well as the level of democracy in a particular state, and has already been discussed in Chapter 4. The fiscal decentralisation index is constructed by using the share of a local Panchayat's own revenue in total expenditures of the Panchayat. This is a legitimate indicator of fiscal decentralisation, since it measures the autonomy of Panchayati Raj Institutions (PRIs) to meet the expenditures of their locality or say the fiscal capacity of PRIs to meet their expenses. This also shows the fiscal dependency of PRIs on top authorities like the central and state governments. Since the detail on PRIs' own revenue and expenditures are not available from the Finance Commission database after 2005, we have taken a period from 1990–2005 for 16 major states of India for which the data is readily available. The measured indices of decentralisation are finally used to find out their impact on two important MDGs or sustainable development goals relating to health outcomes, namely, infant mortality rates (IMR) and under-5 mortality rates (U5MR).[12] These dimensions of decentralisation are further used to evaluate the efficacy of health spending in improving the health outcomes.

Status of decentralisation

The results show that different states performed differently in securing score values representing the level of decentralisation in the state. The status of decentralisation, the devolution of health-related funds, functions and functionaries (3F) powers to PRIs (DIH) are found to be high in Kerala, West Bengal, Karnataka and Tamil Nadu, and low in high-income states like Punjab and Gujarat, as well as in low-income states like Bihar (Figure 5.1). The variation and low value of devolution index (DIH) may be because of the unbalanced nature of the devolution of 3Fs powers to PRIs. For instance, Figure 5.2 reveals that in some of the states, functions have not been fully transferred. Activity mapping[13] was to be carried out to clarify the role of PRIs at different levels. This also has not been carried out in some states. States like West Bengal, Assam, Karnataka and Maharashtra have scored high values in functions devolution, but the score values are noticed to be low in finance devolution, indicating that the SFCs in these states devolved low funds to meet the requirement of the functions which have already been assigned to PRIs. Assigning more functions with low funds certainly may hamper the degree of autonomy to PRIs in determining

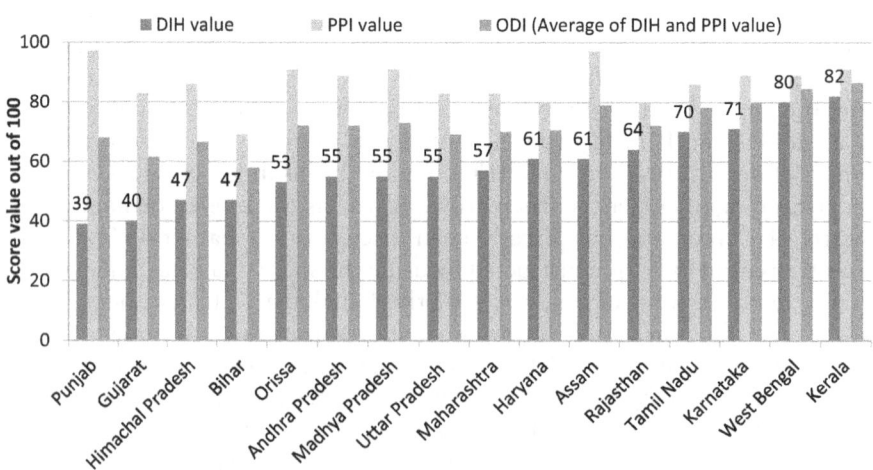

Figure 5.1 Extent of decentralisation in India across states: 2006

Source: Author's estimates, using information on indicators presented in Table 5.1

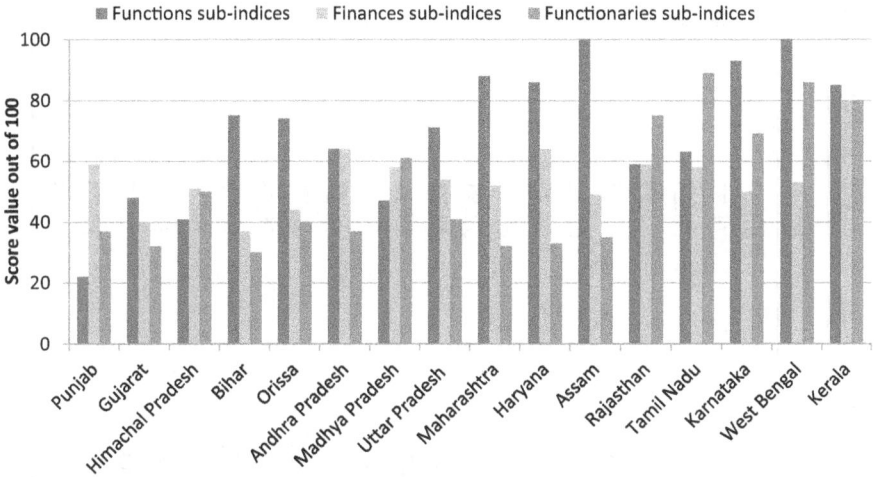

Figure 5.2 Nature of devolution of 3Fs powers to PRIs across states: 2006
Source: Author's estimates, using information on indicators presented in Table 5.1

their spending priorities for different functions. This may mean that most of the revenue raising and expenditure allocation priorities are with the state governments, and PRIs are left with meagre resources. The other reasons for low level of finances sub-indices include low spending by PRIs on core services that are planned and budgeted by the state governments, inappropriate criteria of SFCs for funds devolution from state to PRIs, etc. (Appendices 5.1, 5.2 and 5.3). The performance of functionaries' sub-indicators also shows high variability across states. The devolution index to Panchayats around 3Fs power also varied considerably across states in 2013–2014. The value of overall index varies between 25 and 75 across states. This indicates that uniformity in different sub-indices dimensions is lacking in many states. Such unbalanced nature of different dimensions undermines the functioning of the intergovernmental transfer system. It can be argued that unless the imbalance is corrected through greater fiscal and administrative decentralisation, Indian states are unlikely to evolve effective PRIs. In short, in order for decentralisation to be effective, it needs to be balanced along the three (3Fs) key dimensions. The recent estimates on the devolution index (Table 5.2) also show high variation in overall devolution values, as well as devolution of 3Fs powers to Panchayati Raj Institutions in the country.

The political participation index (PPI) is high in most of the Indian states (Figure 5.1), and its score value turns out to be more than the DIH value. It may be because political participation in a democratic country like India is much

Table 5.2 Panchayat Devolution Index (PDI) and sub-indices, 2013–2014

State	Framework	Functions	Finances	Functionaries	Capacity building	Accountability	PDI
	D1	D2	D3	D4	D5	D6	D
Maharashtra	74.01	63.26	59.03	78.91	78.24	80.24	70.21
Kerala	72.65	61.61	68.37	71.09	60.70	74.77	68.00
Karnataka	70.08	63.14	61.32	65.43	70.15	70.25	65.75
Tamil Nadu	66.14	53.71	56.88	55.63	60.06	65.99	58.98
Chhattisgarh	69.12	48.24	48.81	53.44	55.24	67.15	55.16
Rajasthan	66.82	51.99	45.41	40.23	69.15	64.82	54.23
West Bengal	62.96	54.67	39.09	38.82	79.24	54.42	52.09
Madhya Pradesh	62.93	50.22	41.43	46.01	57.15	62.77	51.14
Haryana	76.90	34.47	41.53	54.41	45.70	52.91	48.27
Gujarat	54.12	40.24	28.43	56.50	51.15	43.26	42.61
Andhra Pradesh	50.53	11.44	31.97	50.38	62.70	49.11	40.69
Assam	51.77	42.83	26.69	30.86	62.06	44.76	40.26
Odisha	58.74	51.46	42.03	35.43	13.97	42.26	39.95
Uttarakhand	54.87	41.47	21.05	31.07	42.55	58.72	37.87
Himachal Pradesh	50.26	21.58	30.89	38.97	39.09	51.49	36.96
Punjab	60.58	28.08	23.80	30.31	38.76	50.09	35.28
Uttar Pradesh	55.20	41.04	35.74	18.68	29.67	29.73	34.11
Jammu & Kashmir	29.67	19.29	34.53	22.00	56.36	33.16	32.95
Jharkhand	56.61	20.36	12.30	36.40	44.91	31.97	29.40
Bihar	48.21	39.49	16.82	24.45	41.88	22.74	29.15
Goa	44.21	17.78	18.21	43.06	10.30	27.94	24.75

Source: Alok (2014)

easier to achieve than vesting the local bodies with administrative control over significant functions or fiscal autonomy. Thus, our construction of the indices of decentralisation and of political participation reveals that the devolution of powers and responsibilities, and the outcomes of political processes and the speed of implementation, vary across states and within a state through time, depending on the initiatives taken by the respective state governments. This results in variation in decentralisation among the Indian states and low levels of decentralisation in some of the states. With varying degrees of decentralisation, one can expect differential impact on outcomes of health sector, as well as on the effectiveness of health spending, which is investigated in the next section.

Decentralisation and health sector outcomes

A simple trends analysis of the infant mortality rate (IMR) across states reveals that it is declining continuously across all states. The variation in IMR across states, however, reduced significantly after the implementation of decentralisation initiatives under NRHM (Figure 5.3).

The graphical presentation of the association between the extent of decentralisation (DIH) and infant mortality rate of rural area shows a negative relationship (Figure 5.4). The estimated linear regression equation of this bivariate association shows that an increment of one basis point in the value of decentralisation (DIH) reduces the infant mortality rate of rural area by –0.61 and the coefficient is significant at 10% level of significance. The coefficient of determination R^2 value indicates that 19% variation in rural IMR is explained by the level of DIH. Overall, the extent of decentralisation leads to a reduction in the infant mortality rate in rural areas.

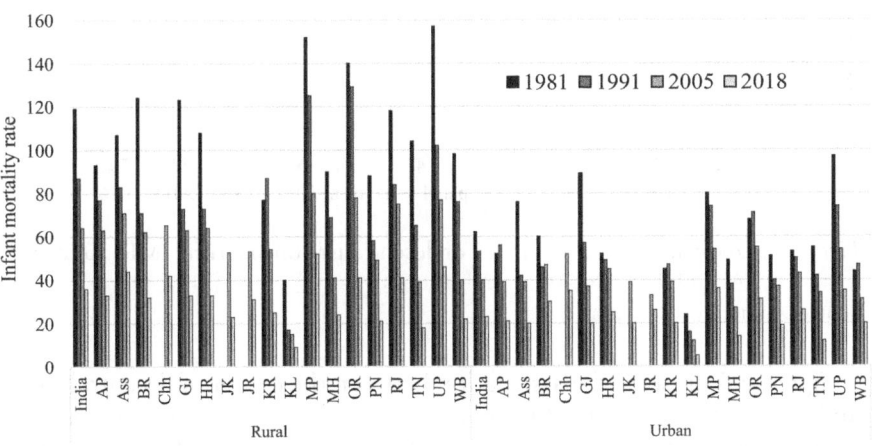

Figure 5.3 Progress in rural and urban infant mortality rates across states of India

Sources: Sample Registration System Bulletins, various year, Office of the Registrar General & Census Commissioner, Ministry of Home Affairs, Government of India

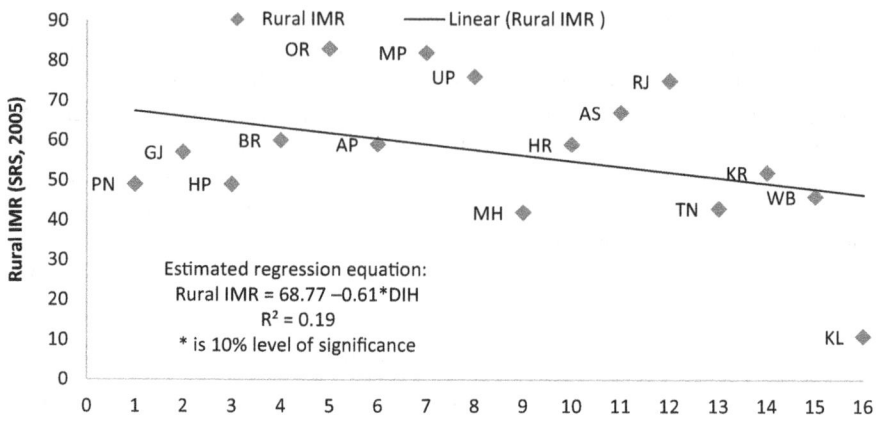

Figure 5.4 Association between extent of decentralisation and rural IMR, 2005–2006
Source: Author's calculations

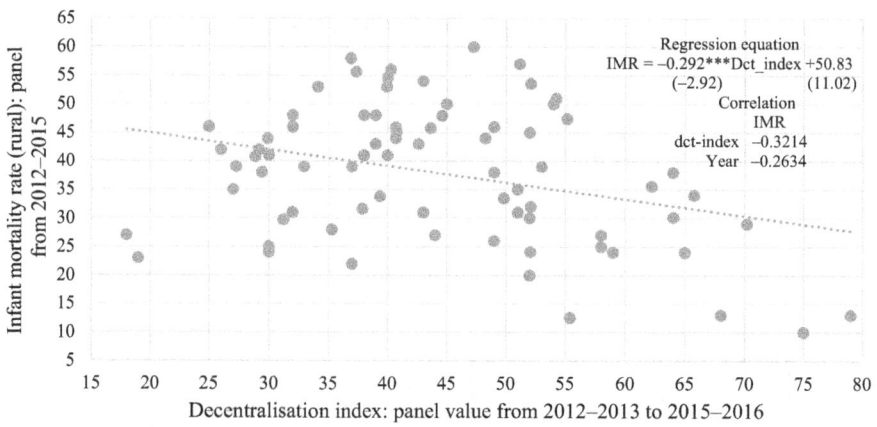

Figure 5.5 Association between index of decentralisation and rural IMR, 2012–2015
           at major states level

Source: Author's calculations

Figure 5.5 presents the association between the extent of decentralisation and infant mortality rate of rural areas. The relationship between these two also turned negative in panel data setting. The estimated linear regression equation of this bivariate association shows that an increment of one basis point in the index of decentralisation reduces the infant mortality rate of rural area by –0.29, and the coefficient is significant at 1% level of signifi-cance. The simple correlation turned out the negative –0.32 between index of decentralisation and rural IMR across the major states of India. Overall, this association reflects that extent of decentralisation leads to reduction of the infant mortality rate of rural India.

Impact of decentralisation on health outcomes: empirical investigation

To evaluate the impact of health expenditure and decentralisation on health outcomes and effectiveness of decentralisation in improving the efficacy of public spending, panel and cross-sectional equation are estimated, controlling for level of development (per capita income), level of female literacy, provisioning of health services, access of drinking water facilities, etc. The estimated equations are as follow.

Panel estimation

$$\ln IMR_s = \alpha + \beta_1 \ln RHE_{st} + \beta_2 (\ln RHE \times DIH)_{st} + \beta_3 \ln IFD_{st} + \beta_4 PPR_{st} + \beta_5 FLR_{st} + \beta_6 LD_{st} + v_s + \varepsilon_{st} \ldots \tag{1}$$

$$\ln IMR_{st} = \alpha + \beta_1 \ln RHE_{st} + \beta_2 DIH_{st} + \beta_3 \ln IFD_{st} + \beta_4 \ln IFD \times PPR_{st} + \beta_5 FLR_{st} + \beta_6 LDst + v_s + \varepsilon_{st} \ldots \tag{2}$$

Where, IMR – infant mortality rate of rural areas of a particular state; RHE – per capita public expenditure on health of rural areas of a state at 1993–1994 prices, which includes expenditure on medical, public health, family welfare and water supply; DIH – devolution index for health – a decentralised governance index; IFD – index of fiscal decentralisation: PRIs' own revenue as a ratio of their total expenditure;[14] PPR – political participation and representative index; LD – level of development (real per capita income of a particular state at 1993–1994 prices); FLR – female literacy rate of rural area; lnIFD × PPR dummy – interaction term of fiscal and political decentralisation, reflecting the effectiveness of political participation in improving the efficacy of fiscal decentralisation. This specifically shows whether high fiscal decentralisation affects the health outcome regardless of the level of political participation; lnRHE × DIH dummy – interaction terms of rural health spending (RHE) and DIH dummy variables. This shows the effectiveness of DIH in improving the efficacy of health spending to have its significant on health outcomes.[15] The v – state-specific residual; ε – wtandard residual with the usual assumption of zero mean, uncorrelated with v and other explanatory variables, and homoscedasticity; s – wtate (16 major states of India); t – time period (1990–2005).

Cross-sectional estimation

$$U5MR_i = \alpha + \beta_1 RHII_i + \beta_2 RHII \times DIH_i + \beta_3 FLRi + \beta_4 UI_i + \beta_5 DW_i + ui \ldots \tag{3}$$

Where, U5MR – rural under-5 mortality rate of a district; RHII – index of health infrastructure in rural areas,[16] used as a proxy for health expenditure;

DIH – devolution index to health, used in dichotomous form (0 for low DIH value and 1 for high – higher than average value); RHII × DIH dummy – interaction term of health infrastructure and decentralisation dummy, reflecting the effectiveness of decentralisation in improving the efficacy of rural health infrastructure; FLR – female literacy rate of rural area (2011); UI – index of maternal and child health (MCH) care use;[17] DW – percentage of households using safe drinking water (2011);[18] i – number of observations: here it is the number of districts (504) across 19 major states of India.

Equation 3 is estimated by applying ordinary least squares (OLS). The panel equations (Equation 1 and Equation 2) can be estimated as 'between effects-BE', 'fixed effects-FE' and 'random effects-RE' models, depending on the assumptions we made about the distribution of v_s and ε_{st}. In the BE specification, the coefficients will be estimated using only the cross-sectional information on the means of the dependent and explanatory variables over time. In the FE model, also known as 'within effect', v_s is assumed to be fixed and the coefficients of the parameters will be estimated using the time series information in the data.[19] This implies that time-invariant variables will not be considered. This means that the model allows for different constant for each group/state. In order to allow for different constants for each group/state, it includes a dummy variable for each group/state. This is known as the least squares dummy variable (LSDV) method of estimating fixed effects in panel regression. Thus, FE model has some weaknesses, as: a) it ignores all explanatory variables which do not vary over time. By this, we mean that it does not allow us to use other dummies in the model, which is particularly inconvenient when we have reasons to consider including such dummies; b) if one uses state dummy, the model is inefficient in the sense that it estimates a very large number of parameters, leading to loss in degree of freedom; and c) it makes it very hard for any slowly changing explanatory variables to be included in the model, because they will be highly collinear with the effects. Thus, even if the F-test (like the Hausman test) suggests, the FE model may not be used, or the model may have to be specified very carefully. In order to avoid the limitations of FE model, the study employs RE model. The random effects model takes v_s as a random variable and assumes v_s not to be correlated with the other explanatory variables. Then it takes a weighted average of the between and the fixed estimates (Greene, 2008). The advantage of RE is that it treats constants for each section not as fixed, but as random parameters. That is, RE assumes individual effects are uncorrelated with the explanatory variables, which is one of the necessary conditions for applying the weighted least square method. Thus, RE estimates measure the impact of decentralisation and health expenditure on rural infant mortality by considering the information across states and within a state, and assume that individual effects are uncorrelated with explanatory variables. Equation 1 and Equation 2, therefore, are estimated with random effect.

Results of the impact of decentralisation

A simple correlation between IMR and DIH turns out to be highly significant (at 5% level of significance), with a negative coefficient value of about –0.43 (Table 5.3). Interestingly, the correlation between rural IMR and general devolution index (DI) turns out to be insignificant with a low coefficient value (Table 5.3). This indicates that a move from general DI to health DI results in lowering the rural IMR more effectively. Further, an examination of the association between different dimensions (sub-indices) of decentralisation and IMR provides more robust results, as it provides a fairly good idea about the importance of a sub-index for better health sector outcomes. The correlation coefficients between these decentralisation sub-indices and IMR show that finances devolution sub-index is negatively associated with IMR (with coefficient value about –0.48) at 5% level of significance. This analysis reflects two important points: a) a move from general devolution of 3Fs powers to devolution of health-related 3Fs powers to PRIs is more significant in lowering the infant mortality rate of the rural areas of India, indicating that sector-specific devolution of powers is more important for better outcomes of that particular sector; and b) of the 3Fs, the devolution of finances powers to PRIs is important in reducing the rural IMR. Similarly, the association between rural IMR and devolution index to PRI show significant negative relation with functionaries devolution sub-index with high coefficient value about –0.46, followed by finance sub-index (–0.42), overall rural decentralisation index (–0.384) and accountability sub-index (–0.34), indicating devolution of different 3Fs powers and accountability and overall index contribute significantly in reducing the rural IMR of India. The capacity building and functions devolution indices also important in reducing the infant mortality of rural area. Most of the indices of rural decentralisation as important for lowering down the rural IMR.

The panel estimation results show that both decentralisation as well as public expenditure on health (RHE) helps in reducing the infant mortality rate of rural area significantly. A 1% increase in real per capita rural health spending reduces the rural infant mortality rate by about 0.045% at 10% level of significance (Model I, Table 5.4). The IMR and expenditure variables are used in log form; the coefficient of expenditure therefore reflects the expenditure elasticity of rural infant mortality rate. The coefficient shows that the expenditure elasticity of rural infant mortality rate is very low. The low coefficient value of health expenditure may be because healthcare spending in India is highly biased towards salary components, while the expenditure on non-salary components (namely, drugs, medicines, machinery and equipment) is low and/or lacking. A low level of spending on non-salary components is an indication of low availability of these facilities with the government hospitals and primary health centres. Such trends limit the health personnel to perform better; it can further reduce faith in public facilities and encourages rural households to use expensive private health

Table 5.3 Correlation coefficient between decentralisation indices and rural IMR

Variables 2007	PPR	Functions DI	Finances DI	Functionaries DI	DIH	General DI#
Rural IMR	-0.09	-0.17	-0.48*	-0.35	-0.43*	-0.36

Variables## 2012–2014	Framework DI	Functions DI	Finances DI	Functionaries DI	Capacity Building DI	Accountability DI	Overall PDI	Year
Rural IMR	-0.033	-0.113	-0.425*	-0.46*	-0.253	-0.344*	-0.384*	-0.15

Source: Author's estimates, using data on IMR and decentralisation indices

Note: * is 5% level of significance. # – Value of General DI is taken from NCAER (2007); ## – the value of decentralisation and sub-indices are taken from Alok (2014) and Vasudevan et al. (2015) and Unnikrishnan et al. (2016)

facilities which are located in the urban areas and purchasing of medicines from outside stores. This may result in high out-of-pocket expenditure and increased financial burden on rural households. Thus, productive and beneficial impacts of public expenditures on health in influencing the performance of the healthcare sector largely depends on how much funds are allocated to the sector and how funds are allocated within the sector.

Estimates show that a 1-percentage-point improvement in the value of the fiscal decentralisation index reduces the infant mortality rate of rural areas significantly (about 0.023%) at 1% level of significance. Similarly, a 1-percentage-point increment in the index of political participation – particularly women's participation – reduces the infant mortality rate of rural area about 0.24% at 1% level of significance. Both the control variables, level of female education and level of state income, turned out to be significant in reducing the rural infant mortality rate across states.

The states with high fiscal and political decentralisation indices have more significant impact in reducing the rural IMR compared to the states that have high fiscal but low political decentralisation indices. Thus, political decentralisation increases the efficacy of fiscal decentralisation in reducing the rural IMR. This may mean that high participation by women in politics is important for better utilisation of local funds, which further leads to better health outcomes in rural areas.

The level of public expenditure on healthcare turned significant in reducing the infant mortality rate of rural areas. The efficacy of public health spending in improving the rural IMR increases with the high level of decentralisation (DIH) in the states. The results show that a 1% increase in per capita public spending in health lowers the rural IMR by 0.052% in states with high decentralisation compared to the low decentralisation states. Thus, decentralisation improves efficacy of rural healthcare spending in reducing rural IMR.

Interestingly, among the different measures of decentralisation – namely fiscal, political and comprehensive measures of health-related decentralisation (DIH) – the comprehensive measure of health-related decentralisation shows greater impact in reducing rural infant mortality rates. The value of the coefficient of comprehensive measure of health-related decentralisation turned out to be even greater than the other socio-economic control variables that are used in the study (Model II, Table 5.4).

The cross-sectional estimates show that availability of rural health infrastructure not only turned insignificant in reducing under-5 mortality rate of rural areas, but its sign also turned positive, which is contrary to our expectation. This may be because of inadequate availability and low quality of health services in rural areas, which are lacking in terms of staffing, medicines and/or equipment. Inadequate availability of healthcare facilities may be one of the factors responsible for not having its significant impact in reducing the U5MR of rural area. Interestingly, however, the availability of health infrastructure turns out to be highly significant in reducing the

Table 5.4 Impact of decentralisation and health expenditure on health outcomes

---

Model I: Panel regression results with random effect

ln*IMR* = 5.48–0.045ln*RHE* – 0.052(ln*RHE*DIH*) – 0.023*lnIFD* – 0.242*PPI* –0.018*FLR* – 0.122*LD*

(34.51)* (–1.89)*** (–2.24)*   (–2.65)*   (–7.43)* (–4.98)* (–4.35)*

R-sq: Within = 0.40; Between = 0.71; Overall = 0.69; Waldchi2(6) = 191.8; Prob >chi2 = 0.00;
sigma_u = 0.23; sigma_e = 0.09; rho = 0.86

Model II: Panel regression results with random effect

ln*IMR* = 6.09–0.084ln*RHE* – 0.204*DIH* – 0.025*lnIFD* – 0.067(ln*IFD*PPI*) –0.017*FLR* – 0.125*LD*

(21.04)* (–4.60)*   (–2.09)** (–2.77)*   (–3.07)*   (–4.59)* (–4.44)*

R-sq: Within = 0.39; Between = 0.75; Overall = 0.73; Waldchi2(6) = 194.2; Prob> chi2 = 0.00;
sigma_u = 0.22; sigma_e = 0.09; rho = 0.85

Model III: Cross-sectional regression results

ln*U5MR* = 5.19 + 0.016*RHII* – 0.11*(IRHI*DIH)* – 0.003*FLR* – 0.696*IU* + 0.0003*DW*

(97.9)   (0.59)   (–3.23)*   (–3.76)* (–11.8)* (0.69)

F(5, 498) = 91.87; Prob> F = 0.00; R-squared = 0.480; Adj R-squared = 0.475

Source: Author's estimates

Note: Models I–II: the figures in parenthesis are z-value; number of obs. = 256; years = 1990–2005; number of states = 16; Model III: Number of observations/districts across major Indian states are 504; figures in parenthesis are t-values; *, ** & *** are 1%, 5% and 10% levels of significance.

under-5 mortality rate in states with high levels of decentralisation (DIH), compared to states with low health-related decentralisation index (Model III, Table 5.4). This indicates that effectiveness of the availability of rural health infrastructure increases with the extent of governance in the health sector, which is measured in terms of devolution index for health (DIH) in the study. Thus, a decentralised delivery mechanism is important for effective delivery of services and better health outcomes. The control variables like, level of female literacy and status of utilisation of maternal and childcare also turn out to be significant in reducing the U5MR of rural area.

These findings confirm that a comprehensive measure of health-related decentralisation, high participation of women in politics and decentralising the budget all improve infant mortality rates of rural areas significantly, both directly as well as indirectly via improving the efficacy of public healthcare spending and infrastructure to have their impact on rural healthcare outcomes. Thus, devolving adequate funds, functions and functionaries powers to local bodies increases the effectiveness of resource utilisation and also significantly reduces the infant and under-5 mortality rates. The results suggest that state governments need to devolve adequate powers, authorities and responsibility to rural local bodies. Some states have devolved adequate powers to PRIs, but some have not. The devolution of 3Fs powers to PRIs also seems to be unbalanced in nature in Indian states. In some states, the finances have devolved but not the functionaries and functions. Some have devolved all the 29 functions but devolved low funds to meet the requirements of these functions. This affects the effective delivery system, particularly healthcare services, in the state. Further, the status of fiscal decentralisation also seems to be low in India. This indicates that there is low revenue-raising capacity (or fiscal autonomy) with the rural local bodies to meet the expenditure requirements of their locality. The share of total expenditure of PRIs in total expenditure of state governments (all states combined) is also very low in India (at about 6–7%), while in most advanced countries, local governments normally account for about 20–35% of total government expenditure (Hooda, 2015). This certainly affects the effective delivery of public services across the Indian states.

Limitation

It is important to note that the analysis in this chapter is based on some qualitative and quantitative indicators that quantify the extent of a comprehensive measure of decentralisation (namely, DIH) across major states of India. The index was constructed using the scaling score method. This method, however, has some limitations, as one can lose information pertaining to institutional settings if one takes a number of binary indicators and combines these with quantitative indicators, after converting the latter into discrete values. For instance, giving equal weights to all functions of the Panchayats or their sources of tax and non-tax revenue and then combining the different dimensions by assigning equal weights can be questioned, as this rules out judgemental factors emerging from field knowledge or experience. However, we could not think of any systematic method to associate different judgemental weights to different functions of the Panchayats or to different sources of their tax and non-tax revenues.

Low revenue of local bodies may reflect not necessarily absence of decentralisation, as we have assumed, but the local body's poor economic base. However, in order to address this limitation, one needs to examine what determines the revenue of local bodies (whether it is poor economic base or low tax base or the number of taxable items on which the PRIs can impose tax, and so on). We have not carried out such an exercise, as it would have taken us much beyond the present scope of our study.

Further, DIH requires broad-based information and content to make it comprehensive in nature. The information on these indicators (presented in Table 5.1) is not readily available for a longer period of time. The DIH, therefore, was constructed at one point of time and then associations with rural health outcomes were presented by considering state, district and cross-sectional units. However, we have used the existing devolution index value for the period from 2012–2013 to 2015–2016 across major states of India and associated them with rural IMR. Additionally, to present robust estimates across space (states) and time, the study has further constructed two (other important measures of decentralisation in governance, discussed previously) time series indices of decentralisation, namely indices of fiscal and political decentralisation for the period from 1990–2005 across major Indian states and values of the other variables collected for the same period.

Exploring data only up to 2005 is, again, a limitation. There are two reasons that restrict us to explore data only up to 2005 for regression analysis. One, the information on PRI revenue and expenditures which are utilised for constructing the index of fiscal decentralisation (IFD) were showing a high jump in the trends of values before and after 2005. Any major distortion in the trends value of a series may very well affect the overall significance of the model, as well as of that particular variable. Even if we were somehow to address the problem of the shift in the trend after 2005 by use of an appropriate dummy variable, as explained in the following paragraph, it was extremely difficult to construct the time series for expenditure on rural expenditure after 2005 required for such an analysis; however, data is available for primary care for later period.

As discussed, the purpose of the present study was not only to examine the effectiveness of decentralisation, but also to evaluate the impact of government spending that is allocated in the rural health sector on health outcomes (not merely of aggregate rural plus urban spending). Getting time series data on rural health spending across states, particularly after 2005, became difficult after April 2005, when the government of India launched the National Rural Health Mission (NRHM). Under NRHM, a structural shift in the routes of transfer of central funds to states was undertaken. Some of the central funds, which were earlier routed through state budgets via centrally sponsored and planned schemes, started bypassing the state budgets after NRHM implementation. Most of the NRHM funds that were allocated in the rural healthcare sector now are implemented through state implementing agencies, as well as decentralised agencies (like the Panchayati Raj Institutions). This changing route of central transfers has made it complex and difficult to work out the expenditure data on health that is allocated in the rural areas, especially after 2005, which enforces us to explore data only up to that year.[20] Since data used in the chapter was from 1990–2005 across major states of India, it therefore provides robust estimates to believe that decentralisation had positive impacts on healthcare sector outcomes and improving the efficacy of rural health spending.

Conclusion

The study finds that government health spending in the rural areas helps in reducing rural infant mortality rates significantly. Interestingly, this expenditure category turned out to be more significant, with a high coefficient value, in reducing the rural infant mortality rates in states with higher levels of decentralisation. Thus, the extent of decentralisation improves the efficacy of rural health spending in its impact in reducing the rural infant mortality rate of India. The extent of decentralisation is associated negatively with rural IMR. Thus, decentralisation ensures better health outcomes via improving the efficiency of resources utilisation.

Fiscal and political decentralisation also plays a significant role in reducing the infant mortality rates of rural areas of India. The effectiveness of fiscal decentralisation in reducing the rural IMR increases with the level of political decentralisation. The regression analysis reveals that states with high fiscal *and* political decentralisation have a greater impact in reducing the rural IMR compared to the states with high fiscal but low political decentralisation. Thus, political decentralisation increases the efficacy of fiscal decentralisation in reducing the infant mortality rates of rural areas of India.

Along with the level, the allocation pattern of health expenditure (particularly more on drugs, medicines, machinery and equipment) is important for the healthcare sector to perform better. Thus, in one sense, the productive and beneficial impact of public healthcare spending in influencing the health sector performance largely depends on how much funds are allocated to the healthcare sector under a more decentralised mechanism and how the funds are allocated within this sector. The impacts of other control variables like female literacy rate and the level of development of the states at the same time cannot be ignored, as they also play a significant role in reducing rural IMRs.

The inadequate availability of rural health infrastructure will not be helpful in improving healthcare outcomes (like the under-5 mortality rates) of rural India. In order to reap the expected outcomes, adequate and comprehensive public health facilities need to be provided across districts and remote rural regions of India. It would be better if these facilities could be provided under more decentralised governance system, as decentralisation improves the efficacy of the existing health facilities in improving the health outcomes. Higher levels of female literacy and status of healthcare utilisation for maternal and child care further add to improving the U5MR of rural areas. Thus, along with other contributing factors, the adequacy of public health facilities and decentralised service delivery mechanisms matter more in improving the health outcomes of rural areas. The adequacy of public health facilities is particularly important in view of the fact that publicly provided health facilities are the single most important source in the rural areas, with private facilities missing.

Overall, the study finds that decentralised governance and public expenditure on healthcare in the rural areas and adequate availability of healthcare facilities are more likely to improve healthcare sector outcomes of rural areas across the Indian states. The role of decentralised governance can be seen as a way to increase the efficacy of resource utilisation, as well as ensuring better health outcomes in the country. The findings demonstrate that both *state interventions* and *institutional change like decentralisation* are important in improving the performance of the rural healthcare sector. These findings are consistent with the theoretical arguments and other empirical findings on the subject, as discussed in the chapter. These factors, therefore, need to be strengthened to reform the Indian health sector. The study specifically recommends that along with the increase in government spending in the rural healthcare sector, Indian states need to devolve adequate powers (at least as prescribed in the 73rd CAA) and authorities over funds, functions and functionaries to rural local bodies so as to improve the performance of the public healthcare system of rural India.

Appendix 5.1

Indicators and criteria used for funds' devolution

	Population/density/rural population	Area	Poverty/level of per capita Income	Illiteracy rate	Population of SC/STs	Population of DDP/DPAP/TAD	Persons per bed in govt. hospitals/IMR/ other health indicator	Road length/sq. km	Financial need	Tax effort	Development criteria	Index of decentral-isation	Lump sum criteria
Andhra Pradesh											Y		
Assam	Y												
Bihar													Y
Gujarat													Y
Haryana													Y
Himachal Pradesh	Y	Y											
Karnataka	Y	Y		Y			Y	Y				Y	
Kerala	Y				Y				Y	Y			
Madhya Pradesh	Y	Y								Y			
Maharashtra	Y	Y											
Orissa	Y												
Punjab													Y
Rajasthan	Y		Y			Y							
Tamil Nadu	Y												
Uttar Pradesh	Y	Y											
West Bengal	Y			Y	Y	Y	Y						

Source: Hooda S. K. (2014) and State Finance Commission Reports, individual states

Note: Y – indicates that criteria are adopted for funds devolution

Appendix 5.2

Value of selected indicators used for devolution index

	Total functions transferred (in no.)	Functions on which activity mapping has been conducted (in no.)	PRIs authority to collect non-taxes (in no.)	PRIs authority to collect taxes/duties/tolls/fees (in no.)	PRIs own revenue as percentage of exp of PRI (avg. of 2000–2004)	PRIs own revenue as percentage of state's own revenue (avg. of 2000–2004)	Real (at 1993–1994 prices) per capita PRI exp on core services (in Rs.) (avg. of 1998–1999 to 2003–2004)	Constitution of State Finance Commission (values are based on scores)	Timely actions on the latest SFC major recommendations (values are based on scores)	Percentage of funds devolved to PRIs that are 'untied' to any scheme (values are based on scores)	Release of Funds to PRIs: compliance of the state government in sending the TFC grant without delay (values are based on scores)	Is the allocation of SFC funds to the PRIs based on an apportionment formula? (values are based on score)	Whether staff transferred	How many functionaries transferred	General support to Panchayats at present: government has specified expert institutions and entities to support PRIs for preparation of Annual Plans and for capacity building	What is the amount of money provided for the training of the PRI's elected functionaries in the state budget?	Has the state's department of Panchayati Raj brought out its Annual Report for the last fiscal year?
AP	12	9	22	16	4	1.02	36	3	3	3	5	5	1	0	1	3	0
Assam	23	23	11	4	99	0.21	638	5	5	1	1	2	4	0	1	1	0
Bihar	25	29	5	0	4	0.16	13	5	1	2	5	1	3	3	1	3	0
Gujarat	15	29	16	5	2	0.41	4	3	1	3	5	1	2	2	1	3	0
Haryana	23	10	5	2	23	0.94	22	5	5	5	5	1	3	2	1	3	0
HP	26	0	7	1	15	0.56	308	5	3	2	4	3	4	1	1	3	5
Karnataka	24	23	10	8	1	0.32	5	5	1	2	5	5	4	3	3	4	5
Kerala	21	19	11	15	13	2.76	3	5	5	4	5	5	5	3	5	4	0

MP	23	20	7	0	30	1.88	370	3	1	3	5	4	4	1	1	3	5
Maharashtra	12	23	8	2	9	2.06	125	5	1	1	5	3	2	2	1	3	0
Orissa	20	10	4	2	5	0.07	6	3	3	4	5	2	4	2	1	3	0
Punjab	20	0	8	2	58	1.03	137	5	5	5	1	1	4	1	1	2	5
Rajasthan	29	25	9	1	2	0.40	68	5	5	4	5	4	3	3	3	4	5
TN	29	29	11	9	12	0.35	671	5	3	4	5	2	1	5	5	4	5
UP	23	27	6	2	11	0.41	0	5	1	5	5	3	3	1	0	3	5
West Bengal	23	23	7	6	10	0.37	205	5	1	2	5	5	3	2	5	3	5

Source: Hooda (2014)

Appendix 5.3

Criteria adopted for funds devolution by SFCs to address horizontal and vertical inequalities

| State | *Devolution recommended* | | |
	SFC-I	*SFC-II*	*SFC-III*
Andhra Pradesh	39.24% of state revenue from tax and non-tax	40.92% per annum of the tax and non-tax revenues of the government, including the share of central taxes to local bodies	No information
Assam	2% per annum of tax revenue of the state; and fixed amount of grants-in-aid: 1996–1997: Rs. 36.89 crore; 1997–1998: Rs. 37.15 crore; 1998–1999: Rs. 37.02 crore; 1999–2000: Rs. 37.02 crore	1. 3.5% per annum of aggregate tax revenue of the state to local bodies 2. Grant-in-aid of Rs. 10 crore per annum for urban local bodies	1. No devolution for the year 2006–2007; 2. 10% of non-loan gross own tax revenue receipts after deducting actual collection charges for the year 2007–2008; 3. 25% of non-loan gross own tax revenue receipts after deducting actual collection charges for the year 2008–2011
Bihar	No information	No information	3% of net proceeds from state
Gujarat	Additional taxation of Rs. 293.09 crore per annum	No information	Not constituted
Haryana	1. 20% of royalty on minerals be devolved to the urban local bodies and Gram Panchayats	1. 20% of annual income from royalty on minor minerals to Gram Panchayats and municipalities;	4% of the net tax revenue to local bodies

State			
	2. 7.5% of net receipts under 'stamp duty and registration fees' be devolved to PRIs 3. Tax on motor vehicles 20%; entertainment tax 50% to urban local bodies	2. 3% of the net receipts from 'stamp duty and registration fees' to PRIs; 3. 65% of the net proceeds of LADT to PRIs; 4. 50% of the entertainment tax; 20% of motor vehicle tax and 35% of LADT to urban local bodies	
Himachal Pradesh	Rs. 138.75 crore devolved to local bodies	Rs. 53.19 crore devolved to the local bodies	1. Cess on liquor to be transferred to local bodies 2. Incentive fund at the rate of Rs. 10 crore to local bodies 3. Gap filling grant of Rs. 228.28 crore 4. Grant-in-aid to LSGIs and maintenance expenditure for roads
Karnataka	36% of non-loan gross own revenue receipts to the local bodies	40% of non-loan net own revenue receipts to the local bodies; Rs. 5 crore to be common purpose fund each year	1. 33% of state's own revenue receipts to be devolved to PRIs and urban local bodies in the ratio of 70:30 2. Salary component of officials; working in the PRIs should be delinked while working out the total share of PRIs and urban local bodies
Kerala	1. 25% surcharge on stamp duty be levied on behalf of urban local bodies. The surcharge on stamp duty as well as basic tax collected from Corporation area be transferred to them on collection basis	1. Government may devolve to the LSGIs, plan funds (excluding state sponsored schemes) not less than one-third the annual size of state plan as fixed by government from time to time	25% of the total state tax revenue of the year 2003–2004 be transferred to local bodies during the year 2006–2007. For subsequent years, annual growth rate of 10% may be applied for transfer of funds to the local bodies

(Continued)

(Continued)

| State | Devolution recommended | | |
	SFC-I	SFC-II	SFC-III
	2. Land tax be doubled and 60% of the additional income generated there from be given to block Panchayats and balance to district Panchayats	2. 5.5% of the annual own tax revenue of the state government may be devolved to the LSGIs as grants-in-aid for maintenance of assets under control of the LSGIs, including the transfer of assets 3. 3.5% of the own tax revenue of the state government based on the figures certified by the accountant general could be devolved to LSGIs as general purpose grant, in lieu of assigned taxes, shared taxes and various statutory and non-statutory grants-in-aid, both specific purpose and general purpose	No information
Madhya Pradesh	2.91% of total tax and non-tax to PRIs and 0.514% share of the divisible pool to urban local bodies; specific grant Rs. 67.66 crore to PRIs	2.93% of total tax and non-tax to PRIs and 1.07% to urban local bodies. Assignment of taxes to local bodies after deduction of 10% collection charges; establishment grant Rs. 28.40 crore to PRIs and Rs. 5 crore to ZPs for training	

Maharashtra	1. 10% of the professional tax collected by the state should be given to local bodies 2. 66.67% of the demand of land revenue and cess thereon should be given to PRIs as advance grants 3. Irrigation cess grant equal to 66.67% of the demand should be given to Zilla Parishads as advance grants 4. 25% of net income from motor vehicle tax be given to urban local bodies	40% of state's tax, duties and tolls proceeds to the local bodies	No information
Orissa	Government is bearing the full salary and other recurring and non-recurring cost of staff deployed by various line departments in PRIs. The quantum of money to be provided for salary of the staff of Panchayat Samities should be treated as direct devolution of funds to RLBs	10% of average of state's gross own tax revenue from 1999–2000 to 2001–2002 be devolved to local bodies. 10% of the state's gross own tax revenue for the year 2002–2003 minus devolvable amount was recommended as grants in-aid for various specific purposes	15% of the average gross tax revenue of the state for the years 2005–2006 to 2007–2008 at Rs. 896.17 crore per annum be devolved to the local bodies
Punjab	20% of five taxes (i.e. stamp duty; motor vehicle tax; electricity duty; entertainment tax; cinema shows tax) be devolved to the local bodies (both urban and rural)	4% of net proceeds from all state taxes be devolved to the local bodies	4% share of net proceeds of all state taxes be devolved to the local bodies
Rajasthan	2.18% of net tax proceeds of the state to be devolved to the local bodies	2.25% of net tax proceeds to the local bodies; entertainment tax 15%; royalty on minerals 1%	50% of net own tax proceeds of the state; entertainment tax 100%; royalty on minerals 1%

(Continued)

State	Devolution recommended		
	SFC-I	*SFC-II*	*SFC-III*
Tamil Nadu	No information	The share of SOTR after excluding entertainment tax of local bodies has been recommended as under: a) 2002–2004: 8%; b) 2004–2006: 9%; and c) for 2006–2007: 10%; 5% of the central devolution should also be passed on to the local bodies; 10% of SFC devolution may be used for capital works in municipalities and corporations, 15% by town Panchayats and 20% by village Panchayats	10% of the state's own tax revenue be devolved to the local bodies; specific purpose grant shall be at 0.5–1% of the state's own tax revenue
Uttar Pradesh	4% of net tax proceeds to PRIs; discontinued grants-in-aid; 7% of net tax proceeds to urban local bodies	5% of divisible pool to PRIs; 7.50% of state's net proceeds of tax revenue to urban local bodies; grants-in-aid: nil	6% of net tax proceeds to PRIs and 9% to urban local bodies, which is under consideration
West Bengal	Entertainment tax: 90%; roads and public works cess: 80%	Annual untied funds of Rs. 350 crore; entertainment and amusement tax 90% to local bodies; cess on road and public works 80%	Untied fund of Rs. 850 crore from 2009–2010 with annual increase of 12% on a cumulative basis for the subsequent years

Source: Hooda (2014)

Notes

1 This chapter is a revised version of my previously published work S. K. Hooda. 2014. Health Expenditure, Health Outcomes and the Role of Decentralized Governance: Evidences from Rural India. *Journal of Indian School of Political Economy*, Vol. XXVI (January–December).

2 This index covers four broad categories: economic management, structural policies, policies for social inclusion and equity, and public sector management and institutions. Countries are rated on several performance criteria with scores ranging from 1 (poor performance) to 5 (high performance).

3 For instance, Mahal et al. (2000) study in Indian context used states that have moved towards decentralisation during the period 1970–1994 as a measure of decentralisation which is identified by knowing the frequency of rural local body election (a proxy of decentralisation) and decentralisation is used in dummy variable form.

4 Like, Asfaw et al. (2004) uses share of local expenditure in the total state government expenditure, the total local expenditure per rural population and the share of local own revenue from the total local expenditure for the period of 1990–1997. Using these indicators an index of decentralisation – named as fiscal decentralisation, was created. This study also used political decentralisation index measured by taking into account the indicators on total voter's turnout, women's participation in polls and the number of polling stations per elector for 14 major states of India. But the comprehensive dimensions of decentralisation have not been utilised.

5 The committee involves the representatives from the community such as educated villagers, village school principals, women, SC/ST/OBC/ minority communities, etc., and headed by village Sarpanch/Pardhan. The government provides an amount of Rs. 10,000 to these committees to help poor women during health emergencies or during pregnancy and control of disease. Financial incentives to women from priority populations is also provided to improve the institutional delivery. However, it may be noted that VHSC can work on diverse issues like healthcare, education, gender discrimination, etc.

6 Under this Act, from a political standpoint, there is provision of three tiers of Panchayats – namely, at village, intermediate and district levels. This Act not only gave discretionary political power to states to devolve power to Panchayati Raj Institutions (PRIs), but also sought to protect the political rights of hitherto neglected groups such as scheduled castes, tribes and women by providing them reservation in politics. This involves the provisions for greater participation of vulnerable sections of the society in decision making.

7 The SEC helps to ensure improved democracy by ensuring regular, free and fair elections at the local level every five years.

8 The SFC is constituted, every five years, to govern the distribution and devolution of financial resources so as to improve the financial position of the Panchayats across the districts within a state.

9 The DPC is involved in planning processes and the plans of the Panchayats and urban local bodies in a district consolidated by DPCs. All Panchayats are to engage in economic development and social justice planning processes under the mandatory action of the constitution. Plans of the Panchayats and urban local bodies in a district are to be consolidated by the District Planning Committees (DPCs). If the constitutional mandate were to be operationalising, minimally, such bodies should be formed and appropriately resourced.

10 The Gram Sabha, or village council, has been envisioned as the foundation of the Panchayati Raj system, as it ensures community participation.

11 The functions are ranging from drinking water, agriculture, poverty alleviation programmes, health and family welfare, education, libraries and cultural activities, maintenance of community assets, etc.

12 In literature, these mortality indicators are considered superior to life expectancy, an alternative measure of health status. It reflects the infant, child and maternal health, in addition to the state of health development within the society. Further, variables like IMR are based on actual data, whereas life expectancy figures are based on extrapolations from child mortality data and assumed life tables. Second, rural infant and under-5 mortality rates are more sensitive to policy reforms such as decentralisation and the levels and allocation patterns of public spending on healthcare in rural areas than any other health outcomes like life expectancy.

13 The assignment of duties to functionaries across PRIs should be based on detailed activity mapping, as activity mapping is a way of unbundling subjects into component activities and mapping them against functions devolved to the Panchayats by law. Thus, inclusion of activity mapping in indices analysis is the first step towards high 'quality' of devolution and strengthens the index of decentralisation.

14 Further, to check the robustness of the result, an index of fiscal decentralisation is also constructed, using share of PRIs' own revenue in total expenditure/revenue of PRIs and in total revenue of the state. The estimated results of these indices show just minor changes in the coefficient values, but their signs and significance remained unaffected. However, these results were not reported in the text in order to avoid confusion in reporting the impact of fiscal decentralisation and to avoid reporting more estimated equations.

15 The dummy of DIH takes 0 for low and 1 for high index value (higher than average). This index is constructed for the year 2006, but the dummy value is used for the period from 1990–2005. This is because states with high DIH value have also taken adequate initiative to implement the decentralised concept from the inception of the 73rd CAA from 1992–1993 (Hooda, 2014).

16 Health expenditure data at district level are not available; this variable therefore is used as its proxy. The infrastructure index is constructed by using numbers of CHCs, PHCs and SCs in rural areas per 100,000 population across districts using principal component analysis (PCA).

17 The status of MCH care use is expected to improve U5MR. This is estimated by using women receiving three or more ANC visits, women receiving two TT injections and child immunization coverage rate by applying PCA for the year 2003–2004.

18 This is because most disease is caused by unsafe drinking water and are the causes of child death at early age. It is expected that a high percentage of use of safe drinking water in a particular district helps in reducing the under-5 mortality rate.

19 As the number of years of observations used here is small, it is obvious that the least squares dummy variable (LSDV) method of estimating fixed effects panel regression is not possible in our case. Not only that, but even individual state-wise regressions (for Equation 1 and Equation 2) were not worth estimating, as the number of years for which data were available was 15 (1990–2005) and 5–6 explanatory variables were to be introduced. Thus, even in this case, the degrees of freedom (*d.f.*) would be very low. A low *d.f.* decreases the chance of rejecting the null hypothesis and increases the probably of accepting the false hypothesis (Gujarati, 2003, Chapter V).

20 Estimates between 2005 and 2008 show that on average, over 60% of all central government health allocations are now allocated under NRHM, which, however, fluctuate across the years. Out of these NRHM allocations, around 69% bypasses the state budgets, and the rest of the funding (31%) flow through the state treasuries and is reflected in the state health budget (Berman and Ahuja, 2008). The Ministry of Health and Family Welfare (MOHFW) NRHM expenditure statement, however, compiles 'total' central funds that are allocated in various NRHM schemes. But, of the total, 31percent NRHM funds (as mentioned previously) are also reflected in the state budget document. Thus, there is a

problem of overlapping of 31% central funds both in MOHFW and state budget documents, which are allocated under various health schemes. Similarly, state governments also allocate funds in NRHM schemes and some of the funds are reported in both state budgets and in NRHM expenditure document statements of MOHFW. Thus, to work out the total rural healthcare spending, a detailed examination of individual schemes is required, which would be a separate study.

References

Acemoglu, D., Johnson, S., Robinson, J. A. 2002. Reversal of Fortune: Geography and Institutions in the Making of the Modern World Income Distribution. *The Quarterly Journal of Economics*, Vol. 117, No. 4, November, pp. 1231–1294. https://doi.org/10.1162/003355302320935025

Alok, V. N. 2014. *Measuring Devolution to Panchayats in India: A Comparison across States Empirical Assessment – 2013–14.* IIPA, New Delhi, August 2014.

Arthur, E., and Oaikhenan, H. 2017. The Effects of Health Expenditure on Health Outcomes in Sub-Saharan Africa (SSA). *African Development Review*, Vol. 29, No. 3, pp. 524–536. https://doi.org/10.1111/1467-8268.12287

Arun, A., and Ribot, J. 1999. Analyzing Decentralization: A Framework with South Asian and West African Cases. *Journal of Developing Areas,* Vol. 33, No. 4, pp. 473–502.

Asfaw, A., Frohberg, K., James, K. S., and Jutting, J. P. 2004. *Modeling the Impact of Fiscal Decentralisation on Health Outcomes: Empirical Evidence from India.* ZEF-Discussion Paper on Development Policy (No.87, June), Centre for Development Research, Bonn.

Azfar, O., Kahkonen, S., Lanyi A., and Meagher, P. 1999. Decentralization, Governance, and Public Services: The Impact of Institutional Arrangements, Working Paper no. 255, September. University of Maryland, IRIS Center, College Park.

Bardhan, P. 1989. The New Institutional Economics and Development Theory: A Brief Critical Assessment. *World Development*, Vol. 17, No. 9, pp. 1389–1395. https://econpapers.repec.org/article/eeewdevel/v_3a17_3ay_3a1989_3ai_3a9_3ap_3a1389-1395.htm

Bardhan, P. 2002. Decentralization of Governance and Development. *Journal of Economic Perspectives,* Vol. 16, No. 4, pp. 185–205.

Barenberg, A. J., Basu, D., and Soylu, C. 2016. The Effect of Public Health Expenditure on Infant Mortality: Evidence from a Panel of Indian States, 1983–1984 to 2011–2012. *Journal of Development Studies*, Vol. 53, No. 10, pp. 1765–1784. http://doi.org/10.1080/00220388.2016.1241384

Berman, P., and Ahuja, R. 2008. Government Health Spending in India. *Economic and Political Weekly*, Vol. 46.

Berman, P., and Bitran, R. 2011. Health Systems Analysis for Better Health System Strengthening. Health, Nutrition, and Population (HNP) discussion paper 08, World Bank. https://openknowledge.worldbank.org/handle/10986/13593

Bossert, T. J., and Beauvais, J. C. 2002. Decentralization of Health Systems in Ghana, Zambia, Uganda and the Philippines: A Comparative Analysis of Decision Space. *Health Policy and Planning*, Vol. 17, No. 1, pp. 14–31.

Breman, A., and Shelton, C. 2001. *Structural Adjustment and Health: A Literature Review of the Debate, Its Role-players and Presented Empirical Evidence.* www.eldis.org/document/A29545

Cassel, A. 1995. Health Sector Reform: Key Issues in Less Developed Countries. *Journal of Health and Population*, Vol. 7, No. 3, pp. 329–347.

Chang, H.-J. 2007. *Institutional Change and Economic Development*. United Nation University Press. https://unu.edu/publications/books/institutional-change-and-economic-development.html#overview

Chaudhury, N., Hammer, J., Kremer, M., Muralidharan, K., and Rogers, F. H. 2006. Missing in Action: Teacher and Health Worker Absence in Developing Countries. *Journal of Economic Perspectives*, Vol. 20, No. 1, pp. 91–116.

Collins, C., and Green, A. 1994. Decentralization and Primary Health Care: Some Negative Implications in Developing Countries. *International Journal of Health Services*, Vol. 24, No. 3, pp. 459–475.

Ebel, R., and Yilmaz, S. 2002. *On the Measurement and Impact of Fiscal Decentralisation*. Policy Research Working Paper 2809, Economic Policy and Poverty Reduction Division, World Bank Institute. World Bank. https://doi.org/10.1596/1813-9450-2809

Eggertsson, T. 1997, August. The Old Theory of Economic Policy and the New Institutionalism. *World Development*, Vol. 25, No. 8, pp. 1187–1203.

Farag, M., Wallack, Stanley, Hodgkin, Dominic, Gaumer, Gary, and Erbil, Can. 2013, March. Health Expenditure, Health Outcomes and the Role of Good Governance. *International Journal of Health Care Finance and Economics*, Vol. 13, No. 1, pp. 33–52.

GBD. 2018. Measuring Performance on the Healthcare Access and Quality Index for 195 Countries and Territories and Selected Subnational Locations: A Systematic Analysis from the Global Burden of Disease Study 2016. GBD 2016 Healthcare Access and Quality Collaborators, June 2018. *Lancet*, Vol. 391, No. 10136, pp. 2236–2271. https://doi.org/10.1016/ S0140-6736(18)30994-2

Gilson, L., Kilima, P., and Tanner, M. 1994. Local Government Decentralization and the Health Sector in Tanzania. *Public Administration and Development*, Vol. 14, pp. 451–477.

Gilson, L., and Mills, A. 1995. Health Sector Reforms in Sub-Saharan Africa: Lessons of the Last 10 Years. *Health Policy*, Vol. 32, pp. 215–243.

Government of India. n.d. *NRHM Expenditure Statement*. Ministry of Health and Family Welfare. Government of India, New Delhi.

Greene, W. H. 2008. *Econometric Analysis*, 5th Edition. Pearson Education, Published by Dorling Kindersley Pvt. Ltd., New Delhi.

Gujarati, D. N. 2003. *Basic Econometrics*, 4th Edition. McGraw-Hill Education (Asia), New York.

Gupta, S., Tiongson, E., and Verhoeven, M. 2001. *Public Spending on Health Care and Poor*, IMF Working Papers 01(01/127), January 2001. https://doi.org/10.5089/9781451854985.001

Gwatkin, D. R. 1999 & 2000. Health Inequalities and the Health of the Poor: What Do We Know? What Can We Do? *Bulletin of the World Health Organisation*, Vol. 78, No. 1, pp. 3–18. https://doi.org/10.1590/S0042-96862000000100002

Habibi, N., Huang, C., Miranda, D., Murillo, V., Ranis, G., Sarkar, M., and Stewart, F. 2001. *Decentralisation in Argentina*. Discussion Paper No. 833. Economic Growth Centre, Yale University, New Haven, CT.

Hall, R. E., and Jones, C. 1999. Why Do Some Countries Produce So Much More Output per Worker than Others? *Quarterly Journal of Economics*, Vol. 114, No. 1, pp. 83–116.

Hanmer, L., et al. 2003. Infant and Child Mortality in Developing Countries: Analysing the Data for Robust Determinants. *Journal of Development Studies*, Vol. 40, No. 1, pp. 101–118. https://doi.org/10.1080/00220380412331293687

Hoffman, B., and Kaiser, K. 2002. *The Making of the Big Bang and Its Aftermath. Can Decentralization Help Rebuild Indonesia?* Andrew Young School of Policy Studies, Georgia State University, Atlanta, Georgia.

Hooda, S. K. 2014, January–December. Health Expenditure, Health Outcomes and the Role of Decentralized Governance: Evidences from Rural India. *Journal of Indian School of Political Economy*, Vol. XXVI.

Hooda, S. K. 2015. Government Spending on Health in India: Some Hopes and Fears of Policy Changes. *Journal of Health Management*, Sage, Vol. 17, No. 4.

Johan, J., and Jacob, M. 2016. *Local Governments and the Public Health Delivery System in Kerala: Lessons for Collaborative Governance.* Cambridge Scholar Publishing. https://books.google.co.in/books?id=Wu9TDgAAQBAJ&printsec=frontco ver#v=onepage&q&f=false

Kaufmann, D., Kraay, A., and Zoido-Lobatón, P. 2002. *Governance Matters II: Updated Indicators for 2000/01.* World Bank Policy Research Department Working Paper No. 2772, Washington, DC. http://www.worldbank.org/wbi/governance/ pubs/govmatters2001.htm

Khaleghian, P. 2003. *Decentralisation and Public Services: The Case of Immunization.* World Bank Policy Research Paper, No. 2989, March. https://openknowledge. worldbank.org/handle/10986/19159

Kolehmaine-Aitken, R.-L., and Newbrander, W. 1997. *Decentralizing the Management of Health and Family Planning Programs.* Management Sciences for Health, Newton.

Lieberman, S. 2002. *Decentralisation and Health in the Philippines and Indonesia: An Interim Report.* World Bank, Washington, DC.

Litvack, J., Ahmad, J., and Bird, R. 1998, September. *Rethinking Decentralisation in Developing Countries.* World Bank Sector Studies Series, World Bank, Washington, DC.

Litvack, J., and Seddon, J. 1999. *Decentralization Briefing Notes.* World Bank Institute, WP No. 37142, World Bank, Washington, DC.

Mahal, A., Srivastava, V., and Sanan, D. 2000. Decentralisation and Its Impact on Public Services Provision on Health and Education Sectors: The Case of India. In J. Dethier (Eds.), *Governance, Decentralisation and Reform in China, India and Russia.* Kluwer Academic Publishers and ZEF, London.

Makuta I and O'Hare, B. 2015. Quality of governance, public spending on health and health status in Sub Saharan Africa: a panel data regression analysis, *BMC Public Health*, Vol. 15, No. 932. DOI 10.1186/s12889-015-2287-z

Maruthappu, M., Bonnie Ng, K. Y., Williams, C., Atun, R., and Zeltner, T. 2015. Government Health Care Spending and Child Mortality. *Pediatrics*, Vol. 135, No. 4, pp. e887–e894. https://doi.org/10.1542/peds.2014-1600

Mills, A., Vaughan, J. P., Smith, D., and Tabibzadeh, I. 1990. *Health System Decentralization: Concepts, Issues and Country Experiences.* World Health Organization, Geneva.

Mishra, P. 2015. Medical Ethics in a Public Health Emergency Ebola Virus Disease. *Economic and Political Weekly*, Vol. 50, No. 25.

Montoya Aguilar, C., and Vaughan, P. 1990. Decentralisation and Local Management of the Health System in Chile. In A. Mills, et al. (Eds.), *Health System Decentralisation.* World Health Organization, Geneva, pp. 55–63.

Nagarajan, H. 2017, March 2. *Democratization and Health Care in Rural India.* Presentation Made at NCAER. www.ncaer.org/uploads/photo-gallery/files/1489750144Health_HKN-NCAER.pdf

NCAER. 2007. *An Index of Devolution for Assessing Environment for Panchayati Raj Institutions in the States.* Draft Report, National Council of Applied Economic Research (NCAER), New Delhi, March.

North, D. C. 1990. *Institutions, Institutional Change and Economic Performance.* Cambridge University Press, Cambridge.

North, D. C. 1997. Prologue. In John N. Drobak and V. C. John Nye (Eds.), *The Frontiers of New Institutional Economics.* Academic Press, New York.

NRHM. 2005. *Mission Documents of the National Rural Health Mission (NRHM).* Government of India. http://mohfw.nic.in/nrhm.html

Oates, W. 1994. Federalism and Government Finance. In J. Quigley and E. Smolensky (Eds.), *Modern Public Finance* (Chapter 5). Harvard University Press, Cambridge, MA, pp. 126–151.

Peabody, J. W., Rahman, M. O., Gertler, P. J., Mann, J., Farley, D. O., and Carter, G. M. 1999. *Policy and Health: Implications for Development in Asia.* Cambridge University Press, Cambridge.

Pokharel, B. 2000. *Decentralization of Health Services.* World Health Organization. Regional Office for South-East Asia, New Delhi.

Prud'homme, R. 1995. *On the Dangers of Decentralisation.* Policy Research Working Paper No. 1252. World Bank, Washington, DC.

Przeworski, A. 2005. Democracy as an Equilibrium. *Public Choice,* Vol. 123, No. 3/4, pp. 253–273. https://www.jstor.org/stable/30026687

Rahman, M. M., Khanam, R., and Rahman, M. 2018. Health Care Expenditure and Health Outcome Nexus: New Evidence from the SAARC-ASEAN Region. *Globalization and Health,* Vol. 14, No. 113.

Rajkumar, A. S., and Swaroop, V. 2008. Public Spending and Outcomes: Does Governance Matter? *Journal of Development Economics,* Vol. 86, No. 2008, pp. 96–111.

Robalino, D. A., Picazo, O. F., and Voetberg, A. 2001. *Does Fiscal Decentralisation Improve Health Outcomes? Evidence from a Cross-country Analysis.* Policy Research Working Paper No. 2565. World Bank, Washington, DC.

Rodrik, D., Subramanian, A., and Trebbi, F. 2004. Institutions Rule: The Primacy of Institutions over Geography and Integration in Economic Development, *Journal of Economic Growth,* Vol. 9, No. 2, pp. 131–165. https://www.jstor.org/stable/40212696

Schmid, A. A. 1978. *Property, Power and Public Choice: An Equity into the Law and Economics.* Prager Special Studies, New York.

Tandon, A. 2005. *Attaining Millennium Development Goals in Health: Is n't Economic Growth Enough?* ERD Policy Brief Series No. 35, Asian Development Bank, March. https://www.adb.org/sites/default/files/publication/28094/pb035.pdf

Treisman, D. 2000. The Causes of Corruption: A Cross-National Study. *Journal of Public Economics,* Vol. 76, No. 3, pp. 399–458.

Unnikrishnan, P. V., Palanithurai, G., et al. 2016. *Devolution Report 2015–16: Where Local Democracy and Devolution in India is Heading Towards?* Ministry of Panchayati Raj, Government of India and TISS, Mumbai.

Vasudevan, U. P., Prabhu, S., Bakshi, A., and Gupta, S. D. 2015. *Devolution Report 2014–15. How Effective is Devolution across States: Insights from the Field.*

Ministry of Panchayati Raj, Government of India. New Delhi, and Tata Institute of Social Sciences, Mumbai.

Wagstaff, A., and Claeson, M. 2004. *Rising to the Challenges: The Millennium Development Goals for Health*. World Bank, Washington, DC.

Williamson, J. 1990. *The Washington Consensus as Policy Prescription for Development*. www.piie.com/publications/papers/williamson0204.pdf

Yee, E. 2001. The Effects of Fiscal Decentralisation on Health Care in China. *Undergraduate Journal of Economics*, Vol. 5, No. 1. www.econ.ilstu.edu/UAUJE

6 Decentralisation, access and service delivery[1]

Recent health reform initiatives argue that healthcare service delivery mechanisms can be made effective through the participation of local governments and communities in policy making, planning and services delivery. The advocates of decentralisation argue that it brings decision makers closer to the people, which would increase the responsiveness of local officials to needs that may not be served by the central government far away (Oates, 1994; Prud'homme, 1995). It removes layers of bureaucracy and incorporates local information into decision-making processes and planning (Bardhan, 1996)[2] through the involvement of local communities and government (Litvack and Seddon, 1999; Lieberman, 2002), which further results in effective delivery of health services.

The important assumption behind undertaking the decentralisation in service delivery is that local communities have better knowledge of local needs and conditions, and can make better decisions if they are granted the authority to manage resources and organise and supply health services. Decentralisation is intended to promote accountability and participation of the local people, make health service providers accountable to the local community and boost the responsiveness of the providers to the local demand for services. Decentralisation is therefore expected to improve the efficiency, equity and quality of healthcare services delivery and management (Tidemand, 2010).

The overall argument is that decentralisation improves the healthcare system performance by bringing decision making closer to service delivery. Several studies have made attempts to investigate whether decentralisation actually improves the health system. Other studies have tried to explore the conditions that enable it to be effective. In this context, it emerges that improperly designed and implemented decentralisation policy may pose risks and challenges which further may lead to deterioration in provisioning of healthcare services – and consequently, to poor health outcomes (Lieberman, 2002). Sometimes, local elites and dominant individuals may hijack the decentralised power and authority to pursue their own interests and may not promote efficiency and equity (Collins, 1989; Mills et al., 1990). It is also possible that local bodies may not necessarily reflect the interests

DOI: 10.4324/9781032108438-8

and developmental priorities of the community that they represent. The problem can be more severe if the expected participation of the community has not materialised at the local level. Sometimes, the confrontation and unwillingness or half-hearted tendency from the central or state/regional body to delegate power and authority to local bodies may also undermine the effects of decentralisation on the delivery of efficient, responsive and qualitative health services at lower levels (Gilson and Mills, 1995; Pokharel, 2000). Even if the central authority devolves adequate decentralised power, the bottom authority may not take effective initiatives to implement these powers in their locality. Decentralisation may also aggravate inequalities in service access between rich and poor persons and areas, if not implemented effectively and perceived at local level.

This chapter starts with a notion that the gain from decentralisation initiatives – to a large extent – depends on properly designed and implemented decentralised policy at ground level. The magnitude of Panchayat support and priorities of healthcare and coordination between local agents and health functionaries are very important to materialise the greater gains from decentralisation. The gains from decentralisation can be enhanced through devolving more health-related functions, funds, management, regulation and policy making powers to local Panchayats and communities. In order to evaluate their effectiveness, first we captured the degree of local agents' participation and extent of decentralisation in health and then measured their impact on healthcare service access and health-seeking behaviour of rural households and healthcare system functioning.

Decentralisation reform initiatives in India

Besides having several challenges before decentralisation, several countries, including India, have embarked on the process of decentralisation in their policy agendas. India has placed the strength of decentralisation in planning and implementation of schemes for economic development and social justice in general, and healthcare services in particular. The political reforms on the one side and healthcare policies reforms on the other have paved the way for decentralisation of healthcare services delivery in rural parts of India. The political reforms give strength to decentralisation that started with the implementation of the 73rd Constitutional Amendment Act in 1992–1993, as discussed in Chapter 5. This Act strengthened direct democracy at the local level via shifting of powers and resources from central, state and regional authorities to lower-level grass-roots institutions (local governments). It ensures the participation of local communities and local agents in planning and implementation of social and healthcare services through the introduction of a concept called Gram Sabha (GS) in the village. Considering the sensitivity of class and caste divisions of society of India, a clear mandate about the reservation of Panchayat representatives (women, minority groups and other social categories like scheduled castes/tribes and other backward castes; SCs/

STs/OBCs) is provided especially to eliminate the power dimension from local politics. In addition, the state-specific Panchayati Raj Acts, clearly define the functions and duties of Panchayats in specific areas. It also define the authority of Panchayat involvement and intervention in the healthcare sector. The specific functions and duties relating to health activities include implementation of programmes on rural sanitation, public health and family welfare, and for women and child development, etc. These acts also define the role of Panchayats in improve the functioning of village healthcare centres through supervision and monitoring.

Within the health-related policies/initiatives, the approach to involve local communities goes back to the Bhore Committee of 1946, which recommended community involvement for better delivery of primary care. After independence, India formulated a Community Development Programme in 1952 as a part of the First Five-Year Plan (1951–1956) for overall rural development. Community development initiatives refers to those which 'create conditions of economic and social progress for the whole community with its active participation and the fullest possible reliance upon the community's initiative' (GOI, 1951, p.21). Several other committees on health in the 1960s and 1970s emphasised the role of community participation in health. Around 1977, under 'placing people health in people hands', a Community Health Volunteer/Village Health Guide (VHG) Scheme was initiated (Strodel and Perry, 2019), VHG was to be a person from the village, most of them women, who was imparted short-term training and a small incentive for the work. The health policy documents (1983 and 2002 NHP) of India envisioned the role of decentralisation (local government and community) in the healthcare sector. A closer review of these policy documents, however, reveals that they are lacking in defining the decentralisation policy agendas clearly. The National Population Policy 2000,[3] however, affirms that the Panchayati Raj institutions are an important means of furthering decentralised planning and programme implementation. It emphasised that in order to realise their potential, they need to be strengthened by further delegation of administrative and financial powers, including powers of resource mobilisation and talk about the formation of committees represented by elected women to promote a gender-sensitive, multisectoral agenda for population stabilisation, that will 'think, plan and act locally, and support nationally' (GOI, 2000: 7). They may identify an area's specific unmet needs for reproductive health services, and prepare need-based, demand-driven, socio-demographic plans at the village level, aimed at identifying and providing responsive, people-centred, integrated, basic reproductive and child healthcare. Panchayats demonstrating exemplary performance in the compulsory registration of births, deaths, marriages, and pregnancies universalised the small family norm, increasing safe deliveries, bringing about reductions in infant and maternal mortality, etc. Their suggested decentralisation model implemented half-heartedly at the ground level. A government document (MoHFW, 2007) on 'Health Sector Reforms in India: Initiatives from States' stressed the role of institutions to reform the healthcare sector. Some policy measures suggested are reorganisation and restructuring of the existing government healthcare system, involving communities in healthcare service delivery and provision, health management information systems, quality of care, financing methods, decentralisation, public-private partnerships, contracting or outsourcing, granting of autonomy, human resources management through supervision and monitoring, etc.[4] However, clear policy guidelines for local government and community participation are better framed under the National Rural Health Mission (NRHM), which was launched in April 2005. Of the several previously discussed decentralisation and community participation initiatives, those proposed under the NRHM were more effective, as least in framing and implementation at ground level.

The primary focus of the mission was to improve access to equitable and affordable primary healthcare to the rural population. Reducing IMR and MMR through promoting infant care, child immunisation, antenatal care, institutional delivery, post-natal care, etc., are some of the important goals of the mission. The foundation of the mission was built upon the involvement of local communities in drawing up village health plans under the auspices of the Village Health and Sanitation (Nutrition) Committee (VHSC), making rural primary healthcare accountable to the community and giving authority to the District Health Mission to implement the intersectoral District Health Plan, including provisions on drinking water, sanitation, hygiene and nutrition. Under the mission, the interface between the community and the public health system at the village level is entrusted through a female Accredited Social Health Activist (ASHA), a health volunteer who receives performance-based compensation for the promotion of universal immunisation, referral and escort services for reproductive and child health (RCH), construction of household toilets and other healthcare delivery programmes. To promote institutional delivery, the cash incentive programme of Janani Suraksha Yojana (JSY) has been made an integral component of NRHM (DLHS-3), along with some other concepts called Rogi Kalyan Samiti (RKS) and Sakshar Mahila Samooh (SMS), etc., for planning and implementation of health programmes that involve community.

The VHSC envisioned local Panchayat and community people taking leadership in the management of the healthcare system and its related matters. This committee involves the representatives from the community which includes ANM, ASHA workers, Gram Sabha members, educated villagers, village school principals, women, NGOs, SCs/STs minority community women and those headed by village Sarpanch/Pardhan. The government provides an amount of Rs. 10,000 to these committees to help poor women during health emergencies or to help poor women during pregnancy and control of disease. The financial incentives (JSY) to women from priority population also provided to improve the institutional delivery. VHSC can work on diverse issues related to health, education, gender discrimination, etc.

Further, ASHA workers, women from minority communities in the villages, have been asked to provide as well as to spread awareness about the importance of basic health programmes and facilities in their villages. This also helps in ensuring pre-pregnancy registration, institutional delivery of children, pre-natal and post-natal care, and child immunisation in the villages. It is proposed that there would one ASHA worker for each 1000 population in the village. The ASHA would act as an interface between the community and the public health system, and would be accountable to the Gram Panchayat.

This discussion conveys that the decentralisation process in the country involves both political and healthcare policy reform initiatives, and they converge with each other. Some of initiatives that involve decentralisation in healthcare policy reforms are presented in Box 6.1. These initiatives explained a sustained process of decentralisation that involve communities, local agents and local governments for effective delivery of healthcare services in rural India. This chapter started with a notion that gains from decentralisation can only be realised with the proper implementation of this concept at ground level, failing which the likely impact would be low. That is, we believe that to evaluate the impact of these decentralised policy initiatives, one needs to assess how these initiatives have been implemented at ground level and have helped in improving the health service delivery system in rural areas. These initiatives involve various dimensions of community and local agents' participation; therefore, evaluating their impacts are not straightforward. In order to fully understand the gain from various dimensions of decentralisation, first the degree of community participation/ engagement and the extent of decentralisation in the healthcare sector are worked out, and then their impacts are assessed on healthcare service delivery, particularly in improving the access to maternal and child healthcare utilisation for which these initiatives were commenced. As reported, due to the sensitivity of a class-and-caste–divided society, the Constitution of India provides a clear mandate about the reservation of women and other social categories in Panchayat representation; therefore, these are also incorporated in the analysis.

This chapter aims to address the question: has the extent of decentralisation in healthcare, nature and degree of community participation, involvement of VHSC and ASHA workers, and representation of village by women and minority groups been able be make any significant differences in improving the utilisation of maternal and child healthcare (such as the ANC, PNC, institutional delivery and child immunisation) in rural India and improve the overall functioning of health system? This also addresses whether these factors lead to access to healthcare utilisation and influence the choice of healthcare facility (public and private), controlling for others confounding factors like socio-economic background of the households and village-level characteristics. This chapter uses District Level Household Survey (DLHS-4) and field survey data conducted in Haryana. DLHS-4 is the only recent

Box 6.1   Reform initiatives promoting decentralisation in India

- Political reforms
  - The 73rd Constitutional Amendment Act (1992–1993)
    - Devolution of funds, functions and functionaries powers to PRIs in 29 functional areas and their involvement in planning, approval, execution and monitoring of these functions
    - Free and fair Panchayat elections every five years
    - Reservation of seats for women and marginalised groups in Panchayat elections
    - Establishment of Gram Sabhas; the Panchayat would be accountable to the GS
  - The Panchayati Raj Acts of state(s): Haryana
    - Whether medicine reached to village health centre, purchase of medicine, if shortfall, visit of village's Sarpanch for monitoring, supervision, to check data record, to know about health centre condition; like availability of water supply, sanitation and equipment, and other problems, if any

- Health sector reforms
  - Pre-NRHM period: first (1983) and second (2002) National Health Policy (NHP)
    - While specifying 'why health sector of India could not perform well in the past', the Second NHP (27) concluded that decentralisation initiatives have not been implemented effectively, and as a result, the healthcare sector could not perform well in the country – but this policy itself failed to describe what said decentralisation initiatives must include and how they should be designed
  - The NRHM decentralisation initiatives
    - Introduction of VHSC – the NRHM defined the number, composition, functions, funds and training for VHSC
    - Appointment of ASHA – workers from village communities to improve antenatal care (ANC) registration, institutional delivery, post-natal care (PNC) and child immunisation, etc.; accountable to GS
  - Post-NRHM
    - Health sector reform documents of states: monitoring and supervision powers to PRIs

Source: Panchayati Raj Act of Haryana, National Health Policy 1st & 2nd, NRHM-2005 Mission document

data set available in the public domain that captures the status of maternal and child healthcare, as well as involvement of decentralisation in planning, monitoring, implementation and evaluation of healthcare services through village-level surveys by interviewing the Panchayat representatives of the villages. This capture presents some important dimensions of decentralisation in healthcare.

The case of Haryana

Along with presenting the decentralisation implementation status and its impact on service delivery system at a nationwide level, the detail evidences are provided from Haryana. Identifying the role of decentralisation in a state like Haryana, where unregulated Panchayat (*Khap Panchayat*; organised local community) seems to be an active phenomena, can be of great significance for decentralisation policy, especially how they (community, local agents and elected Panchayats) are involved in health service delivery in the villages and whether they have made any significant impact on service access. The secondary data do not capture some important dimensions relating to extent and nature of community participation that influences the village-level health programmes and planning, the extent of Panchayat involvement and intervention in the implementation of healthcare-related functions like the authority of the Panchayat in provisioning of healthcare finances, management and regulation of functionaries through supervision and monitoring, healthcare services organisation and policy making. These are important dimensions to understand the extent (and implementation quality) of decentralisation in health and the degree of community participation for impact assessment. The success of the implementation of all these dimensions depends on how village Panchayats are involved and the magnitude of Panchayat support on these issues. The priorities and coordination between Panchayats and health departments is another important dimension that needed to be captured. All these dimensions are captured through a field survey conducted in some selected villages of Haryana in 2011, when NRHM was about to complete its first phase.

The villages are selected from culturally, geographically, socio-economically and endemicity diversified three districts of Haryana namely Rohtak, Mahendargarh and Yamunanagar.[5] The selection of these districts, out of total 21 districts of Haryana, is based on level of health infrastructure, female literacy rate and health outcome (under-5 mortality rate) criteria[6] (Box 6.2). The infrastructure and literacy are considered important factors for influencing the health outcomes in literature. A comparative picture of districts around these three indicators shows significant variation in health outcomes with same or different levels of female literacy and availability of health infrastructure, indicating that some other factors influence the health sector outcomes. The other factors can be institutional factors (like active involvement and intervention of Panchayat and community in health-related activities) and other can be socio-economic-demographic factors. Our survey is designed to capture the role of institutional factors, while controlling for the others.

Of the three districts, a total of 12 villages (four from each district) representing different Panchayat backgrounds are selected (Box 6.2) from different blocks of the district, especially to capture the diversity across villages. The selection of different Panchayat representatives is based on the justification indicated in the 73rd CAA that highlights the reservation of women and disadvantaged (scheduled caste and tribe); groups in Panchayat representation is not only important for empowering them politically, but they can address issues of equity in access to healthcare utilisation across low socio-economic strata. Based on the understanding from the literature discussed in the previous chapters, we have postulated that women Panchayat members expectedly feel the importance of healthcare facilities for women and children, and can take greater interest in monitoring healthcare facilities. They may ask the health workers (particularly the female staff) to regularly visit in the village to provide basic healthcare to women and children. Thus, the dimensions of decentralisation need to be understood across gender categories (male/female and reserved/unreserved) representing Panchayat villages.

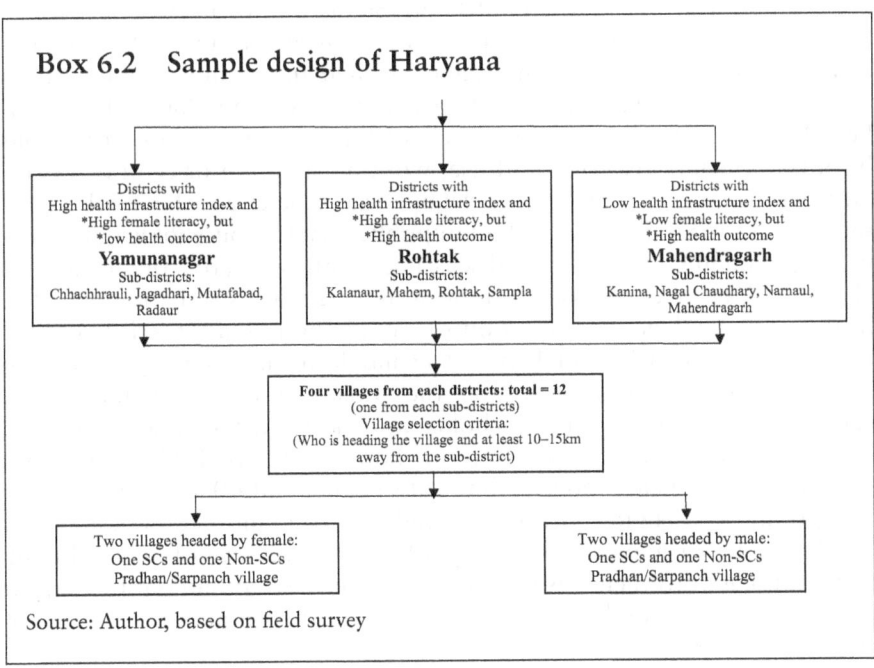

Box 6.2   Sample design of Haryana

| Districts with High health infrastructure index and *High female literacy, but *low health outcome **Yamunanagar** Sub-districts: Chhachhrauli, Jagadhari, Mutafabad, Radaur | Districts with High health infrastructure index and *High female literacy, but *High health outcome **Rohtak** Sub-districts: Kalanaur, Mahem, Rohtak, Sampla | Districts with Low health infrastructure index and *Low female literacy, but *High health outcome **Mahendragarh** Sub-districts: Kanina, Nagal Chaudhary, Narnaul, Mahendragarh |

Four villages from each districts: total = 12
(one from each sub-districts)
Village selection criteria:
(Who is heading the village and at least 10–15km away from the sub-district)

| Two villages headed by female: One SCs and one Non-SCs Pradhan/Sarpanch village | Two villages headed by male: One SCs and one Non-SCs Pradhan/Sarpanch village |

Source: Author, based on field survey

As previously reported, effectiveness of decentralisation in healthcare depends on how Panchayats and local-level agents are involved in health-care-related functions, provisioning of finances, management and regulation of functionaries, healthcare service organisations, policy making and addressing the issues of equity and accessibility at ground level (Bossert, 1998; Bossert and Beauvais, 2002). It also depends on the magnitude of Panchayat support and priorities, community participation and coordination of both Panchayats and health departments. Most of these dimensions have been initiated in a health policy and political reform process in India which requires a careful investigation that needs to be gathered from different stakeholders, such as health functionaries, Panchayat representatives and Sarpanch, VHSC and ASHA members, and households. To capture all the dimensions, the interview schedules are designed and filled out across all these stakeholders, especially from health functionaries (doctors, ANM, ASHA, VHSC members) of the village's healthcare centre, Panchayat representatives (Sarpanch/Pardhan) and households. The interview schedule captured the decentralisation dimensions that are mentioned in health policy (NRHM), 73rd CAA and PRIs Act documents and some of the important issues that are discussed in the dominant literature.

From health functionaries and Sarpanch, information about their awareness, involvement, intervention (monitoring, supervision, etc.), quality and working conditions of health centres, health centre management, and coordination between Panchayat and health functionaries is worked out. The information about functioning of Gram Sabha and their level of involvement in healthcare-related issues are covered. The involvement of VHSC and ASHA in healthcare system management, their functioning and initiatives taken at ground level are covered from a discussion with VHSC/ASHA members. From household schedules, we elicited their views and concerns about healthcare facility selection and use, working situation of central (Janani Suraksha Yojana; JSY) and state-level financial protection schemes that promote institutional delivery of child in public facility, household/community participation in Gram Sabha in discussing health issues, role of village Panchayat and their awareness/involvement in programmes/activities related to health in the village. For selection of sample household, the list of total number of women who had delivered a child during last 365 days was taken from the village health centre. From the available list, 12 households from each village (a total of 144 households) are selected for interview purposes, which is based on a proportionate method. Of the total, 60% from SCs category having below poverty line (BPL) cards and 40% from Non-SCs background households are selected randomly from most corners/streets of a village. The basic idea of selecting a higher percentage of SC (including BPL) household women was that we were interested to find out the impact of decentralisation and benefit of NRHM schemes on poorer segments of the society at ground level.

Implementation status of decentralisation in health

Involvement and interventions of VHSC and GS/Panchayat

The finding from the village-level survey of DLHS-4 2012–2013 reveals that only 57% of the 8550 villages had VHSC and 43.5% of 708 Haryana villages were found to have VHSC. This survey captured information on involvement and interventions of VHSC in ten healthcare-related issues. Around 50% of the village's VHSC were found to be engaging in spreading awareness about essential health programmes in all reported states under DLHS (Figure 6.1). This percentage for Haryana is 79%. The profile of their involvement in all survey states and Haryana is reported to be around 46% and 67% in developing village health plans, village-level nutritional awareness activities (44%/59%), estimation of annual expenditures incurred for management of healthcare plans (32.7%/43%), overseeing the work of health and nutrition functionaries (40%/62%), taking into consideration the problems in the community, discussing every maternal death or neonatal death that occurs in the village, suggesting necessary action to prevent such deaths, getting deaths registered at Panchayat level and managing the village health funds (Figure 6.1). The involvement and intervention of VHSC in all ten health issues in Haryana villages was found to be lower than in all other states (here reported as India). The role/intervention of VHSC in at least in

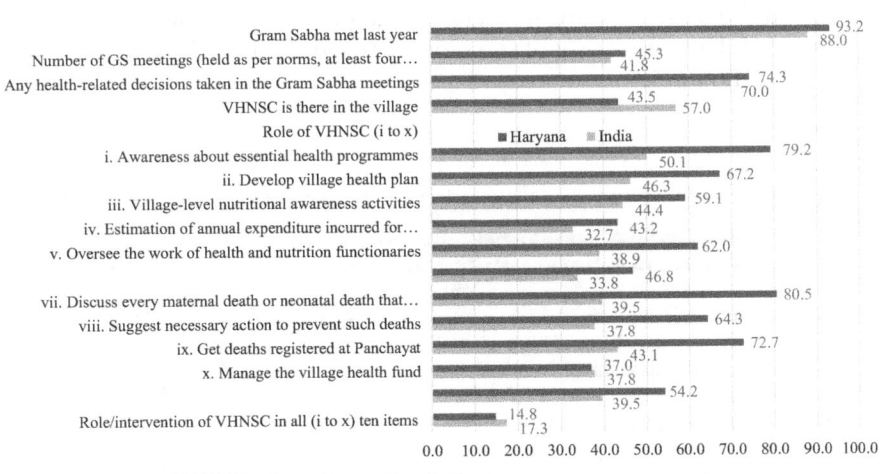

VHSC/GS involvement in percentage of villages

Figure 6.1 Involvement and intervention of VHSC and GS in health: India and Haryana

Source: Estimated using DLHS-4 (village file) unit-level data 2012–2013

Note: Number of obs. for India = 8550 & Haryana = 708; VHSC exist in HR villages = 308 (percentage of i to x is out of 308)

five of the reported ten items was found to be around 39.5% at reported states level, while this percentage was 54.2% in the case of Haryana. The intervention of VHSC in all the ten items found to be low – around 17% villages of India and only in 14.8% villages of Haryana, indicating that even if the VHSC exist in the village, there is no guarantee that they are engaging effectively in health-related issues at the village level where they are entitled to play active roles.

The comparison of intervention of VHSC in some selected states show a considerable variation ranges from 50% in Kerala to 13% in West Bengal. The involvement of VHSC in all the ten functions was reported to be very low in Haryana when compared with the other states (Figure 6.2).

In order to find out the level of decentralisation in health (LDH) in select villages of Haryana, the information collected through the field survey is combined. This includes visit of Panchayat members or Sarpanch at village healthcare centres for supervision or monitoring or other purposes; the number of meetings, composition and the specific initiatives taken by VHSC to improve the health of the villagers; issues related to health raised in Gram Sabha; participation of women and minority groups in the meeting (GS and VHSC) to capture the functioning of Gram Sabha; appointment of ASHA from low socio-economic strata; and the quality of health centre in terms of availability of basic instrument, medicine, etc. Information related to these dimensions is captured through almost 19 variables and by using subjective scaling score (between 0 and 4) method, the LDH status is measured. The score value 4 refers to high decentralisation in health and 0 otherwise. The rationality of the score is based on the existing guidelines reported in Box 6.3.

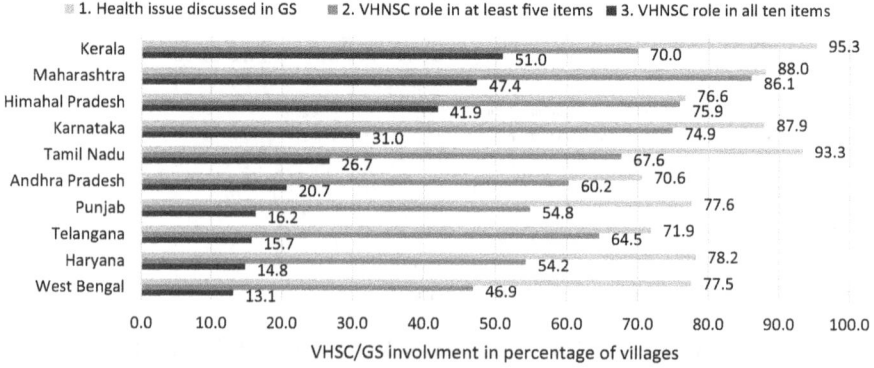

Figure 6.2 Involvement and intervention of VHSC and GS in health: a comparison between states

Source: Estimated using DLHS-4 (village file) Unit level data 2012–2013

Box 6.3 Decentralisation in health: measurement and indicators, Haryana

1. No of VHSC meeting during last one year – If ≥24 = 4; If 12–23 = 3; If <12 = 1; If no meetings = 0
2. Composition of VHSC attend

   – If proposed member (like, teachers, health staff/AWW/ASHA, educated youth etc.) with high share of women (about ≥25 women) attend = 4
   – If Pradhan of such meeting and a high share of women (about 15–24 women) attend = 3
   – If Pradhan, health staff and low a low share of women (<15 women) attend = 2
   – Otherwise = 0

3. Who plays major role in VHSC meetings

   – Health educators, health staff or Pradhan = 4
   – If villages' women and social activists = 3
   – If village Sarpanch or PRIs members = 2
   – Others = 1

4. Plan finalised or discussed on strategy to spread awareness in VHSC

   – If MCH care, FW programmes, NRHM guideline and other disease programmes discussed = 4
   – If any two programmes discussed from these = 3
   – If sanitation, sewerage and hygienic issues discussed = 2
   – If female feticides, dowry or other social issues discussed = 1

5. No of ASHA workers attending VHSC meetings

   – If all = 4; If >half = 3; If half = 2; If <half = 1

6. No of AWW workers attending VHSC meetings

   – If all = 4; If >half = 3; If half = 2; If <half = 1

7. Do women Sarpanch or Panch attend VHSC meetings?

   – If yes = 4; If sometimes = 2; If no = 0

8. Who appoints ASHA?

   – If VHSC = 4; If Sarpanch = 3; If health staff and Sarpanch just put signature = 2; Other = 1; If ASHA exist = 0

9. No of training programmes for ASHA

   – If >2 = 4; If = 2 = 3; If <2 = 2; If no training = 1

10. No of ASHA appointed from priority population

    – If all (100 %) ASHA is appointed from SCs/BPL family = 4
    – If 75–99% are from SCs/BPL family = 3
    – If 2/3 to < 75 % from SCs/BPL family = 2
    – If < 2/3 from SCs/BPL family = 1

11. Who helps in organising the training programme for ASHA

    – If VHSC = 4; If Panchayat = 3; If health staff = 2; If other/NGOs = 1

12. Role of ASHA

    – If effectively help in pregnancy identification + ID improvement + go for PNC = 4; If any two of these items = 3; If sometimes helps in all items = 2; If sometimes helps in any two items = 1; If no role = 0

13. Role of PRIs in primary health centre (PHC)

    – If PRIs role new construction, land provision, and approval = 4; If maintenance from own source = 3; If supervision and monitoring = 2; Other = 1; No role = 0

14. Role of PRIs in MCH care use, FW programmes, NRHM implementation and immunisation

   – If yes in all items = 4; If yes in NRHM and immunisation = 3; If yes in NRHM = 2; If yes FW = 1; Other = 0

15. Role of PRIs in health and sanitation

   – If yes in items (like [i] ensure and checked whether medicine reached to health centre, [ii] to ensure the distribution of medicine among needy persons, [iii] campaign to remove environmental, sanitation and communicable diseases from village, [iv] help in construction and maintenance of open drains for disposal of wastewater, [v] maintenance/repair of public stand post, etc.) = 4
   – If yes in any four items = 3; If yes in three items = 2; If yes in two items = 1; If yes in <2 items = 0

16. No of PRIs visit at health centre

   – If ≥ average visit of all villages taken together = 4
   – If < average visit of all villages taken together = 2
   – If no visits = 0

17. Purpose of PRIs visit at health centre

   – If yes for supervision, for monitoring, for checking health data record, to check the data, to discuss health-related problem or prevailing disease in the village; to discuss status of MCH care use, to know health centre problem) = 4
   – If yes in any 6–7 items = 3; If yes in 4–5 items = 2; If yes in 2–3 items = 1; If <2 = 0

18. If any type of problem exists, disciplinary action taken by PRIs

   – If no problem exists = 4; If yes, complain to DPC/ZP or setup health monitoring committee to improve the situation after discussing the issue in GS = 3; Complain to COM = 2; Write confidential report and send to concerned authority = 1; No action taken = 0

19. Number of times health-related issues (especially about health centre functioning) discussed in (last 2–3) GS meetings

   – If discussed in ≥average meetings of all villages taken together = 4; If discussed in <average meetings = 2

Source: Field survey

The estimated score of LDH does not only capture the community, Panchayat and local level agents' involvement and intervention in the healthcare sector for planning and decision making, but also captures the NRHM decentralised indicators and other indicators related to coordination between Panchayat and healthcare functionaries for the better functioning of village health centres. Panchayat involvement in the healthcare sector includes visits of Panchayat members or village Sarpanch at health centres for supervision or monitoring or other purposes, VHSC functioning (like number of meetings, composition of members and initiative taken by these committees to improve the health of the villagers) and Gram Sabha activeness (like number of time health-related issues discussed in GS, participation by women in the meeting, etc.). This measure promotes the intersectoral coordination and community participation, and increases accountability and improves the implementation of health programmes; this in turn is expected to affect the delivery of healthcare services and ultimately health outcomes. The score of the level of decentralisation in health (LDH) is recorded about 2.78 out of the maximum score value 4. There exists a variation in the level of decentralisation in healthcare across districts. Its level was recorded as high in Rohtak district (around 2.85) compared to the other districts (Table 6.1).

The level of decentralisation in healthcare was recorded as high in male-headed Panchayat villages compared to female-headed Panchayat villages (Table 6.1). Low scores of LDH in female-headed villages is opposite to our expectation. We had expected that the women Panchayat members expect-edly feel the importance of health facilities for women and children, and can take greater interest in monitoring the healthcare facilities. They may ask the healthcare workers to regularly visit in villages to provide the healthcare services, and may take steps to start the training programmes for untrained dais (traditional birth attendants) or ASHA workers to improve the health of the village's women and children. The other village's women may also have greater autonomy to raise their voices for health requirement in VHSC and GS, particularly in women-headed Panchayat villages, but the low score value of LDH in women-headed Panchayat villages confirms that they are less active in ensuring the better delivery of healthcare services in their villages compared to the male-headed Panchayat villages. During the survey, we observed that though the election is fought in the name of females, while most of the executive work is handled either by the husband or by the son of that female Sarpanch. The score value of LDH in SCs Sarpanch-headed Panchayat villages is recorded as high compared to non-SCs–headed Panchayat villages.

Table 6.1 Score of different dimensions of decentralisation

	Background	Level of decentralisation in healthcare (LDH)	Degree of community participation and awareness (DCPA)
Districts	Yamunanagar	2.68	2.59
	Mahendargarh	2.81	2.49
	Rohtak	2.85	2.16
Village's Sarpanch sex	Male Sarpanch	2.86	2.35
	Female Sarpanch	2.69	2.47
Village Sarpanch category	Non-SCs Sarpanch	2.70	2.39
	SCs Sarpanch	2.85	2.43

Source: Estimated from field survey data

Involvement and interventions of Gram Panchayat and GS

From DLHS-4 data, we observed that in around three-fourths of the village in Haryana, health-related issues are discussed in Gram Sabha meetings, indicating high involvement of local stakeholders GS where Panchayat members and members of the village community are present. This data set, however, provides information whether any health issues are discussed in GS, but it is interesting to know to what extent Panchayat is involved in all 29 functions, as well as healthcare-related functions that are devolved to them under the 73rd CAA. This Act divides these functions into core, welfare, economic and health functions. It is not so easy to arrive at the status of involvement of a Panchayat, as there is no hard and fast method to show their involvement. To avoid any complexity, we have used the guideline of the 73rd CAA that defines the involvement of Panchayat in a function. This Act mentioned that the Panchayat could be involved in planning, approval, execution and/or monitoring of a function. Therefore, status of Panchayat involvement (SPI) in provisioning of the 29 functions is measured using these four dimensions. Equal weight is assigned to each dimension (one can think of giving different weight) to avoid complexity in measuring the SPI score, like if involved in planning = 1; if involved in approval = 1; if involved in execution = 1; if involved in monitoring = 1 and for non-involvement, the weight 0 is assigned. The 'State of Panchayat Report' of Haryana reveals that government has devolved all the 29 functions to Panchayat. Therefore, one can expect 4 score values of Panchayat involvement in each function, a lower score will show the low level of involvement of Panchayat in that particular function.

The estimated score value shows that the average score recorded as high for core functions (about 1.80), followed by health (1.40), welfare (about 0.83) and economic (about 0.39) functions,[7] indicating low level of involvement of Panchayat in planning, approval, execution and monitoring of these functions (Figure 6.3).

The SPI varies considerably across sample districts. In core functions, Mahendargarh district was high as compared to Yamunanagar and Rohtak districts (Figure 6.4). A high level of involvement of Panchayats in Mahendargarh is not surprising because of early starting of decentralised planning in the district. Drinking water is a part of core function and the Panchayats in this district are highly involved in drinking water supply, because of major drinking water problem in the area. The drinking water supply remains, in most cases, a political issue in the district, and Panchayats of the villages' influence the political party, as well, on this issue. Therefore, the score of core functions in this district is high. The average score of SPI in health functions (which includes health and sanitation, including hospitals, primary health centres and dispensaries, family welfare, and women and child development) is also recorded high in Mahendargarh district compared to the others (Figure 6.4).

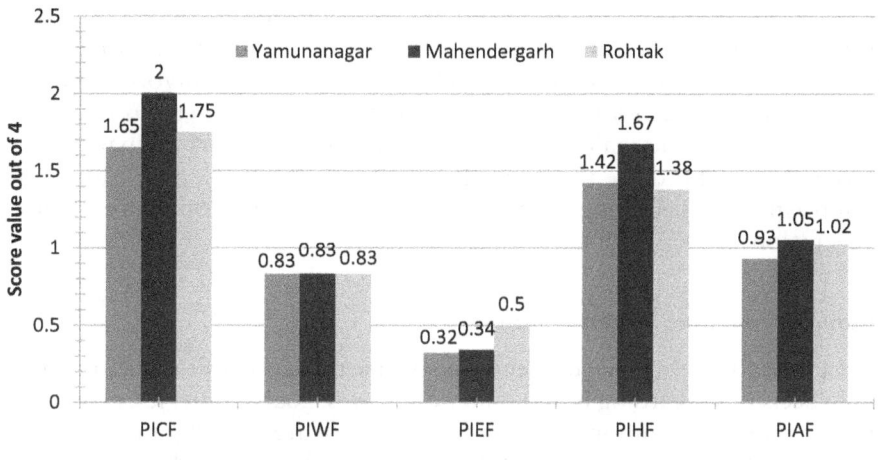

Figure 6.3 Status of involvement of Panchayat in core, welfare, economic and health functions in sample districts

Source: Field survey

Notes: Panchayat involvement in core functions (PICF), welfare functions (PIWF), economic functions (PIEF), health functions (PIHF) and in all 29 functions (PIAF)

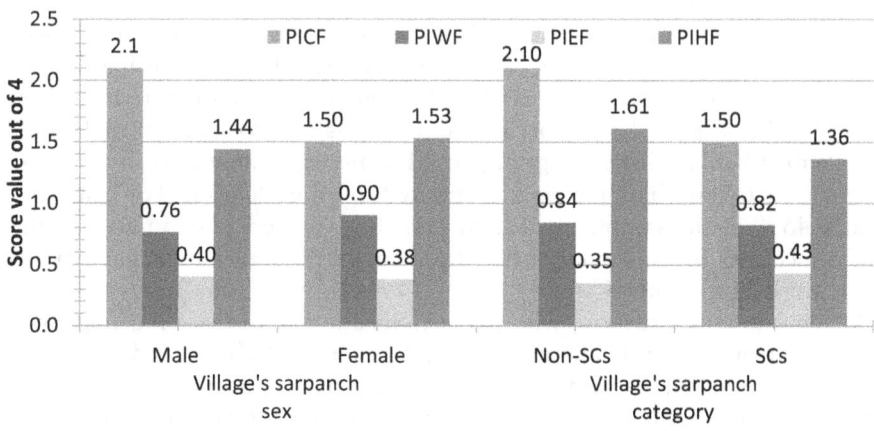

Figure 6.4 Status of Panchayat involvement in core, welfare, economic and health functions by Sarpanch background

Source: Field survey

Notes: Panchayat involvement in core functions (PICF), welfare functions (PIWF), economic functions (PIEF), health functions (PIHF) and in all 29 functions (PIAF)

Interestingly, the status of involvement in Panchayat of women and/ or SCs-headed villages did not meet our expectations, as the score value in these villages was found to be low in most of the functions compared to their counterparts (Figure 6.4). The variation in the involvement in health function across these Sarpanch categories was very low. Overall, we observed the male Sarpanch and non-SCs category Sarpanch are more active or hold the power in the planning, approval, execution and monitoring of these functions in the village, which is opposite of our expectations.

Degree of community participation

Decentralisation is expected to enhance the participation of local communities in decisions regarding health policy objectives, goals, strategies, planning, financing, implementation and monitoring, which are important to improve delivery of healthcare services and access to healthcare at the local level. Therefore, it is important to capture the nature and degree of community participation and awareness (DCPA), especially to capture the community and local agents' participation, interventions and involvement in decision making through different committee meetings (like VHSC, Gram Sabha and Gram Panchayat). While estimating the DCPA, both household and village-level information that facilitate in improving the degree of community participation are used (Box 6.4). DCPA is measured using the subjective scaling scores method. The identification of possible indicators is based on the consensus provided in Metzger (2001; see Welschhoff, 2006 for detail[8]; Murthy and Klugman, 2004).

The estimated score value of DCPA shows that their involvement in various decision-making committees and meetings was 2.40 out of the maximum value of 4. The value was high (2.59) in Mahendargarh as compared to other districts (Table 6.1). This is because not only is the presence of male and female members in GS meetings high in Mahendargarh, but also all villagers are quite active in these meetings compared to other districts. For instance, nearly 45% of the sample household says that villagers play an active role in GS meetings in Mahendargarh district, compare to Yamunanagar (about 9%) and Rohtak (only 5%).

When one looks at those who play significant role in these meetings, we found that out of total general category households (who attended the GS meeting), about 39.1% said that they played active roles in GS meeting and have also given instructions in the meetings. This percentage, however, is very low (about 7.3%) among SC/BPL households. About 63.4% of households (out of total who have attended the GS meeting) from SC/BPL background said that they sit quietly in the GS meetings. In order to find out what factors determine the community participation, we have extended this section to arrive at a specific conclusion.

Box 6.4 Indicators to measure the degree of community participation and awareness: DCPA

---

1. Do you (male as well as female separately) know about GS and VHSC/SMS meetings? If yes = 4; If no = 0
2. Do you or your family member(s) attend such meetings? If yes = 4; If no = 0
3. How many GS and VHSC/SMS meetings have been held during last one year? The score value is: number of meetings/average number of meetings in sample area
4. How many GS and VHSC/SMS meetings have been attended by you during last one year? The score value is: number of meetings attended/average number of meetings attended by households in sample area
5. Household involvement by nature of participation in such meetings like, if play active role = 4; If give instructions = 3; If ask questions and sometimes give instructions = 2; If households attend the meeting but sit quietly = 1
6. Who plays the major role in these meetings? If role played by villagers = 4; If role played by villagers and Gram Panchayat = 3; If role played by village's Panchayat or NGO who represents villagers interest or by youth club = 2; If role played by fellow official (BDPO) or powerful client in case of GS and Pardhan of such committee/samooh in case of VHSC/SMS = 1
7. Do you know that any health programmes running in the village? If yes = 4; If no = 0
8. What is the level of involvement of Panchayat and VHC/SMS in these programmes by their nature of participation?: If active involvement = 4; Neutral involvement = 2; No involvement or Do not know about PRIs involvement = 0
9. Your or any household member's involvement in these programmes by nature of participation: If active involvement = 4; Neutral involvement = 2; No involvement = 0

Source: Field survey

The dominant literature argues that participation of community generally depends on educational standards, as education is most important for questioning or their role in meetings. The communication and information transfer, interest in participation, motivation and sustainability are also considered as the guiding principles of community participation (Metzger, 2001).[9] The identification of such factors is considered as useful tools for prerequisites of successful community participation (see Murthy and Klugman, 2004; Metzger, 2001; Green, 1992; Rifkin, 1996).

More participation is positive if it generates more information. It is an additional tool which can enhance efficiency and rationality of planning for local provisions. We have assumed that the prerequisites of successful community participation probably depend on information and education standards, socio-economic conditions of the community and, more importantly, on who represents the village Panchayat (i.e., reserved category or women Sarpanch, etc.). Furthermore, community participation also depends on democratic level of the village's Panchayat. The democratic level of Panchayat, however, is based on many indicators like level and composition of Gram Panchayat (GP) and Gram Sabha (GS); PRIs office and PRIs financial authority, which are the measure of access, service organisation and governance rule; and nature of involvement of community in decision making and planning, etc.

The factors that determine the successful participation of a community are measured by taking into account the multinomial logit regression model (presented in Equation 1). The multinomial logit model (MLM) is generally used in cases when the dependent variable takes categorical (multiple) responses. In general, when the dependent variable is qualitative (categorical responses), dichotomous response models like linear probability model (LPM), logit or probit or tobit (censored regression) models have been adopted. Because of non-normality of u_i, heteroscedasticity of u_i, possibility of $\hat{Y}_i$ lying outside the 0–1 range, and the assumption of $P_i = E(Y = 1|X)$ increases linearly with X – that is, the marginal or incremental effect of X remains constant throughout – the LPMs are not considered. The logit model (including two response categories) has advantages over it. The MLM is a straightforward extension of simple logit model and allows us to incorporate multiple (more than two) categorical responses (Maddala, 1993; Greene, 2008). In the case of simple logit model, the dependent variable takes an odd ratio of two probabilities. In MLM, the dependent variable takes three probabilities. In our case, nature of community participation (NCP) is taken as dependent variable. The nature can be of three types: sitting quietly, asking questions and playing an active role. Thus, NCP takes three categories of participation and therefore is used to indicate three probabilities: 1 = is sitting quietly, which indicates a lower nature of community participation; 2 = is asking questions, which is a mediocre level of community participation; and 3 = is playing an active role and giving instructions, which is a high degree of community participation. The NCP1 is used as base category in our MLM regression model. The MLM equation is as follows.

$$NCP = \alpha + \beta_1 Age + \beta_2 EDU + \beta_3 PA + \beta_4 SS + \beta_5 ES + \beta_6 SSD + \beta_7 SCD + \beta_8 DDP + u \ldots \tag{1}$$

The estimated equation takes a log ratio of two probabilities (i.e., [P_NCP2/NCP1]:[P_NCP3/NCP1]) and corresponds to two equations in each case. This equation is estimation for both male and female participation in Gram Sabha and VHSC/SMS meetings separately.

Where, Age – is the age of the household (continuous variable); EDU – education status of household members who attend the meeting (continuous variable and rank is given from low education standard = 1 to high education standard = 4); PA – any member of the household having political association (if yes = 1, 0 otherwise); SS – social status (SC = 1, Non-SC = 0); ES – economic status of the household, which is determined by the interaction variable of log of MPCI in rupees and land possession per person in acre (an index is created using these variable using PCA method). After predicting the score, the dummy variable for ES is created, 1 for score value greater than or equal to average scores value and 0 otherwise. SSD – Sarpanch sex dummy (1 = female; 0 = male); SCD – Sarpanch category dummy (1 = SC Sarpanch, 0 = non-SC Sarpanch); DDP – is the democratic decentralised Panchayat score and used as dummy variable (1 = high democratic decentralisation [higher than average score value] and 0 for low DDP). The score for democratic decentralised Panchayat (DDP) is measured using scaling score method from 0–4. A higher score value of DDP shows that higher participation of local agents with more powers in decision making with highly democratic process in the village.[10] This measure is assumed to affect the prerequisites of successful community participation in a village.

The results show that the likelihood of asking questions and playing an active role in CP meetings increases with education standard of the households who have attended the meeting. The households which have any political association also play more active roles compared to those who do not have any association, which is quite expected. SC/BPL households have little to say in these meetings, as the coefficient of social status turned out to be insignificant. The households which have high economic status (measured through level of income and land possession) play significant active roles in CP meetings rather than sitting quietly, and accordingly influence village-level policy and planning. Further, the probability of asking questions, as well as playing an active role in different GS/VHSC meetings, is high in SCs-headed Panchayat villages. The people in high democratic decentralised areas do not play any significant role in the village-level meetings, which is opposite of our expectation (Table 6.2).

A further description on community or Panchayat involvement in health-related functions (particularly in health-related programmes/activities running in the village) is that we found the village Panchayat is more active in drinking water supply, sanitation and garbage management and sewerage and cleanness of drainage in Mahendargarh district compared to other two districts, as per household observations. The active involvement of Panchayats in disease control programmes, immunisation and in organising health camp, however, is negligible in all the districts, whereas the active involvement of VHSC/SMS in these activities was higher in Yamunanagar and Rohtak districts than in Mahendargarh. The community/

186   *Institutional reforms*

Table 6.2 Factors of successful community participation: multinomial logit model estimation

Independent variable	A. Male participation in Gram Sabha		B. Female participation in VHSC/SMS	
	Eq-I: log (P_CP2/P_CP1)	Eq-II: log (P_CP3/P_CP1)	Eq-I: log (P_CP2/P_CP1)	Eq-II: log (P_CP3/P_CP1)
Age: used as continuous variable	0.004 (0.13)	0.03 (0.93)	-0.02 (-0.74)	-0.04 (-0.82)
Education status: used as continuous variable	**0.79*** (**1.82**)	0.34 (1.27)	0.13 (0.42)	0.40 (1.08)
Household member political association dummy (1 = yes, 2 = no)	-0.05 (-0.05)	0.49 (0.72)	1.23 (1.30)	**3.39**** (**2.24**)
Social status: SC = 1, Non-SC = 0	-0.28 (-0.25)	-0.32 (-0.33)	0.04 (0.03)	-1.66 (-1.20)
Land possession and lnMPCE dummy: (1 for high value [higher than average score] & 0 for low)	0.55 (0.40)	**1.76*** (**1.65**)	1.22 (0.70)	**4.27*** (**1.84**)
Sarpanch sex dummy (1 = female; 0 = male)	0.04 (0.05)	0.12 (0.18)	-1.46 (-1.45)	0.35 (0.27)
Sarpanch category dummy: (1 = SC Sarpanch, 0 = non-SC)	**1.82*** (**1.79**)	-0.06 (-0.06)	0.51 (0.45)	**2.77*** (**1.64**)
DDP dummy: high DDP = 1, Low DDP = 0	-1.78 (-1.4)	-0.72 (-0.78)	-1.44 (-1.27)	-1.08 (-0.72)
Constant	-3.99 (-1.39)	-2.99 (-1.40)	-0.08 (-0.05)	-3.26 (-1.10)

Source: Author's estimation, using field study data

Notes: P_CP is probability of community participation (CP1) – sit quietly and indicate lower nature of community participation. This is used as base category. CP2 – ask questions, a mediocre level of community participation. CP3 – play active role and give instructions; ***, ** & * indicate 1%, 5% and 10% level of significance, respectively; The figures in parenthesis are z-test values; The no. of observation in A = 64 and in B = 52

household awareness about these health-related functions is higher in all the districts. About three-fourths of households said that they do not have any involvement in these activities. About 80% of households (which attended GS meetings) reported that in most cases, street cleanness, IAY, BPL identification, plot distribution to BPL family, water supply, villagers' dispute, sanitation and PDS are discussed. In VHSC/SMS meetings, nearly 60% of women say that in most cases, MCH care, NRHM guidelines, family welfare programmes and female feticide issues are discussed. On average, 30 women attend such groups and committees. The proposed members in VHSC, as per guidelines (educated youth/women, teachers, etc.), do not attend the meeting in most of the villages; therefore, these findings corroborate with the DLHS-4 results that VHSC role in ten listed health-related functions was very low in the case of Haryana (as reported in Figure 6.1).

Decentralisation and health system functioning

The village-level reporting from DLHS-4 indicates that decentralisation components, like the active engagement of VHSC and GS in health-related issues, plays a significant role for better functioning of village health centres and implementation of health programmes in the village. The improved source of drinking water, availability of drainage facilities, accessibility of SCs/PHCs throughout the year, implementation of ICDS scheme, accessibility of ICDS throughout the year, availability of ASHA workers in the villages and as per norms, undertaking of cleaning and fogging drives in the village, improvement in village health facility, functioning of village health centres all around, utilisation of untied funds for multipurposing, implementation of JSY scheme and implementation of mid-day meal and sanitation programmes were reported to be high in villages where VHSC actively engaged in at least five items and if any health issue discussed in the Gram Sabha relative to the villages where VHSC is not actively playing role and where health issues are not discussed in the village GS. The role of VHSC and GS seems to be effective in villages of Haryana, as well as all Indian states reported in DLHS-4 data (Table 6.3).

The probability of implementing the health programmes related to sanitation, nutrition, drainage, cleanness and water supply increase with the active intervention/involvement of VHSC and GS in the village. The probability of improving the village health centre, as well as their accessibility throughout the year, increase with the active engagement of VHSC and GS. The NRHM initiatives like the utilisation of untied funds for multiple purposes, appointment of ASHA and schemes like JSY found were to be implemented effectively in villages where VHSC/GS are active relative to their counterpart villages (Table 6.4).

Table 6.3 Decentralisation and health system functioning between villages

	India				Haryana			
	Health issue discussed in GS		Role of VHNSC		Health issue discussed in GS		Role of VHNSC	
	Yes	No	At least in five items	In fewer than five items	Yes	No	At least in five items	In fewer than five items
Improved/protected source of drinking water	87.5	82.0	90.1	85.5	94.1	95.9	95.6	94.1
Drainage facility available in the village	62.2	50.4	67.5	58.3	98.9	97.3	98.3	99.3
SHC accessible throughout the year	55.2	49.5	61.1	47.7	40.3	41.5	28.9	44.7
PHC accessible throughout the year	72.7	66.9	77.9	64.7	76.2	68.7	70.6	77.6
Integrated Child Development Scheme (ICDS) implemented	87.6	85.1	91.5	84.6	83.1	81.0	83.3	83.6
ICDS (anganwadi) accessible throughout the year	38.1	34.1	47.3	32.5	4.0	2.7	4.4	5.9
Availability of ASHA in the village (staying/visiting)	76.9	79.9	79.2	79.1	96.6	95.9	100.0	96.7
Number of ASHA as per norm (have at least one per 1000 population)	43.1	37.3	47.8	39.9	60.6	62.6	65.6	58.6
During the last six months, how many times cleaning drive was undertaken in the village (at least one)	58.7	32.4	82.0	68.2	33.1	21.1	60.6	53.3
During the last six months, how many times fogging drive was undertaken in the village (at least one)	37.1	16.2	51.6	38.8	12.2	8.8	22.2	22.4
Any improvement in the health facilities, i.e. sub-centres/PHCs/CHCs in your area (very good and good)	83.0	63.6	87.3	76.2	78.5	57.1	89.4	75.7
Health centre located in your area provides healthcare services/treatment daily all the year round	69.8	52.6	75.0	58.3	79.1	66.0	87.8	78.9

Aware of untied funds provided by government for improvement of health and sanitation	66.0	42.2	78.8	61.0	49.6	27.9	73.9	52.6
Untied funds utilised for multitasking (like hiring transport facilities, arranging camps, other purposes): at least one item	32.4	20.5	41.4	31.1	23.4	9.5	31.1	32.9
Janani Suraksha Yojana implemented	94.4	87.5	97.6	91.1	96.6	95.9	98.3	96.1
Janani Shishu Suraksha Karyakram implemented	68.4	49.4	79.6	55.6	88.0	87.1	94.4	90.8
Rogi Kalyan Samiti been constituted in the PHC of your area	43.3	21.7	54.5	34.6	49.6	27.2	63.3	55.3
Mid-day Meal Programme implemented	89.4	86.7	91.9	86.4	96.2	95.9	97.2	96.1
Sanitation Programme (SP) implemented	61.2	45.3	73.5	55.8	58.6	61.9	66.1	51.3
Kishori Shakti Yojana implemented	55.3	37.1	67.9	57.0	63.7	59.2	78.3	60.5

Source: Estimated using DLHS-4 (village file) unit-level data, 2012–2013 (DLHS-4, 2012–13)

Table 6.4 Impact of decentralisation on health system functioning and implementation of programmes: logistic estimation using village-level data

Dependent variables	Independent variables (estimated equation)		Constant	No. of obj.
	Role of VHNSC at least in 5 items = 1, otherwise = 0)	Any health issue discussed in GS (yes = 1, no = 0)		
Availability of ASHAs in the village (staying/visiting) (yes = 1, no = 0)	0.009	0.113	1.16	4995
	0.81	1.19	11.79	
Number of ASHAs as per norm (have at least one per 1000 population = 1, otherwise = 0)	0.269***	0.265**	-0.046	3851
	3.78	2.93	-0.54	
Drainage facilities available in the village (yes = 1, no = 0)	0.295***	0.387***	0.106	4993
	4.62	4.86	1.41	
Improved/protected sources of drinking water (protected source = 1, otherwise = 0)	0.367***	0.082	1.763	4995
	3.91	0.69	16.20	
Aware about untied funds provided by the government for improvement of health and sanitation (yes = 1, no = 0)	0.751***	0.635***	0.016	4994
	11.10	7.71	0.21	
Untied funds utilised for multitasking purposes (hiring transport facilities, arranging camps, other purposes): (more than one item = 1, otherwise = 0)	0.226***	0.188*	-0.347	3845
	3.16	2.02	-3.81	
During the last six months, how many times cleaning drive was undertaken in the village (at least one = 1, otherwise = 0)	0.521***	0.604***	0.564	4881
	6.92	6.76	6.88	
During the last six months, how many times fogging drive was undertaken in the village (at least one = 1, otherwise = 0)	0.261***	0.671***	-0.719	4769
	4.09	8.03	-8.92	

Health centre located in your area provides healthcare services/ treatment daily all the year round (yes = 1, no = 0)	0.682*** 10.42	0.482*** 5.94	-0.001 -0.01	4995
Any improvement in health facilities i.e. sub-centres/PHCs/CHCs in your area (very good = 1, good = 2, no improvement = 3, base) (multinomial logit model is applied here) Very good-1/base3	0.549*** 5.25	1.122*** 8.07	-1.108 -8.43	4990
Good-2/base3	0.534*** 6.40	0.608*** 6.34	0.622 7.22	
Sanitation Programme (SP) implemented (yes = 1, no = 0)	0.698*** 10.80	0.327*** 4.02	0.035 0.46	4994
Janani Suraksha Yojana implemented (yes = 1, no = 0)	1.201*** 8.09	0.695*** 4.55	1.923 15.33	4997
Janani Shishu Suraksha Karyakram implemented (yes = 1, no = 0)	0.983*** 14.62	0.622*** 7.54	-0.154 -2.02	4997
Mid-day Meal Programme implemented (yes = 1, no = 0)	0.536*** 5.44	0.269*** 2.26	1.664 15.52	4996
Integrated Child Development Scheme (ICDS) implemented (yes = 1, no = 0)	0.602*** 6.39	0.331** 2.94	1.466 14.53	4997
National Food for Work Programme (NFFWP) implemented (yes = 1, no = 0)	0.247** 2.81	0.023 0.21	-1.888 -17.65	4996

Source: Estimated using DLHS-4 (village file) unit-level data, 2012–2013 (DLHS-4, 2012–13)

Decentralisation, access and service delivery

The NRHM in 2005 was launched specifically to address the MCH care demand and reduce inequality in service access among the rich-poor and rural-urban divides. The mission initiated economic resources, as well as institutional and decentralisation reforms. If one looks at the access to maternal and child healthcare, one would observe a significant improvement after the launch of NRHM. Figure 6.5 presents the performance of the healthcare sector over time for ANC and PNC received, institutional birth and child immunisation. After the launch of NRHM, not only did the gap between rural and urban reduce, but overall MCH care use increased. The institutional birth status of a child was 31% in rural areas and 69.4% for urban areas in 2005–2006 which increased to 90.5% for rural areas and 96% for urban areas in 2017–2018, a sign of reducing the institutional birth gap between rural and urban areas. Institutional births in public facility were 18% in 2005–2006, which increased to 52.1% in 2015–2016. Childbirth in public facilities was recorded 48.3% for urban areas and 69.2% for rural areas 2017–2018. The breakup of institutional birth in public facilities among rich and poor provides an interesting insight. In 2017–2018, birth in public facilities was 62.1% among urban poor (Q1), relative to that of only 19.3% among urban rich (Q5). Similarly, 74.4% of rural poor had institutional birth in public facility, while for rural-rich it was 57% (NSS, 2019). This indicates that these economic and institutional reforms have been able to address the demand for rural and poor people.

Figure 6.6 presents progress in institutional delivery in rural and urban regions across states. The year-wise progress of institutional delivery reveals a decline in variation across states; the decline in variation seems to be much faster in urban areas than in rural areas. However, the rural-urban gap is reducing over time.

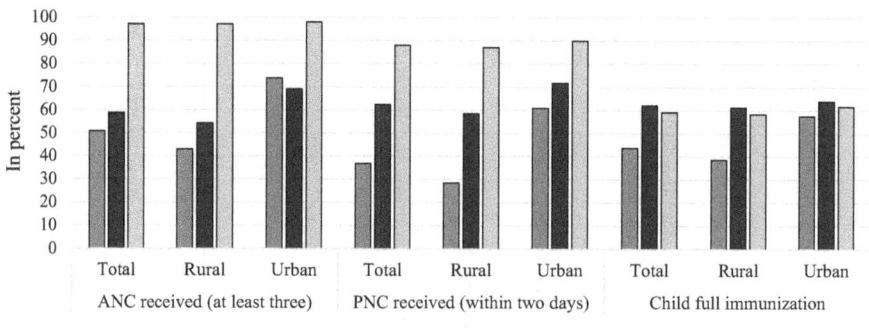

Figure 6.5 Status of utilisation of health facilities for MCH care in pre- and post-decentralised initiative phase, 1992–2018

Source: NFHS-3 & 4; values for 2017–2018 are from NSS-2019

Institutional delivery of live births (in percent)

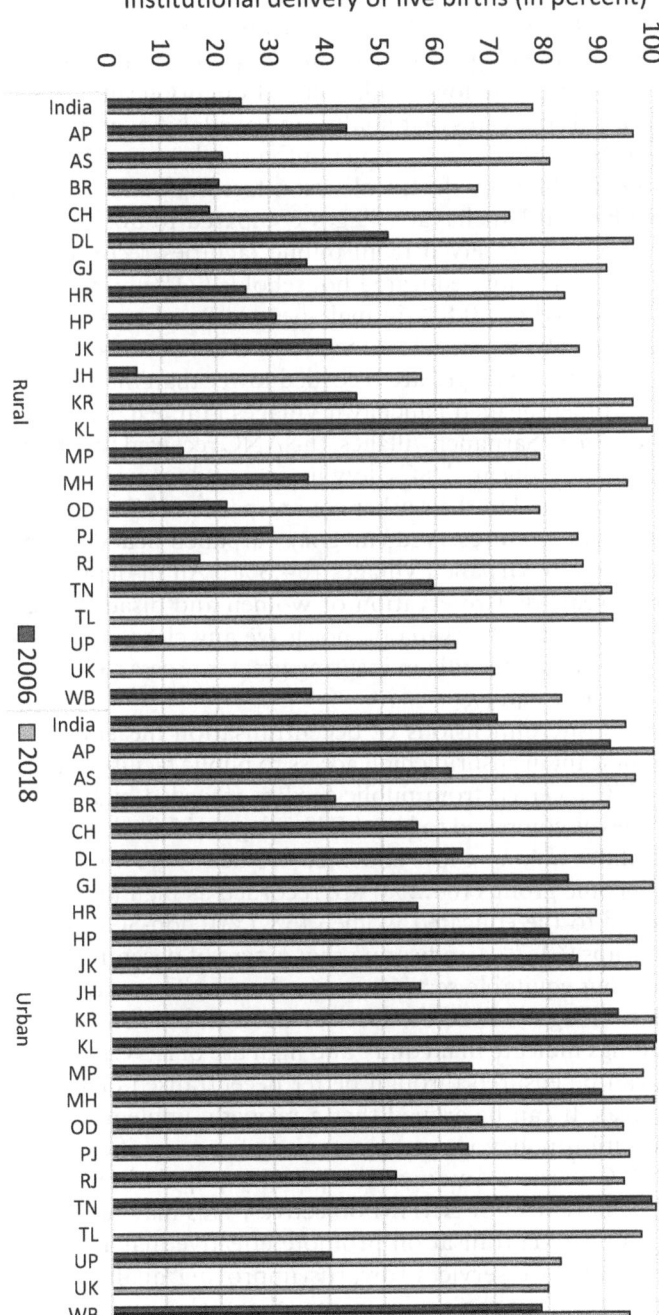

Figure 6.6 Progress in institutional delivery: declining gap between rural-urban and states

Source: Sample Registration System, Office of the Registrar General, Government of India

The field survey findings suggest that ANC received from public facilities is high amongst the low socio-economic strata as compared to their other counterparts. The use of ANC services from public facilities are even much higher (62.2%) in villages where quality of public health facilities were better as compared to the low availability of quality health facilities (58.6%) (Table 6.5). This indicates that quality and availability of public health facilities do matter more for ANC usage in the rural areas. ANC received status from public facilities by decentralisation factors found to be high (65.4%) in women-headed Panchayat villages compared to 56.3% in male-headed villages. The ANC received from public facilities recorded as even much higher amongst the low-educated households (71%) in women-headed villages as compared to 60.8% in male-headed Panchayat villages. The ANC services among SCs women, low income and households living in low-QHC (quality healthcare) villages are recorded lower than their other counterpart groups in women-headed Panchayat villages (Table 6.5). In the caste-based reserved-category Sarpanch villages, the ANC received was found to be high amongst the low-educated, SCs, low income and women living in low-QHC villages as compared to their other counterparts. ANC received status found to be low (56.8%) in reserved-category Sarpanch-headed villages compare to the unreserved Sarpanch villages (64.3%). An in-depth examination of field data reveals that reservation of women and disadvantaged groups in Panchayat politics in Haryana do not leave any clear message whether reservation plays a greater role in insuring greater access to healthcare services that can promote equity.

The composite dimensions of decentralisation measured through LDH turned significant in ensuring high access to public facility with greater equality. The ANC received from public facility recorded high (63.3%) in high-LDH villages as compared to low-LDH villages (55.9%). ANC received from public facilities amongst low-educated women (69.6%), SCs/BPL (65.7%) and low-income groups (64.2%) are recorded as high in high-LDH villages as compared to the educated women (58.1%), non-SCs (59.2%) and high income groups (61.7%), indicating that extent of decentralisation does matter in ensuring equitable services in rural areas. These trends, however, are reversed in villages where the level of decentralisation is low (Table 6.5). These findings indicate that equity and high use of ANC services from public facilities can be ensured through better decentralised delivery mechanisms in rural areas. It can be argued that a properly implemented and designed decentralisation policy in healthcare can play a significant role in providing the ANC services amongst the priority population in rural area and facilitate achievement of NRHM objectives. This may mean that composite dimensions of decentralisation promote effective management of publicly provided healthcare services towards improving quality of these services that in the end affect the choice, rather than using any one specific tool of local governance. The findings are consistent with the earlier study (Nagarajan, 2017), which showed that overall, local governance matters more for

Table 6.5 Decentralisation and ANC received and child delivery in public facilities (percentage)

Decentralisation dimensions	Low-educated women	High-educated women	SC/BPL	Non-SC	Low-income (Q I–III)	High-income (Q IV–V)	Low infrastructure area	High infrastructure area	Total (%)
ANC received status									
Male Pradhan villages	60.8	53.1	57.1	55.2	60.8	50.6	45.8	60.5	56.3
Female Pradhan villages	71.0	61.5	64.6	66.7	63.8	69.0	64.4	67.4	65.4
Unreserved Pradhan villages	70.2	60.1	63.3	65.7	65.3	62.8	51.1	70.2	64.3
Reserved Pradhan villages	60.7	54.0	58.4	54.4	59.4	52.0	62.5	46.0	56.8
Low LDH	56.4	55.6	50.7	62.3	59.1	50.0	54.7	59.0	55.9
High LDH	69.6	58.1	65.7	59.2	64.2	61.7	63.1	63.3	63.2
ANC from public facility	65.7	57.1	60.9	60.4	62.4	57.8	58.6	62.5	60.7
ANC from private facility	11.5	26.9	16.4	26.6	19.1	23.0	18.2	22.7	20.5
ANC not received	22.8	15.9	22.8	13.0	18.5	19.2	23.2	14.8	18.8
TP in number	67	95	96	66	101	61	77	85	162
Child delivery status									
Male Pradhan villages	45.7	30.6	43.8	27.8	40.4	32.4	25.0	41.7	36.9
Female Pradhan villages	53.1	37.0	41.7	46.7	44.4	41.7	49.1	32.0	43.6
Unreserved Pradhan villages	60.0	34.7	53.1	34.3	49.0	39.4	30.8	51.7	45.2
Reserved class Pradhan villages	37.5	32.6	31.9	38.7	36.0	32.1	47.1	11.1	34.6
Low LDH	55.0	27.8	41.9	32.0	44.4	25.0	46.3	13.3	37.5
High LDH	46.8	37.3	43.1	39.0	41.5	41.5	36.1	44.3	41.5
Child delivery in public facility	47.8	34.7	42.7	36.4	42.6	36.1	41.6	38.8	40.1
Child delivery in private facility	14.9	36.8	24.0	33.3	20.8	39.3	29.9	25.9	27.8
Home delivery	35.8	29.5	33.3	30.3	36.6	24.6	28.6	35.3	32.1
TD in number	67	95	96	66	101	61	77	85	162

Source: Estimated using field survey data, 2011

Notes: TP – Total number of pregnant women delivered a child during last 365 days; TD – Total number of (public + private + home) deliveries

effective service delivery. It is interesting to note that despite initiating several measure relating to the awareness of the importance of PNC through ASHA/ ANM and VHSC/GS, the total number of PNC received found very low in the study area, which restricted us not to present PNC results.

As far as the place of child delivery is concerned, on average around 40.1%, 27.8% and 32.1% child delivery took place in public facilities, private facilities and at home, respectively, in the sample villages (Table 6.5). The share of institutional delivery of children in public facilities (out of total deliveries) was reported as high among low socio-economic background households. The percentage of child delivery in public facilities remained high among low literate women, SC-BPL and low-income group women compare to high literate, non-SCs and high-income groups. This shows a better health sector functioning in rural Haryana.

The analysis of child delivery by decentralisation factors shows that child delivery in public facilities recorded as high (43.6%) in women Sarpanch– headed villages compare to male Sarpanch–headed villages (36.9%). Child delivery across socio-economic groups shows that low literate and low-income group women enjoy more public facilities compare to the high-literate and high-income groups in women-headed Panchayat villages, which is comparatively higher than in male-headed Panchayat villages. Child delivery among SCs households, meanwhile, is recorded lower (41.7%) as compared to the non-SCs households (46.7%) in women-headed Panchayat villages. Class divisions were addressed properly by women Sarpanches, but caste division in service utilisation remained unresolved. There is no clear visibility in addressing these issues in reserved and unreserved category Sarpanch-headed villages. The equity in healthcare utilisation for child delivery is properly addressed in highly decentralised villages. That is, the level of LDH does not only address the issue of equity in healthcare utilisation, but also ensures high use of public facilities for child delivery among low-literate and SC-BPL women as compared to high-literate and non-SC women. The high quality and availability of public infrastructure in areas ensures high shares of child delivery in public facilities among low-income, low-educated and SC/BPL as compared to low-infrastructure villages. The findings indicate that along with strengthening the decentralised delivery mechanism of healthcare services, government needs to provide adequate and quality health facilities in rural areas.

With regards to the child immunisation, those of the low socio-economic strata receive high immunisation in female-headed villages. Immunisation status among these groups was high in both low-LDH and high-LDH districts (Figure 6.7). The results on immunisation status more or less remained inconclusive in the study area. This may be because the decentralisation factors do not matter for child immunisation, as it was observed during the field survey that hardly any discussion happened relating to that. It is the household's individual awareness that matters more for child immunisation. However, an effective awareness can be ensured through the health workers or community health workers (like ASHAs) available at the local level. This

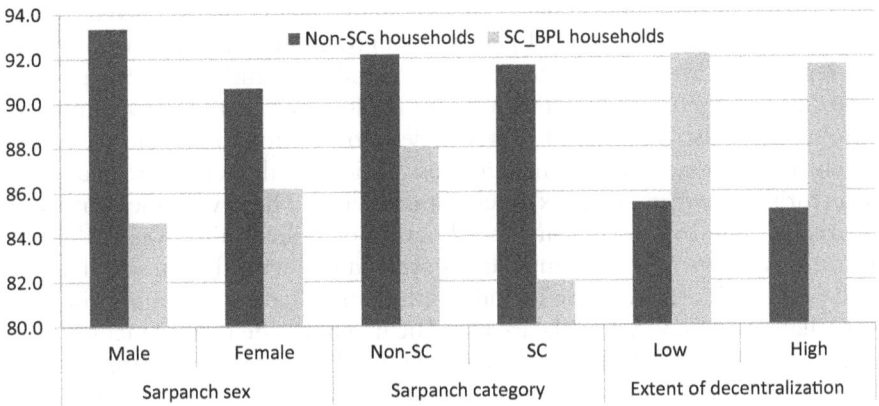

Figure 6.7 Decentralisation and child immunisation status

Source: Estimated using field survey data, 2011

Note: Average of child immunisations received for BCG, polio, DPT, measles, vitamin doses (A and B) and food supplement are reported

can be an effective instrument to generate awareness among individuals and households.

Data from NFHS (2016) reveals that about 14%, 14% and 11% of the women came in contact an auxiliary nurse midwife (ANM) or a lady health visitor (LHV), an anganwadi worker (AWW), or an ASHA in last past three months, respectively. A higher percentage of women met with ASHA workers from low-income households, SC/STs, low-educated and rural areas as compared to their counterparts, indicating it can be an effective instrument of spreading awareness amongst the lowest socio-economic stratum group households in India. In Haryana, around 29% of the women came with a contact with a health worker, which is higher than the national average of 23.9%. Among women who met with a health worker in the past three months, 63% met with a health worker at home, 60% met with a health worker at an anganwadi centre, and 41% met with a health worker at a health facility or camp (NFHS, 2016). The percentage of women who visited a healthcare facility or health camp in last three months was 9.8% at the national level, while it was 16.7% in case of Haryana – indicating that the women in the state are more actively participating in health camps organised by the healthcare sector or village Panchayats, but the percentage is still low.

Decentralisation and health facility preference

The section empirically measures the impact of decentralisation dimensions on healthcare facility choice for child delivery and ANC/PNC received, controlling for other socio-economic and demographic characteristics of households and availability and quality of health centres in the village. The important factors that influence the choice of health facility can be categorised into four components: a) predisposing; b) enabling; c) cost of care; and d) need factors (as reported in Stephenson and Tsui, 2002; Andersen and Aday, 1978; Young et al., 2006; He et al., 2007). Further, ANC/PNC received and child immunisation status is also presented by level of decentralisation in health.

The predisposing factors include those which are demographic and social structural in nature (age, sex, social status, etc.). These variables have low degree of mutability with any social action or policy initiatives and affect healthcare usage. The enabling factors are mutable with shift in social norms and policy initiatives. These include both demand-side and supply-side factors that can promote healthcare use. The demand-side factors include individual and household characteristics like household size, work status, level of education, type of house, land possession and household per capita income and expenditure. These factors show the household or individual capabilities that promote the demand for healthcare. The other part of enabling factor are the supply-side factors. These include access to, availability and quality of healthcare and the institutional structure of service delivery (like decentralised delivery of healthcare services). These factors can have significant impact on household healthcare facility selection and use, and influence healthcare use particularly amongst the priority population. The cost of healthcare and need factors (nature of illness or burden of disease, etc.) also affects household choices of healthcare facility use, but have been outside from the analysis due to the lack of availability of data.

It is postulated that supply-side enabling factors – particularly the availability and quality of healthcare facilities and decentralised delivery structures – play a significant role in influencing the choice of care. This presumption is based on the notion that decentralisation first brings decision makers closer to the people and enhancing the participation of community in the decision making and implementation processes, and in turn improves the equitable access to healthcare.

To examine the factors that determine the choices of healthcare, the household preference model provided in Andersen and Aday (1978) is used. In case of choice of facility for child delivery, the information is available in discrete form with multiple responses. In case of discrete dependent variable with multiple responses (more than two), the multinomial logit (ML) model is preferred over the other conventional models (which are applicable up to two responses), logit or tobit models (Maddala, 1993). The ML model proposes two equations which talk about the probability of selecting one choice over the other (the base category) choice. In case of three choices (like, 1, 2 or 3), if we take choice 3 as base category, then the ML model proposes the probability of choice 1 over 3 and the probability of choice 2 over 3.

The nested multinomial logit (NML) model is preferred over the ML model if choices are not straightforward and when partitions are made in groups ('nests'). In NML model, a choice is made first between 1 and (2, 3) and then, if (2, 3), a choice is made between 2 and 3. The NML model can be generalised to various nesting levels by grouping the alternatives within such a nest in sub-nests, and so on (Heiss, 2002).[11]

In our case, the data on choices of health facility usage for child delivery is available in nest form, like the non-institutional (home = 1) and institutional (public = 2 or private = 3) delivery of a child. This requires application of NML model. In NML model, the choices are made first between 1 and (2, 3), and then choice is made between 2 and 3. The estimated equation that derived from the random utility maximisation (RUM) model (Heiss, 2002) is as follows.

$$C = \alpha + \beta_1\,AGE + \beta_2\,FL + \beta_3\,SC + \beta_4\,lnMPCI + \beta_5\,QHC + \beta_6\,PVT \\ + \beta_7\,LDH + \beta_8\,DCPA + \beta_9\,SSD + \beta_{10}\,SCD + u$$

Where: C – choice of health facility for child delivery (public, private or home); AGE – age of female is used as continuous variable, as choice of health facility usage changes with the age; FL – female literacy level, which is used as a continuous variable i.e., 1 = illiterate, 2 = primary, 3 = secondary, and 4 = higher education. An educated woman is assumed to have better understanding of the need for services and prefer institutional delivery compared to home delivery; SC – a woman from a scheduled caste background having BPL card (SC = 1, non-SC = 0). Women in this category are considered to be economically deprived and are expected to have less access to healthcare services, as suggested in literature; lnMPCE – log of monthly per capita income of the household. The better-off (higher income) households are expected to have greater access to healthcare and they may use differential (probably private rather than public) healthcare services, in face of affordability. This variable is used as continuous variable. QHC – availability/quality of public health facilities in the village and expectation of good quality public facility promote institutional delivery. This is used as dummy variable 1 for good and 0 for poor quality. The quality is assessed through: does the facility open regularly, and does it have beds, BP machines, weight scales, safe delivery kits, skilled birth attendants, a referral network, residence facilities, etc. As per the Indian Public Health Standard (IPHS), these services are considered as basic services at a health centre to promote service access. PVT – availability of different types of private facilities (including dais) in the village with their better performance in service delivery in the village (yes = 1, no = 0); LDH – level of decentralisation in health (higher than average – high = 1 and low = 0); SSD (Sarpanch sex dummy) – village Sarpanch's gender (female = 1, male = 0). SCD (sarpanch caste dummy) is the social category of village Sarpanch (SC = 1, Non-SC = 0).

Bivariate analysis confirmed that choice of health facility is highly influenced by availability and quality of care and institutional and decentralisation factors. How much these factors matter after controlling for other socio-economic and demographic characteristics of households is presented through multivariate analysis using NML regression technique. The NML model allows us to examine the factors that impact the likelihood of institutional (public and private) delivery over the non-institutional (at home) and

Table 6.6 Choice of health facility for child delivery: nested multinomial logit model estimation

	Institutional vs. home delivery (home delivery is base)		Public vs. private delivery (delivery at private facility is base)	
	Coeff.	Z-value	Coeff.	Z-value
Female age: continuous variable	0.10*	1.74	–0.12*	–1.67
Female literary: continuous variable	0.34	0.81	–1.81**	–2.85
SCs/BPL dummy: SC = 1, non-SC = 0	0.37	0.87	–0.81	–1.27
Log of MPCI: continuous variable	0.61**	2.10	–0.53	–1.51
Quality of public health facility: good = 1, poor = 0	1.45***	3.34	1.43***	2.87
Availability of private facility: good = 1, poor = 0	–0.17	–0.41	–1.43**	–2.31
LDH dummy: high = 1, low = 0	1.07**	2.43	0.88*	1.70
DCPA dummy: high = 1, low = 0	0.30	0.80	0.23	0.48
Sarpanch sex: female = 1, male = 0	0.34	0.90	0.30	0.61
Sarpanch category: SC = 1, Non-SC = 0	–0.14	–0.31	–1.22**	–1.97
Inclusive value parameters				
Non-institutional_tau	1		Pub._tau 1	
Institutional_tau	0.85		Pvt._tau 1	
Log-likelihood	–164		–56	
Number of cases	162		110	

Source: Estimated using field survey data, 2011

then likelihood of child delivery within institutions (public or private). The NML regression results show that the probability of institutional delivery of a child over non-institutional increases with the age of the mother and household income (Table 6.6). The likelihood of institutional delivery of a child over non-institutional delivery is high in villages where quality of public facilities is good. The extent of decentralisation also influences the choice of health facility significantly and promotes institutional delivery.

The likelihood of choice of institutional delivery of a child (public over the private) decreased with the age of the women. This may mean that use of private facility increases with the age of the mother, which is opposite of our expectation. The probability of child delivery in public facilities decreases significantly with the level of education of a female. The scheduled caste factor does not play significant role in influencing the household choice of health facility selection and use. The probability of using public facilities for child delivery is recorded as significantly high in villages where quality of public facility is available. This indicates that the quality of public facilities does matter more for promoting institutional delivery. The availability, along with the quality of public health facilities, is one of the guiding factors that influences the utilisation pattern among different socio-economic strata. It is observed that the quality of public facilities helps in restoring the reputation of service providers at the village health centres. The findings of the present study are similar to some earlier studies (Ager and Pepper, 2005; Haddad et al., 1998) that have mentioned that reputation in terms of perceived quality has been one of the main determinants of utilisation of a particular healthcare provider. Patients generally first judge the quality of services and then make the choice of those health services.

The reservations of women and disadvantaged groups in politics do not matter in influencing the choice of either institutional or non-institutional delivery or public or private facility for child delivery. This may be because in a class/ caste- and male-dominated society, the forward class/caste and males of Haryana generally do not allow the women even to take active part in Panchayat work, even if they are Sarpanch of the village. Similarly, the disadvantaged groups Sarpanches are unable to deliver service effectively, as many times, their activities and ideas are opposed by the dominant caste/class society in the village.

The extent of community participation, measured through DCPA, shows that the likelihood of using public as opposed to private facilities for child delivery is recorded as high if the level of community participation is high in the village. The coefficient, however, was insignificant. However, properly implemented decentralised policy, which includes indicators on active involvement/interventions of local agents (ASHA, VHSC and PRIs members in health policy making, supervision, monitoring, actions taken and fund utilisation, etc.), plays a greater role in influencing the choice of a cost-effective public facility over a private facility. This indicates that the individual factors of decentralisation – like merely given the reservations of women and disadvantaged sections of the society in Panchayat politics – either does not statistically significantly tend to provide unexpected results, but comprehensive dimensions of decentralisation taken together are important for affecting the choice of care. This may be because the collective dimensions effectively manage the publicly provided healthcare services, which in turn affects the choice of care. These findings suggest that rather than relying on a specific tool or dimension of local governance and decentralisation, the extent of decentralisation that includes several of its dimensions is important for effective delivery of healthcare in rural areas of India.

The all-states level results from DLHS-4 data reveals that the probability of receiving ANC and PNC services increases if health issues are discussed in GS, if VHSC is active in at least five items (as reported in this chapter), if distance to health facility is less than 15 km, if healthcare facilities improved over time, if ANM/ASHA is available in the village, and when women receive financial (JSY) benefits. These variables were found to be important in influencing the probability of ANC/PNC received in case of Haryana, but the relationship in some cases was found to be little weak (Table 6.7). These

Table 6.7 The role of decentralisation and the public health system in influencing the preference of facility for child delivery and ANC/PNC received status: India and Haryana

	India (N = 33,697)				Haryana (N = 3583)			
	Dependent variable, place of child delivery: Public = 1, Private = 2, Home = 3							
	Facility choice: 1 over 3 (base)		*Facility choice: 2 over 3 (base)*		*Facility choice: 1 over 3 (base)*		*Facility choice: 2 over 3 (base)*	
	Coeff.	z-value	Coeff.	z-value	Coeff.	z-value	Coeff.	z-value
Choice of health facility for child delivery								
Any health issue discussed in GS	0.075*	1.85	0.236***	5.24	-0.252**	2.08	-0.103	-0.76
Active role of VHNSC at least in five items out of the listed ten items	0.486***	14.81	0.454***	12.80	0.074	0.85	0.217**	2.26
if distance of government facility less than 15 km = 1	0.521***	13.09	0.734***	17.83	0.588***	3.51	0.559***	3.13
if Sarpanch marked that health facility improved significantly = 1, rather than marginal or no improvement	0.323***	8.08	0.388***	8.81	0.057	0.50	-0.119	-0.97
if received any financial support like the JSY	2.032***	44.24	0.108**	1.93	1.518***	8.92	-0.880***	-3.15
availability of ASHA in village as per norm of population	0.194***	6.16	0.455***	13.35	-0.306***	-3.43	-0.223**	-2.28
Availability of ANM in the village	0.435***	11.91	0.548***	13.45	-0.290	-2.24	-0.304**	-2.19
Constant	-0.634	-12.30	-1.292	-21.99	0.949	5.13	0.535	2.67

ANC and PNC received status

	ANC received (Yes = 1; No = 0)		PNC received (Yes = 1; No = 0)		ANC received (Yes = 1; No = 0)		PNC received (Yes = 1; No = 0)	
Any health issue discussed in GS	0.004	0.080	0.229***	6.510	0.175*	1.630	−0.297**	−2.800
Active role of VHNSC at least in five items out of listed ten items	0.219***	5.850	0.293***	10.410	−0.312***	−3.880	−0.009	−0.110
if distance of govt. facility less than 15 km = 1	0.466***	9.990	0.275***	8.770	0.036	0.260	0.171	1.300
if Sarpanch marked that health facility improved significantly = 1, rather than marginal or no improvement	0.055	1.190	0.101**	2.830	−0.024	−0.230	−0.182*	−1.810
if received any financial support like the JSY	0.703***	14.010	0.198***	6.640	0.191	1.390	0.651***	4.870
availability of ASHA in village as per norm of population	0.037	1.030	0.206***	7.740	0.012	0.150	0.197**	2.580
Availability of ANM in the village	0.374***	9.130	0.365***	11.320	0.285**	2.600	0.141	1.310
if institutional birth = 1, otherwise-home 0	1.561***	42.560	2.417***	68.240	1.338***	16.440	1.706***	19.870
Constant	0.139	2.410	−2.315	−42.220	−0.373	−2.160	−0.913	−5.300

Source: Estimated using unit-level data of DLHS-4 (2012–13)

Table 6.8 Impact of decentralisation and public health system on OOP expenditure for institutional delivery

Dependent: log of OOP expenditure per child delivery

Independent variables	India (N = 19837; Adj-R2 = 0.29)			Haryana N = 1005; Adj-R2 = 0.36		
	Coeff.	Std. Err.	t-value	Coeff.	Std. Err.	t-value
Any health issue discussed in GS	-0.036*	0.021	-1.70	0.126	0.094	1.35
Active role of VHNSC at least in five items out of listed ten items	-0.072***	0.017	-4.36	-0.306***	0.069	-4.41
If place of delivery is government relative to that of private	-1.339***	0.016	-81.72	-1.491***	0.071	-20.93
If distance of government facility less than 15 km = 1	-0.166***	0.017	-9.51	-0.152	0.115	-1.32
If Sarpanch marked that health facility improved significantly = 1, rather than marginal or no improvement	-0.003	0.020	-0.17	-0.141**	0.070	-2.02
If received any financial support like the JSY	-0.075***	0.018	-4.240	-0.488***	0.123	-3.95

Source: Estimated using unit-level data of DLHS-4 (2012–13)

decentralisation and health system variables turned out to be highly significant in influencing institutional delivery, especially the choice of healthcare facility from public and private facilities relative to that of home delivery at the India-wide level. Except for variables like health issues discussed in GS and availability of ANM/ASHA in village, all these variables contributed positively in influencing the institutional delivery as opposed to the home delivery in Haryana, as well (Table 6.7).

Another important dimension of healthcare system performance is to find out whether it has been able to reduce the out-of-pocket burden from households. Under the recent health policy dialogues, especially under the universal health coverage, reducing OOP is an important goal even under the sustainable development goals. In the case of OOP expenditure for child delivery, we observed that both decentralisation dimensions and healthcare system functioning influence OOP expenditure significantly. We found OOP expenditure on child delivery low in villages where healthcare issues are discussed in GS and VHSC play an active role in at least five functional areas at all-state level. The healthcare system variables – like distance to the health facility and improvement of the health facility – significantly reduce the OOP expenditure for child delivery. The OOP spending was also low if delivery takes place in a government hospital and if women had received financial support of JSY (Table 6.8). Except for the variable of whether health issues were discussed in GS, all other variables relating to the healthcare system, decentralisation, and financial support play significant roles in reducing the OOP expenditure for child delivery in case of Haryana, as well (Table 6.8).

Conclusion

The study finds that properly implemented and designed decentralisation policy can ensure utilisation of public facility for maternal and child healthcare. The extent of decentralisation also addresses the issues of access of public facilities with greater equity in healthcare utilisation across different socio-economic groups as compared to the areas where decentralisation concept has not been implemented effectively. The issue of equity, however, remained inconclusive in women-headed and SCs-headed Panchayat villages. This reflects the reservations of some women and disadvantaged groups in local politics not necessarily meant to improve health services delivery systems in a state like Haryana where dominant class/caste/males capture most of the decentralisation powers. Such structures even have resulted in low degrees of community participation in the states which further affected the effectiveness of DCPA in promoting service utilisation. The properly implemented decentralised policy at the ground level turns significant in improving the access to health utilisation in an equitable manner (across different socio-economic strata) and in influencing the choice of health facility and institutional delivery. It is not that who is heading the village, but it is the active involvement of a local agent (captured through extent of decentralisation and VHSC interventions) that makes a significant difference in improving the status of healthcare utilisation amongst the priority population from cost-effective public facilities and in reducing the OOP payment burden on households.

We observed that gains from decentralisation increase with the devolution of health-related functions, provision of funds, management and regulation of functionaries, and policy making powers to Panchayat. The magnitude of Panchayat support, priorities and coordination between local agents and health functionaries adds up to materialise more gains from decentralisation. The quality and availability of public healthcare infrastructure also influences the household choice of healthcare use for maternal and child health higher, as well as from public facilities. Thus, it can be argued that effective implementation of decentralised policy/planning in the healthcare sector can promote the effective delivery of health services and results in improving healthcare sector performance in rural Haryana. One can expect such positive impact of decentralisation dimensions in other parts of rural India.

Between 2006 and 2016, no doubt, one can see a substantial jump in institutional delivery, which increased from 39% to 79% during the period. However, about two-thirds (67%) of women reported at least one problem for themselves in obtaining medical care. One-fourth of women cite money as a problem. Thirty percent of women cite the distance to a health facility, and 27% cite having to take transport as a problem. Thirty-seven percent of women report concerns that no female health provider is available. Forty-five percent of women report concern that no provider is available, and 46% that no drugs are available (NFHS, 2016), which needs to be addressed.

Notes

1 This chapter draws from certain arguments and data in my previous work originally published in S. K. Hooda. 2016. Effectiveness of Local Government and Community Participation in Health Service Delivery in Rural Haryana. *International Journal of Rural Management*, Vol. 12, No. 1, pp. 27–50 Copyright 2016 © Institute of Rural Management. All rights reserved. Reproduced with the permission of the copyright holders and the publishers, SAGE Publications India Pvt. Ltd, New Delhi.
2 This study argues that not only do local governments have more and better information regarding their constituents, but they may be better able to enforce and coordinate policies and programmes, if a stable structure of government is in place. Being in close proximity to those in charge also enables citizens to better monitor the responsible parties' performance and hold them accountable.
3 https://nhm.gov.in/images/pdf/guidelines/nrhm-guidelines/national_population_policy_2000.pdf
4 The initiatives taken by some states are reported in Appendix 5.4.
5 MNREGA scheme was implemented through decentralized planning in 100 selected poorer districts of India. Among them, two poorer districts – Mahendargarh and Sirsa – were identified from Haryana. Mahendargarh geographically is in the south and touches the Rajasthan border. Rohtak has high per capita income

with high quality of health infrastructure and is located in the centre of the state. Yamunanagar is situated in north of the state.

6 Rohtak has high infrastructure, female literacy and health outcomes; Yamunanagar has high infrastructure and literacy, but low outcomes; and Mahendargarh has low infrastructure and literacy, but better outcome.

7 It may be noted that the village Panchayat have no involvement in seven types of functions (that is, those numbered 10–12, 24–26 and 28).

8 To examine the extent of participation, one needs to know: a) to what extent the population is interested in participation; b) how much participation is possible with the actual educational status of the population; c) what possibilities exist for communication and information transfer for the implementation of participation; and d) how can motivation for participation be made sustainable (Metzger, 2001).

9 To examine the extent of participation, one needs to know: a) to what extent the population is interested in participation; b) how much participation is possible with the actual educational status of the population; c) what possibilities exist for communication and information transfer for the implementation of participation; and d) how can motivation for participation be made sustainable (Metzger, 2001).

10 The score value of DDP recorded low in Rohtak compared to the other districts. Interestingly, however, the score value recorded high in women-headed and SCs Sarpanch-headed Panchayat villages compared to their male and non-SCs counterparts. The higher level of DDP in reserved and female-headed Panchayat villages can be explained by the reasoning that in these villages, a high share of SCs and BPL household attend the GS/VHSC meetings. For instance, the data reveals that out of total 142 households, about 45% attended the GS meetings, of which about 64.1% are from SC/BPL households. These villages further expected to influence the community participation in the village. But the interesting point is that how the villagers play a role in the GS meetings, and what factors determine their participation needs to be examined. This measure is used as an independent variable and is expected to influence the nature of community participation.

11 Heiss (2002) specifies that the NML model can be derived from a structural model of random utility maximization. In that model, agents are assumed to choose the alternative from which they drive the highest utility.

References

Ager, A. and Pepper, K. 2005. Patterns of Health Service Utilization and Perceptions of Needs and Services in Rural Orissa. *Health Policy and Planning*, Vol. 30, No. 3, pp. 176–184.

Andersen, R., and Aday, L. 1978. Access to Medical Care in the US: Realized and Potential. *Medical Care*, Vol. 16, No. 7, pp. 533–546.

Bardhan, P. 1996. Decentralized Development. *Indian Economic Review*, Vol. XXXI, No. 2, pp. 139–156.

Bossert, T. 1998. Analyzing the Decentralization of Health Systems in Developing Countries: Decision Space, Innovation and Performance. *Social Science and Medicine*, Vol. 47, pp. 1513–1527.

Bossert, T., and Beauvais, J. 2002. Decentralization of Health Systems in Ghana, Zambia, Uganda and the Philippines: A Comparative Analysis of Decision Space. *Health Policy and Planning*, Vol. 17, No. 1, pp. 14–31.

Collins, C. 1989. Decentralization and the Need for Political and Critical Analysis. *Health Policy and Planning*, Vol. 4, No. 2, pp. 168–171.

DLHS-4. 2012–13. *District Level Household Survey-4*. Unit Level Data, IIPS India. https://nrhm-mis.nic.in/SitePages/DLHS-4.aspx

Gilson, L., and Mills, A. 1995. Health Sector Reforms in Sub-Saharan Africa: Lessons of the Last 10 Years. *Health Policy*, Vol. 32, pp. 215–243.

Government of India. 1951. *The First Five Year Plan, Planning Commission of India*. Government of India, New Delhi.

Government of India. 1983. *First National Health Policy, 1983*. Ministry of Health and Family Welfare Government of India, New Delhi.

Government of India. 2000. *National Population Policy, 2000*. Ministry of Health and Family Welfare, Government of India, New Delhi. https://nhm.gov.in/images/pdf/guidelines/nrhm-guidelines/national_population_policy_2000.pdf

Government of India. 2002. *Second National Health Policy, 2002*. Ministry of Health and Family Welfare, Government of India, New Delhi.

Green, A. 1992. *An Introduction to Health Planning in Developing Countries*. Oxford University Press, New York.

Greene, W. H. 2008. *Econometric Analysis*, 5th Edition. Pearson Education, Published by Dorling Kindersley Pvt. Ltd., New Delhi.

Haddad, S., Fournier, P., Machouf, N., and Yatara, F. 1998. What Does Quality Mean to Lay People? Community Perceptions of Primary Health Care Services in Guinea. *Social Science and Medicine*, Vol. 47, No. 3, pp. 381–394.

He, Wan, Sengupta, M., Zhang, K., and Guo, P. 2007. *Health and Health-care of the Older Population in Urban and Rural China: 2000*. Census Bureau, International Population Reports, Government Printing Office, Washington, DC.

Heiss, F. 2002. Structural Choice Analysis with Nested Logit Models. *STATA Journal*, Vol. 2, No. 3, pp. 227–252.

Lieberman, S. 2002. *Decentralization and Health in the Philippines and Indonesia: An Interim Report*. World Bank, Washington, DC.

Litvack, J., and Seddon, J. 1999. *Decentralization Briefing Notes*. World Bank Institute, WP No. 37142, World Bank, Washington, DC.

Maddala, G. 1993. *Limited Dependent and Qualitative Variables in Econometrics*. Cambridge University Press, New York.

Metzger, U. 2001. *Dezentralisierung in Entwicklungsländern finanzielle Dezentralisierung und Sustainable Human Development*. Ergon Verlag, Würzburg.

Mills, A., Vaughan, J. P., Smith, D., and Tabibzadeh, I. 1990. *Health System Decentralization: Concepts, Issues and Country Experiences*. World Health Organization, Geneva.

MoHFW. 2007. *Health Sector Reform: Initiatives from States*. Ministry of Health and Family Welfare, Government of India, New Delhi.

Murthy, R., and Klugman, B. 2004. Service Accountability and Community Participation in the Context of Health Sector Reforms in Asia: Implications for Sexual and Reproductive Health Services. *Health Policy and Planning*, Vol. 19, No. 1, pp. i78–i86.

Nagarajan, H. 2017, March 2. *Democratization and Health Care in Rural India*. Presentation at NCAER. www.ncaer.org/uploads/photo-gallery/files/1489750144Health_HKN-NCAER.pdf

NFHS. 2006 & 2016. National Family Health Survey (NFHS-3:2005-06; NFHS-4:2015–16). International Institute for Population Sciences (IIPS), Mumbai, India and International Classification of Functioning, Disability and Health (ICF).

NRHM – Government of India. 2005. *National Rural Health Mission (NRHM)*. Government of India, New Delhi.

NSS – Government of India. 2019. *Key Indicator of Social Consumption in India: Health*. 75th Round (July 2017 to June 2018), National Sample Survey (NSS) Office, Government of India, November, New Delhi.

Oates, W. 1994. Federalism and Government Finance. In J. Quigley and E. Smolensky (Eds.), *Modern Public Finance* (Chapter 5). Harvard University Press, Cambridge, MA, pp. 126–151.

Pokharel, B. 2000. *Decentralization of Health Services*. World Health Organization, Regional Office for South-East Asia, New Delhi.

Prud'homme, R. 1995. *On the Dangers of Decentralization*. Policy Research Working Paper No.1252, World Bank, Washington, DC.

Rifkin, S. B. 1996. Paradigms Lost: Toward a New Understanding of Community Participation in Health Programmes. *Acta Tropica*, Vol. 61, No. 2, pp. 79–92.

Stephenson, R., and Tsui, A. O. 2002. Contextual Influences on Reproductive Health Service Use in Uttar Pradesh, India. *Studies in Family Planning*, Vol. 33, No. 4, pp. 309–320.

Strodel, R. J., and Perry, H. B. 2019. The National Village Health Guide Scheme in India: Lessons Four Decades Later for Community Health Worker Programs Today and Tomorrow. *Human Resources for Health,* Vol. 17, No. 76. https://doi.org/10.1186/s12960-019-0413-1

Tidemand, P. 2010. *Draft Note on Health Sector Decentralisation*. Ministry of Foreign Affairs of Denmark.

Welschhoff, A. 2006. *Community Participation and Primary Health Care in India Dissertation der Fakultät für Geowissenschaften der Ludwig-Maximilians-Universität München*. Eingereichtam, 14 February 2006.

Young, J. T., et al. 2006, February. Who Receives Health-care? Age and Sex Differentials in Adult Use of Health-care Services in Rural Bangladesh. *World Health and Population*, Vol. 8, No. 2, pp. 83–100.

Part 3

New financing and policy paradigms

Redefining the role of state

The idea of healthcare as a 'public good' expanded with half-hearted efforts in India. In a parallel process, neoliberal thinking heavily tried to justify the rationale of public sector underfunding and privatisation in the liberalisation phase. A narrative was built in the liberalisation phase that the ability of India's healthcare system to fight infant mortality, communicable diseases and malnutrition is being stretched. At the same time, it faces emerging demands for better service and more attention to chronic diseases. India's underfunded public sector and extensive – but largely unaccountable – private sector cannot hope to meet the country's enormous, growing and shifting healthcare needs. If India continues on its present path, the mismatch between its healthcare system and its health problems will become only more severe. It is advocated that the country needs to promote the private sector and then take advantage of the capacity of private sector to deliver better service for all regions and across socio-economic groups. This neoliberal priority invited opening up of investment opportunities for the private sector, including domestic and foreign corporate players with approval of 100% foreign direct investment in hospital sector. The sector could see relaxation in import duties for importing medical equipment and technology, granting long-term loans at low interest rates to private health institutions, confirmation of the hospital sector with industry status and several other initiatives that encouraged private providers to exploit the Indian hospital market. The state, in the post-liberalisation phase, was seen as facilitator to the private sector through subsidies, credits, insurance and introduction of public-private partnerships.

Over the last decade, it is increasingly being realised that economic gradients of inequality in access to healthcare sharply worsened in many countries, including India, where rural and poor people felt financially squeezed and experienced difficulty in finding services they can afford. This generated a new requirement to find a way to provide financial protection to the needy. Devising a financial protection mechanism has emerged as a central policy tool of achieving universal health coverage (UHC) around the world in recent times. The UHC debate focuses more on devising the strategies to finance healthcare rather than providing the healthcare itself. It suggests developing a

DOI: 10.4324/9781032108438-9

roadmap for developing countries to adapt their financial systems to meet the requirements of universal health coverage. An insurance-based health financing strategy to finance care is advocated whereby all citizens are insured and can utilise healthcare services, regardless of whether they can afford it or not. India launched several public-funded health insurance schemes for poor and informal community workers. They are entirely funded from public (tax) sources. The financing of the insurance-based system entirely from public sources has led to an important shift in the fundamental nature of healthcare financing in the country. Until recently, public investment in healthcare was mostly used for financing public health system for service provisioning; now out of the total health budget, some tax funds will be diverted to finance the insurance-based system.

As a reform initiative, the recent National Health Policy 2017 of India floated a new idea of strategic purchasing of health services from private players promoted through insurance. The policy highlighted that strategic purchasing would ensure access to affordable and quality secondary and tertiary care services from private providers in healthcare services deficit areas. The policy advocates a positive and proactive engagement with the private sector for critical gap filling towards achieving national health goals. It argues that strategic purchasing would play a stewardship role in directing private investment towards those areas and those services for which currently there are no providers or few providers. A proposal has been floated to facilitate the private players in land allotment, special window clearness, providing viability gap funding for improving the financing viability and bankability of the project, and they will be linked with government insurance for coverage reimbursement of referred patients. Thus, insurance-based financing over time became an integral part of healthcare budget and an instrument to promote privatisation in the healthcare sector.

In this context, one needs to understand how the private sector took advantage of these initiatives and grew in terms of size, ownership and location, and how it exploited the Indian healthcare market and resulted in unaffordable treatments and inaccessibility, hindering fulfilment of the national health goals. Second, the currently promoted insurance-based system will get finance in the same way as the public health sector; the difference lies in the fact that the provisioning would now be shifted almost entirely to the private sector. How the changing financing nature has been able to promote access to healthcare and provide financial protection needs discussion. This is important because global experience suggests that countries that have tried to deliver care through the private sector and insurance ended up with costly care systems. How the changing policy and financing paradigms have performed in India is examined in Chapter 7 and Chapter 8.

7 Towards privatising healthcare
At what cost?[1]

Countries across the globe follow different approaches to delivering healthcare to their citizens. Despite several shortcomings in market-based models, the pro-market phenomenon is spreading even to socialist countries like Russia, China and emerging economies like South Africa, Latin America, Asia – including India – and other developing countries (Lefebvre, 2010). The extent and nature of privatisation in healthcare delivery, however, vary widely. The aim of this chapter is to discuss to what extent Indian healthcare market is exposed to the private sector and what factors have contributed to India's journey towards privatising healthcare. We have listed several macroeconomic conditions and policy changes, neoliberal ideology and global debates around reshaping the healthcare system to discuss the emerging role of privatisation. A section in the end briefly touches upon implications of privatisation.

The public system

India's spending on health has always remained lower than the commitments made. The public spending on health historically hovered around 1% (currently 1.23%) of GDP. The current spending level is significantly lower than the required level of resources (2–3% of GDP) and lower than the internationally recommended standard of spending 5% of GDP. Low government spending resulted in deficiency of facilities at primary, secondary and tertiary levels that can meet the growing health needs of the population. Since a detailed discussion around the public system has already been provided in previous chapters, the following sections will describe how macroeconomic conditions and policy changes, as well as pro-market arguments, have placed the role of private sector in health service delivery.

Macroeconomic conditions and pro-market arguments

India has undergone various policy changes at macroeconomic levels, as well as health policy fronts, that influenced its journey towards privatising the healthcare sector. We begin with listing the liberalisation

DOI: 10.4324/9781032108438-10

and macroeconomic policy restructuring of the early 1990s. In the early 1990s, India faced huge economic and fiscal crises, a period known as the beginning an era of liberalisation, privatisation and globalisation which impacted the Indian economy in a big way. An outcome of the macroeconomic restructuring was the implementation of structural adjustment programmes (SAPs). The fiscal stringency induced by the structural adjustment measures affected the central, as well as state, finances significantly. In the restructuring process, a squeeze in spending in social sectors (largely in the healthcare) was observed at national and state levels in India (Chapter 2). No doubt, India had taken almost 35 years to bring its First National Health Policy in 1983. With the announcement of NHP, a rise in public investment in the healthcare sector was also observed as government investment in health increased as a share of total budgetary allocation. This phenomenon of rising public investment in healthcare was short lived, however, starting in the early 1980s and ending well before the start of the liberalisation phase of the 1990s.

In the early 1990s, some international agencies put forward an idea of pro-market ideology. The World Bank brought out a report on 'Investing in Health' in 1993. The report appreciated the role of government's efforts in improving the health outcomes in past 50 years, but at the same time argued that public healthcare systems in developing nations were confronted with several challenges on efficiency and equity grounds. The report insisted upon the limited role of governments' involvement in healthcare, as well as the insurance sector. The report argued that government should limit its role in healthcare and insurance, and it rejected the idea of a healthcare system as a public good. It insisted that healthcare is a matter of individuals and families, due to their strikingly different health needs (Fisk, 2000). The report also argued that when a country develops, a section of its population becomes able and willing to spend its own money on healthcare. At such a point, the state – according to the World Bank – should not retain sole responsibility for a field like healthcare. It should be shared with the private sector, though the public sector can continue with taking responsibilities of healthcare for low income and public health matters. Beyond that, it should use its resources not to deliver healthcare but instead to make it possible for individuals to buy private insurance and healthcare. It could return its obligatory fees for healthcare to individuals and add subsidies to those fees if they are insufficient for buying private insurance. As affluence spreads among citizens, such public sector stimulation of private insurance would create demand sufficient to call forth a brisk supply of private healthcare (World Bank, 1993; Fisk, 2000), a notion to put forwards promoting privatisation in health sector. Another component in reforms suggested by the World Bank was to promote and open up the health insurance sector to private players. Thus, this report laid out a way of thinking to look towards the private sector for service delivery and at the same time denial of free healthcare in the public system.

A similar type of argument was put forwarded in India-specific report of the World Bank entitled 'India: Raising the Sights: Better Health Systems for India's Poor' in 2001. It summarises that India's healthcare system is at crossroads. Its ability to fight with infant mortality, communicable disease and malnutrition is being stretched. At the same time, it faces emerging demands for better service and more attention to the chronic diseases of adulthood. India's underfunded public sector on the one hand, and its extensive but largely unaccountable private sector on the other hand, cannot hope to meet the country's enormous, growing and shifting healthcare needs. If India continues on its present path, the mismatch between its health system and its health problems will only become more severe. The present moment is a decisive one because the government of India is now seeking to define a better health system for the country through the draft report (2001) of Second National Health Policy. The World Bank report highlights that the country needs to promote the private sector and then it can take better advantage of the capacity of the private sector and deliver better healthcare service and improve health outcomes for all regions across different socio-economic groups (World Bank, 2001). The report further stressed that the underfunding and privatisation are actually defensible in the sense that the Indian economy has potential to grow high and at faster rate, leading to increase in paying capacity of masses. Since the public system has largely been inefficient in meeting the population healthcare needs, there would not be any harm to marketising the healthcare sector. Such neoliberal arguments that make cuts in public investment necessary were made familiar to everyone. This was the neoliberal argument to open up investment opportunities for the private sector.

The neoliberal understanding put forwarded in the World Bank's reports tries to justify the public sector underfunding and greater role of privatisation. The decade of the 1990s became a turning point for the Indian healthcare sector. In this period, the reforms in the healthcare sector were piecemeal but incremental in nature, which led to extensive changes in the organisational structure, financing and delivery of healthcare services. An important development was the introduction of user fees in public hospitals and facilities. The implementation of user fees was seen in many states during the late 1990s and early 2000s (Ghosh, 2010).

In the World Bank–suggested reforms, it was argued that the middle-income population is growing, and therefore, the insurance sector should be opened up to private players. India did this in 1999, setting the foreign direct investment (FDI) cap in health insurance at 26%. Such insurance generally promotes hospitalisation care from private providers.

Another major development in the healthcare sector was the introduction of new Drug Price Control Order (DPCO) in 1995. According to the DPCO (1995), only 74 out of 166 commonly used bulk drugs were to be kept under statutory price controls. The impact of these drug policy changes could be seen in spiralling increases in drug prices during the period of 1994–2004 (Ghosh, 2010).

A key factor in realising the neoliberal strategy was opening up of the hospital sector to foreign players in the beginning of 2000. India allowed 100% FDI in the hospital sector through automatic route in 2000, an initiative to invite and attract foreign private players in the hospital sector. Some foreign players pursued independent ventures, while others entered into joint ventures with domestic players. Foreign players made significant strides through FDI which increased to Rs. 3995 crore in 2013–2014 from a meagre amount of Rs. 31 crore in 2001–2002 in the hospital sector (Hooda, 2015). This study showed that the share of FDI equity inflow in hospital sector out of total FDI inflow of health sector increased from 12.8% in 2000 to 25.5% in 2013.

In another initiative, the hospital sector was accorded industry status in the 2003–2004 budget, after which long-term and cheap loans were granted to private healthcare institutions and hospitals (Shah and Mohanty, 2011). Due to industry status, the hospital sector received various benefits such as reduced custom duties on medical equipment (from 100% to 40% during the late 1980s and further to 15% in the 2000s and 7.5% in 2016), subsidised land, cheap loans, income tax exemptions, etc.

The liberalisation phase of the Indian economy brought out a significant change in the healthcare service delivery market in India. One can see a significant rise in private healthcare providers since the 1990s (Figure 7.1). The sector grew at a much faster rate in the first decade of the 2000s, when several liberalisation policies were initiated by the government within the

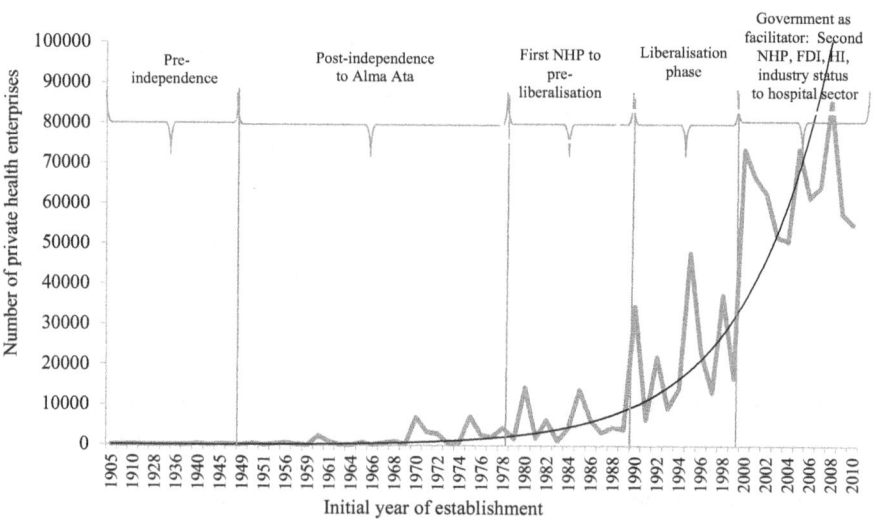

Figure 7.1 Growth pattern of private healthcare providers in India

Source: NSS, Services Sector Enterprises, 2010–2011

healthcare sector. Significantly higher growth was observed in hospital and diagnostics sector (Hooda, 2017).

PPP in public facility

The Indian healthcare sector has been influenced significantly by the ideology put forwarded in the previously discussed independent reports of the World Bank of the 1990s and 2000s. In 2017, the World Bank made a direct intervention in healthcare policy. It helped the NITI Aayog to bring out an agenda of implementing public-private partnership (PPP) within government hospitals (GOI, 2017). No doubt, India's healthcare sector is experienced with several PPP ranging from ambulatory to diagnostic testing to support the public system. The NITI Aayog brought out a document (with the help from Bank) to implement PPP within the district hospitals for care of non-communicable diseases. The guidelines suggest that 50-bed and 100-bed private facilities will be co-located within the district hospitals (DHs) having annual outpatient department (OPD) case loads of 1000 patients per day. Such hospitals will have to allocate 30,000–60,000 square feet of space for a 50-bed facility and a 100-bed facility for setting up PPP. A minimum 75% and 50% of this space, respectively, would be allocated within the existing built-up structure and remain on vacant land within the premises of the hospital. The staff (from attendants at registration desk to the chief medical officer) have to refer patients and facilitate reimbursement of expenditures incurred on referred patients at PPP. The guidelines suggest that the government will facilitate the private players in land allotment, special window clearness, providing viability gap funding (VGF) for improving the financing viability and bankability of the project (Box 7.1). This is a step towards overtaking the land and building of public institutions and engaging their staffs to facilitate them further. Ideally, these well-performing public institutions should have been rewarded and incentivised. The moves of privatising public institutions is indicative towards facilitating the already dominated private players to flourish further.

Box 7.1 The guidelines for PPP model in district hospitals

Establishing PPP in existing district hospitals: various hospital models under the guidelines

- Model I: doctor owner (30–50 beds) (doctor owns one or two specialties)
- Model II: doctor manager partnership-multispecialty (100 beds) (doctor partners with a businessman with multispecialty services)

- Model III: multispecialty (100 beds or more) (funded by corporate or existing hospital chains)

Responsibility of district hospital

- Allocate 30,000 and 60,000 square feet of space for 50-bed and 100-bed facilities for setting up PPP
  - Minimum 75% and 50% of this space, respectively, would be allocated within the existing built-up structure and for the remaining vacant land within the premises of the hospital
- Hospital to share its ambulance services, blood blank, physiotherapy services, biomedical waste disposal system, mortuary services, parking facilities, electricity load, inpatient payment counters and hospital security with the private enterprise running out of its campus
- Hospital to provide freedom to PPP to run its own cafeteria, parking and pharmacy, with authority to upgrade these facilities
- Hospital staff (from attendants at the registration desk to the chief medical officer) have to refer patients to PPP
- Hospital staff to facilitate reimbursement of expenditures of individuals incurred in PPP facilities from Chief Minister wellness funds and/or link state/centre-level financial protection insurance schemes (including PMJAY) for reimbursement

Government interventions to incentivise the private sector

- Facilitate land allotment
- Facilitate various clearness with special window within specific time
- Viability gap funding (VGF) for improving the financing viability and bankability of the project
  - VGF up to 40% of total project cost, gap funding up to 50% of tax on capital cost, restoration of status of hospital as an industry for getting benefits of VGF
- Ensure timely payments for services provided to the referred patients. The reimbursement are to be provided through Chief Minister wellness funds and/or PMJAY and state level financial protection insurance schemes

Ensuring patient load

- Government to ensure fair amount of patient load at DH (preferably, annual average OPD 1000 patients per day) for establishing PPP. It is recommended that this can be achieved by:

- • Establishing a strong downward linkages with CHCs (5624 number of existing) and PHCs (25,650 number of existing) of that and neighbouring districts to where the project is being implemented, for referring patients to HD
  - • A nationwide network of existing 1.58 lakh SCs spread across remotest rural part of the country, can be explored for referring patients
- • Under Ayushman Bharat, of the total number of different centres, 1.5 lakh centres are proposed to be upgraded into HWCs for catering to the prevention and detection of NCDs needs of the community.

Source: GOI (2017)

UHC debate: changing landscape of healthcare financing and the private sector

Universal health coverage (UHC) is important for addressing the equity, accessibility and affordability in a developing country (WHO, 2010). This debate centred on strategies to finance healthcare for achieving UHC. This largely advocates for financial protection measures (through social health insurance or another publicly financed health insurance system) by which all citizens can utilise healthcare services regardless of whether they can afford the services. The World Health Reports suggested a road map for developing countries to adapt their financing systems to meet the requirements of universal health coverage (WHO, 2010, 2013).

A detailed discussion on UHC financing was provided in Chapter 8. Here, we will briefly touch upon how this debate helped in promoting privatisation in health. For instance, India constituted a High-Level Expert Group (HLEG) on UHC in 2010 which submitted its report in 2011 (GOI, 2011). The Steering Committee of the erstwhile Planning Commission, in its review of HLEG report, made in clear that given the major share of personnel, beds and patients, 'the private sector has to be partnered with health care' (Qadeer, 2013: 158). Thereafter, in the name of UHC, the Third National Health Policy (draft 2015) 2017 supplemented the idea of strategic purchasing of secondary and tertiary care services from the private sector to assure universal healthcare. The NHP highlighted that strategic purchasing would ensure access to affordable and quality secondary and tertiary healthcare services from private providers in healthcare services deficit areas. It advocates for a positive and proactive engagement with the private sector for critical gap filling towards achieving national health goals. Strategic purchasing would play a stewardship role in directing private investment towards those areas and those services, for which currently there are no providers or few providers. The report clearly mentioned that India needs to influence the operation and growth of the private healthcare sector and medical technologies to ensure alignment with public healthcare goals, enabling private sector contribution to making healthcare systems more effective, efficient, rational, safe, affordable and ethical. The policy document argues for service purchasing from private players promoted through health insurance – that is, health insurance is considered as a means to finance healthcare expenses of households. It is important to note that due to low uptake of private insurance among individuals (Chapter 8), the policy advocated linking strategic purchasing of services from the private sector through central-funded and state-funded insurance schemes. The launch of a public-funded national health insurance (called Pradhan Mantri Jan Arogya Yojana; PMJAY) with Rs. 5 lakh covering 40% of the population (10.74 crore households) was a major step towards promoting insurance-based financing for availing of healthcare from public or private providers. Considering the fact of high tendency towards availing healthcare from private facilities among those insured, one can expect further growth in the private healthcare sector to exploit the market. It seems from the current policy that the state would ensure access to – but not necessarily provision of – services, at the cost of public money where public funds are utilised to support private insurance and care.

Private sector: the growth dynamics

Inadequate public investment on the one hand, and the liberalisation and privatisation initiatives of 1990s, the neoliberal ideology of the 2000s and the UHC debate of 2010s on the other hand, have contributed significantly towards privatising the Indian healthcare market. However, coupled with these factors, population dynamics, people's awareness and perception about health change in treatment-seeking behaviour, double burden of disease, changing nature of lifestyle diseases, global integration and medical tourism are other possible factors that have encouraged private providers and enterprises and foreign investors to exploit the hospital market in India. These together have resulted in high growth of informal and formal providers ranging from individual practitioners to small clinics to large hospitals to exploit the Indian healthcare market. Such services are generally classified, viz. hospitals, medical and nursing homes, dental care practices, nurses, masseurs, physiotherapists, paramedical practitioners, diagnostic and pathological laboratories, blood banks and others, including independent ambulatory care, Ayurveda, Unani and homeopathy (Table 7.1). NSS data reported to have around 10.4 lakhs of health enterprises in 2010–2011 (Hooda, 2017). Ayurveda service providers were dominant in the 1950s, while allopathic providers and hospitals (with more than five workers) grew faster in the post-liberalisation phase of the Indian economy and became dominant in 2010–2011 with a share of 76%. Diagnostic service providers also grew

Table 7.1 Growth and structure of the private healthcare sector in India

	1905–1950	1951–1960	1961–1970	1971–1980	1981–1990	1991–2000	2001–2010	Cumulative total	GR	% dist.	% of est.	By workers size distribution		
												Small (1)	Medium (2–5)	Large (≥6)
Hospital	187	11	1284	4332	8123	13973	52240	80265	1.13	7.8	66.8	4.1	8.4	53.0
Medical	331	2342	2539	19630	42847	137144	368517	576027	1.12	55.6	21.7	61.1	50.2	18.4
Dental	42	0	201	73	1747	7841	31805	42052	1.16	4.1	65.1	1.8	9.2	0.5
Ayurvedic	504	449	1796	6866	9812	29662	27767	76891	1.08	7.4	17.2	8.0	7.2	1.2
Unani	0	512	477	202	61	6187	9346	16837	1.06	1.6	30.3	1.6	1.9	0.0
Homo	0	23	765	4709	11150	34000	64748	115760	1.16	11.2	18.8	13.2	8.7	0.7
Nursing	0	0	2366	1360	1130	13712	23663	42231	1.07	4.1	12.0	5.2	2.5	0.0
Diagnostic	0	0	32	707	2342	13215	29056	45805	1.18	4.4	61.6	2.2	8.2	9.7
Others	0	0	1239	1053	2591	5688	12931	23856	1.07	2.3	21.8	0.0	0.0	0.1
Residential	289	90	42	429	127	1233	4232	6521	1.05	0.6	76.9	2.5	2.0	1.3
Social	0	1	0	388	800	2270	5783	9252	1.10	0.9	77.1	0.2	0.7	5.4
Total	1353	3428	10741	39749	80730	264925	630088	1035497	1.11	100	28.7	0.2	1.0	9.5

Notes: dist. – overall distribution of services; est. – share of establishment; GR – growth rate. The total is higher than the cumulative add up, as it represents total enterprises up to the year 2010–2011

Source: NSS, Services Sector Enterprises, 2010–2011

Table 7.2 Changing growth dynamics of private health enterprises

	Type of enterprises		Size of enterprises (by no. of workers)				Total
	OAE	Est.	Single (1)	Small (2–5)	Medium (6–10)	Large (>10)	
2001–2002 (57th)	1081325 (81.8)	241106 (18.2)	1009064 (76.3)	276690 (20.9)	25777 (1.9)	10900 (0.8)	1322431 (100)
2005–2006 (63rd)	793032 (72.7)	280469 (25.7)	757227 (69.5)	287611 (26.4)	28629 (2.6)	16819 (1.5)	1090286 (100)
2010–2011 (67th)	738647 (71.3)	296850 (28.7)	659475 (63.7)	327344 (31.6)	30246 (2.9)	18432 (1.8)	1035497 (100)
CAGR (2001–2002 to 2010–2011)	–0.041	0.023	–0.046	0.019	0.018	0.060	–0.027

Source: NSS, Services Sector Enterprises Survey, 2001–2002, 2005–2006, and 2010–2011, Government of India

at a faster rate as compared to the Indian System of Medicines (AYUSH) providers.

The estimates from different Service Sector Enterprises rounds of NSSO reflects that total number of enterprises decreased from 13.2 lakh in 2001–2002 to 10.4 lakh in 2010–2011 (Hooda, 2017). There is a significant reduction in the numbers of own-account enterprises generally run by individuals (Table 7.2). The analysis by size of workers reflects that large-size enterprises (>10 workers) are increasing, while single- and individual-run enterprises are declining. Similarly, the share of own-account enterprises (OAEs) shows decreasing trends, while establishment share increased. This reflects that large-size enterprises are mushrooming in the country, while small providers are vanishing – is it an indication that big fish (large-size enterprises) are eating the small fish (small clinics and individual providers) over time, especially due to pro-market approaches that generally focus on curative or hospital care?

Privatisation: at what cost

The growth in private health enterprises over time resulted in their high presence in the healthcare market. The share of private hospitals increased from 18.5% in 1974 to 74.9% in 2000, and hospital beds from 21.4% to 50.7%. The share of private medical institutions for producing human resources for health increased from 3.6% at the time of independence to 54.3% in 2014 (Figure 7.2). The share of government hospitals, hospital beds and medical institutions has been declining over the period. Due to the dominance of private sector in service provision, they provide majority of

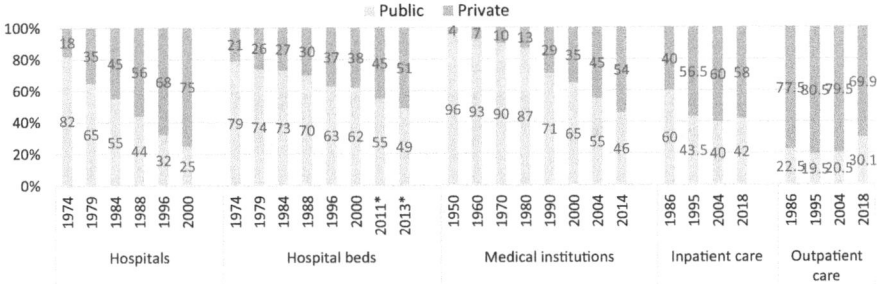

Figure 7.2 Dominance of the private sector in health service provision and delivery

Note: The hospital beds for 2011 and 2013 (indicated with asterisks) represent beds in medical institutions only due to non-availability of hospitals beds data.

Source: Government of India, Health Rounds of NSSO 1986, 1995, 2004, 2014 & 2019 and Hooda, 2017

inpatient (two-thirds) and outpatient (three-fourths) care treatment to the population. The outpatient care treatment received from the private sector, however, is almost constant since 1986–1987, but in providing inpatient treatments, its share increased to 58% in 2017–2018 from a low share of 40% in 1986–1987 (Figure 7.2).

The dominance in service delivery of the private sector also resulted in costly care. A closer look at Figure 7.3 reflects that cost of care in the private sector increased manifold over time – around 10–11 times between 1987 and 2018. The cost of healthcare in the private sector was noticed to be more than four times than the average cost of healthcare in the public sector in 2014, which increased to more than seven times in 2019 (Figure 7.3). This was a time when an insurance-based financing mechanism was functional in most of the Indian states. The cost of hospitalisation in private facilities as compared to public facilities was around 2.3 times higher in rural areas and 3.1 times higher in urban areas in 1986–1987. In 2019, the cost of hospitalisation in a private facility in rural and urban areas increased 6.37 times and 8.03 times, respectively, as compared to the cost in public facility (Figure 7.3).

Amongst the different types of ailments, cancer, cardio and neurological and psychiatric disorders have the highest medical costs. If one compares the average medical expenditure per hospitalisation case in public and private facilities, it is observed that the cost of care in private hospitals was around 3–8 times higher than in public facilities across different diseases and ailments. The cost of healthcare for some of the diseases in a private facility is around 7–8 times higher than that in a public facility (Figure 7.3). This reflects that the cost of hospitalisation in private facilities has increased more significantly than in public facilities, indicating that the private sector

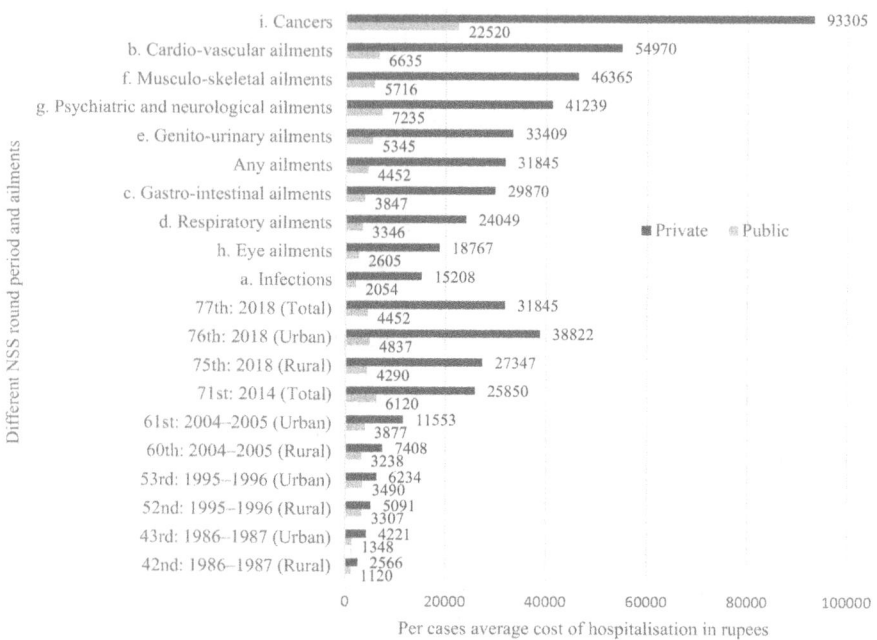

Figure 7.3 Per cases average cost of hospitalisation in public and private facilities
Source: Government of India, Key Indicators of Social Consumption on Health, NSS, 2019.

escalates the cost of care. The costly care results in unaffordable of care to general population and resulted in high burden of OOP payment in the country (Hooda, 2017).

No doubt, the private sector grew at faster rate and has overtaken the hospital market of India, but we did not find any evidence that they are inclined to address the health deficiency gap of the most remote parts of the country. For instance, a large number of health enterprises are found to be located in urban areas, while rural areas remained dominated by individual practitioners (Hooda, 2017). A survey on large private hospitals (IMS-Health survey) conducted in 62 Indian cities in 2012 covering 14,121 hospitals also reflects that out of total surveyed hospitals, almost half (48%) of large private hospitals and two-thirds of the corporate hospitals are located in cities with populations of at least five million, with 16% share of Mumbai alone in all hospitals (Mukhopadhyay et al., 2015). The urban metropolitan areas have high concentrations of organised private and corporate hospitals. The insurance empanelment list of hospitals of RSBY (8697 hospitals), Aarogyasri (2130 hospitals) and ROHINI (Registry of Hospitals in Network of Insurance) (33,000 hospitals) between 2017–2018 reflects that a majority of them found to be located in million-plus cities and urban areas of a few districts of some states (Hooda, 2020). A list of 18,236 hospitals empanelled under PMJAY in 2019 also shows their skewed distribution with their high concentrated in a few pockets (Choudhury and Datta, 2020). Many regions (especially the aspirational districts) face significant facility and capacity gaps as compared to their peer districts (Smith et al., 2019). The national hospital directory reported 30,273 large-size hospitals, including 1048 corporate hospitals, in both the public and private sectors in 2015. Most of the large hospitals (around 76%) were found to be concentrated in only 26% of districts of India. Seven districts of India – Mumbai, Ahmadabad, Bengaluru Urban, Thane, Hyderabad, Pune and Chennai – occupy on average of 20% of India's large hospitals (Hooda, 2017).

Conclusion and discussion

There is no doubt that India has been experimenting with private healthcare since independence, and it has grown and diversified over time. Its growth is noticed to have been faster since the early 1990s, the liberalisation phase of the Indian economy. The private sector attracted greater attention in 2000 when the government of India approved 100% FDI through automatic route in the hospital sector. The hospital sector was accorded industry status in the 2003–2004 budget, following which cheap and long-term loans were provided to private healthcare institutions. The neoliberal ideology enforced by international agencies and other pro-market reform initiatives – along with factors like population dynamics, people's awareness and perception of health, change in treatment-seeking behaviour, double burden of disease, and the changing nature of lifestyle diseases, global integration and medical tourism – have encouraged private providers and enterprises, including foreign investors, to exploit the hospital market in India. Insurance-based financing strategies also contributed towards high growth of the private sector.

The growth of the private sector remained highly heterogeneous, providing a variety of services ranging from hospitalisation, medical, dental, diagnostics, homoeopathic, Unani, Ayurvedic and residential nursing to social services. The allopathic hospitals and diagnostics providers have recorded high growth. The growth of the private sector has largely been urban-centric, while rural areas and several of the most remote districts are suffering from a deficiency of healthcare facilities.

The growth pattern is one of private providers moving from a fragmented market to a concentrated market, and a gradual shift from informal to formal and then to large entities. Interestingly, large and corporate hospitals are emerging, whereas small providers are vanishing – a phenomenon of big fish eating the small fish. The market in India is evolving in a similar way as happened some decades ago in the United States, where privatisation produced monopolies in the healthcare market. A recent post from The American Interest (2016) reflects that monopolists are taking over American healthcare. Over the years, four major hospital chains have controlled 90%

of the market in the United States (Havighurst and Richman, 2011). The present growth pattern in India may lead to a hospital market concentrated in fewer hands. Smaller providers and individual practitioners in these areas are being sucked into large and corporate-run hospital networks, which further creates induced demand.

The high growth of private sector providers resulted in their dominance of the healthcare delivery market. This resulted in costly care, which in turn has increased OOP burden in the country, leading to unaffordability.

No doubt, large-size health enterprises are on the rise in the country, but own-account enterprises run by individuals still constitute the majority share of the total enterprises (about three-fourths of the health entities). Rural areas are dominated with small and individual practitioners, and the majority of such providers are unskilled and without formal degrees (Hooda, 2017).

A large number of health enterprises in India are unregistered under any act or legislation, leading to unhealthy and unethical practices in the country. The global experience, however, suggests that the countries that have followed pro-market approaches to deliver care draw up strong regulatory guidelines for the private sector (Baru, 2006). Registration under the Medical Practitioners Act (MPA) in India was found to be very low (Hooda, 2017). In India, it is the state's prerogative to make appropriate regulations and legislation for the private sector. A review of regulation status of private practitioners at the state level shows that out of 29 states, 16 states did not have any legislation, which makes it mandatory for private establishments to have a licence to function. The remaining 13 states adopted various Acts,[2] but they either are outdated or lack appropriate guidelines and rules, due to which acts could not be enforced properly in many states. For instance, minimum standards related to infrastructure, human resources, patient safety and display of information have not been developed; nor have the issues relating to accountability with respect to quality and price been addressed in states that have enforced such legislation (Phadke, 2016). The service provision and quality norms in many formal facilities are reported to be inadequate. For instance, in West Bengal, around 94 people died in a state-of-the-art corporate hospital on December 9, 2011 simply because the hospital did not follow proper quality and safety rules (Polgreen and Kumar, 2011). Such unhealthy and unethical health practices are serious cause for concern.

The Parliament of India passed a Clinical Establishments (Registration and Regulation) Act, 2010 for all types of healthcare providers covering all clinical establishments owned, controlled or managed by private or government providers, society/trust (public or private), dental clinics, corporations and private practitioners, services of practitioners of recognised systems of medicine (Ayurveda, Unani, Siddha, etc.), all types of laboratories, diagnostic institutions and therapy centres, and so on (GOI, 2010). This is important for infrastructure, human resources, availability of medicines and equipment, including their maintenance for improving the quality of healthcare services (Phadke, 2016). The Clinical Establishment Act 2010 has only been enforced by a few states like Bihar, Jharkhand, Uttrakhand, Himachal Pradesh, Arunachal Pradesh, Sikkim, Pondicherry, Uttar Pradesh, Rajasthan, and Mizoram, despite inadequate form.

Several entities have received subsidised land, loans at low interest, exemptions on income tax and tariff rates, etc., on the condition that they would provide affordable care and serve economically weaker sections of people free of cost and they would prioritise investment in rural/semi-urban areas and fill health service deficient gap. In practice, they do not adhere to such guidelines. Several hospitals are found to register themselves as non-profit entities to receive benefits and exemptions, but they are found violating the aforementioned conditions. They provide medical services at market prices, and thus do not fall under the charitable category any longer (Kurian, 2012).

Some entities even found avoiding tax compliance. For instance, in Delhi, Max Hospital has run into tax trouble and was also found flouting the charity clause (Mehta, 2015). Our regulatory system is weak. The punishment for violating a rule is not adequate in itself. For instance, Delhi Nursing Homes Registration Act, 1953 states that 'whoever contravenes any of the provision of the Act will be punished with a fine of Rs. 100 and in case of continuing offence to a further fine of Rs. 25 in respect of each day on which the offence continues after such conviction', reflecting a lack of adequate and effective regulation.

Notes

1 This chapter draws from certain inferences and data previously published in S. K. Hooda. 2017. Growth of Formal and Informal Private Healthcare Providers in India: Structural Changes and Implications. *Journal of Health Care Finance*, Wolters Kluwer, Illinois, Chicago, Vol. 44, No. 2, Fall 2017 (September–November). References to these instances have been provided at relevant places.
2 Namely, the following: Bombay Nursing Homes Registration Act 1949; West Bengal Clinical Establishment Act, 1950; Delhi Nursing Homes Registration Act, 1953; Jammu and Kashmir Nursing Homes and Clinical Establishments (Registration and Licensing) Act, 1963; Madhya Pradesh Upcharya Griha Tatha Rujopchar Sambandhi Sthampamaue (Registrikaran Tatha Anugyapan) Adhiniyam, 1973; Punjab State Nursing Home Registration Act, 1991; Orissa Clinical Establishments (Control and Regulation) Act, 1991; Manipur Nursing Home and Clinic Registration Act, 1992; Sikkim Clinical Establishments (Licensing and Registration) Act, 1995; Nagaland Health Care Establishments Act, 1997; Tamil Nadu Private Clinical Establishments Regulation Act, 1997; Andhra Pradesh Private Medical Care Establishments (Regulation and Registration) Act, 2002, Rules 2005 and 2007; Karnataka Private Medical Establishments Act, 2007.

References

The American Interest. 2016. *Monopolists Are Taking Over American Healthcare*, 29 September 2016. www.the-american-interest.com/2016/09/29/monopolists-are-taking-over-american-healthcare/

Baru, R. V. 2006. *Privatisation of Health Care in India: A Comparative Analysis of Orissa, Karnataka and Maharashtra States.* A Joint Publication of IIPA, CMRD and UNDP India, New Delhi.

Choudhury, M., and Datta, P. 2020. Health Insurance in Private Hospitals: Implications for Implementation of Ayushman Bharat. *Economic and Political Weekly,* Vol. 55, No. 17.

Fisk, M. 2000. Neoliberalism and the Slow Death of Public Healthcare in Mexico. *Journal of Socialism and Democracy,* Vol. 14, No. 1, pp. 63–84.

Ghosh, S. 2010. *Catastrophic Payments and Impoverishment Due to Out-of-pocket Health Spending: The Effects of Recent Health Sector Reforms in India.* Asia Health Policy Program, Working Paper No. 15, July. Available at SSRN at https://papers.ssrn.com/sol3/papers.cfm?abstract_id=1658573

GOI. 2011. *High-Level Expert Group report on Universal Health Coverage for India, Planning Commission.* Government of India (GOI). http://phmindia.org/wp-content/uploads/2015/09/Plg-Commission-HLEG-Report-on-Health-for-12th-Planrep_uhc0812.pdf

GOI. 2017. *Public Private Partnership for NCDs in District Hospitals 2017.* NITI Aayog, Government of India, New Delhi. https://niti.gov.in/writereaddata/fi les/document_publication/Draft%20Guidelines%20on%20PPP%20in%20NCDs_0.pdf

Government of India. 1987, 1996, 2004, 2014 and 2019. *Health Rounds of National Sample Survey (NSS) Office.* Ministry of Statistics and Programme Implementation, Government of India.

Government of India. 2002, 2007 and 2011. *Unit Level Records of Unorganised Service Sector Enterprises of 57th, 63rd and 67th Rounds of National Sample Survey Office.* Ministry of Statistics and Programme Implementation Government of India, various years.

Government of India. 2010. *Clinical Establishment (Registration and Regulation) Act (CEA).* http://clinicalestablishments.gov.in/cms/Home.aspx

Havighurst, C. C., and Richman, B. D. 2011. The Provider Monopoly Problem in Health Care. *Oregon Law Review,* Vol. 89, No. 847. https://www.antitrustinstitute.org/wp-content/uploads/2018/08/Havighurst.pdf

Hooda, S. K. 2015. *Foreign Investment in Hospital Sector in India: Trends, Pattern and Issues.* Institute for Studies in Industrial Development, Working Paper No 181. http://103.82.220.134/pdf/WP181.pdf

Hooda, S. K. 2017, September–November. Growth of Formal and Informal Private Healthcare Providers in India: Structural Changes and Implications. *Journal of Health Care Finance,* Walters Kluwer, Illinois, Chicago, Vol. 44, No. 2, Fall.

Hooda, S. K. 2020. Penetration and Coverage of Government-funded Health Insurance Schemes in India. *Clinical Epidemiology and Global Health,* Vol. 8, pp. 1017–1033.

Kurian, O. C. 2012. Charitable Hospitals: Charity at Market Rate. *Economic and Political Weekly,* Vol. 47, No. 39, pp. 23–25.

Lefebvre, B. 2010. *Hospital Chains in India: The Coming of Age?* Asie Visions 23, India/South Asia Programme Centre – Asie/Ifri, January. https://halshs.archives-ouvertes.fr/hal-00687105/document

Mehta, Avantika. 2015. Delhi: Max Hospital in Trouble; Found Flouting Charity Clause. *Hindustan Times,* April 5.

Mukhopadhyay, I., Selvaraj, S., Sharma, S., and Datta, P. 2015. *Changing Landscape of Private Healthcare Providers in India*. Paper Presented at International Public Policy Association Conference. Milan, July 2015.

Phadke, A. 2016. Regulation of Doctors and Private Hospitals in India. *Economic and Political Weekly*, Vol. 51, No. 6, pp. 46–55.

Polgreen, L., and Kumar, H. 2011. 94 People Die as Private Hospital in India Burns. *The New York Times*, December 9. https://www.nytimes.com/2011/12/10/world/india-hospital-fire-kolkata-west-bengal.html

Qadeer, I. 2013. Universal Health Care in India: Panacea for Whom? *Indian Journal of Public Health*, Vol. 57, No. 4, pp. 225–230.

Shah, U., and Mohanty, R. 2011. Private Sector in Indian Healthcare Delivery: Consumer Perspective and Government Policies to Promote Private Sector. *Information Management and Business Review*, Vol. 1, No. 2, pp. 79–87.

Smith, O., Dong, Di, and Chhabra, Sheena. 2019. *PM-JAY Policy Brief 3: PM-JAY and India's Aspirational Districts*. Government of India, September. www.pmjay.gov.in/sites/default/files/2019-10/Policy%20Brief%203_PM-JAY%20and%20India%27s%20Aspirational%20Districts%20%28PRINT%29_WB.pdf

WHO. 2010. *The World Health Report: Health System Financing: The Path to Universal Coverage*. World Health Organization, Geneva.

WHO. 2013. *World Health Report 2013: Research for Universal Health Coverage*. World Health Organization, Geneva.

World Bank. 1993. *World Development Report 1993: Investing in Health*. Oxford University Press, New York.

World Bank. 2001. *India: Raising the Sights: Better Health Systems for India's Poor*. World Bank, Washington, DC: HNP Unit-India, Report No. 22304.

8 Changing nature of healthcare financing

Who benefits?

Recently, achieving universal health coverage (UHC) has become an internationally accepted developmental goal. UHC is elaborated that all people receive access to healthcare they need without exposing the user to financial hardship (WHO, 2013). Thus, the paramount issue in health policy circles is which type of health financing mechanism can provide efficient financial risk protection to all people against the cost of healthcare. The emergence of UHC has brought healthcare financing mechanisms to centre stage (Barnes et al., 2017). It advocates for restructuring the financing nature of healthcare to achieve UHC.

In general, two types of healthcare financing approaches are put forward to achieve UHC. One is the tax-funded system to finance health services which are usually provided through a network of public healthcare systems like in the UK, Cuba and Sri Lanka. The other is the society risk-pooling mechanism whereby all individuals share the total cost of healthcare. This is termed as social health insurance (SHI), which argues for a country to develop a risk-pooling mechanism for achieving UHC. The risk-pooling mechanism is indicative of the development of SHI whereby entire populations – ranging from workers, self-employed and enterprises to the government – pays contributions for a social health insurance fund. In the case of workers and enterprises, workers can contribute from their salaries. Employers and enterprises pay a matching premium, while the government may provide contributions on behalf of those who are not able to pay, such as the unemployed, informal sector workers and low-income households. The SHI mechanism pools resources from public sources and from contributions made by employers and beneficiaries (GOI, 2011). The risk-pooling mechanism, however, is not uniform across the world. Countries like the Philippines, Vietnam and Colombia have sought to provide insurance coverage to the poor and informal sector workers through fully subsidised insurance premiums. The non-poor in Vietnam and the Philippines have the option of voluntarily enrolling in the schemes, while non-poor workers and their families are compulsorily enrolled in these schemes in Colombia. A broad-based SHI programme is being prescribed as a key instrument of health financing strategy in Germany, France and Mexico (GOI, 2011). However, whatever

DOI: 10.4324/9781032108438-11

resource-pooling mechanism a country adopts, the insurance-based system has gained popularity for financing care and achieving UHC across the globe including India.

Health insurance and risk-pooling mechanism in India

The history of health insurance in India goes back to the early 1950s, when schemes for formal sector workers (Employees' State Insurance Scheme; ESIS) and for civil servants (Central Government Health Scheme; CGHS) were introduced through contributory – but heavily subsidised – health insurance programmes in 1952 and 1954, respectively (GOI, 2011). These schemes are generally called social health insurance (SHI) schemes.

India introduced a medi-claim policy in 1986 and the insurance sector was opened up for private players in 1999 on a pay-for-premium basis. The uptake of these schemes remained very low, due to high premiums and low paying capacity of the majority of the population, and low willingness of individuals to take on private insurance (Hooda, 2020). These schemes are generally termed as commercial or voluntary health insurance (VHI) schemes.

India has seen some experiments of community-based health insurance (CBHI) schemes since the beginning of the 21st century for informal sector communities. The coverage and uptake were observed to be very low under such schemes, as well (GOI, 2011). The government of India introduced the Universal Health Insurance Scheme (UHIS) in 2003 to provide financial risk protection to people below the poverty line at subsidised premiums. This scheme was also extended to self-help groups in 2004. The uptake under the schemes remained negligible, and only about 3.7 million people were covered by 2008–2009 (Ahuja, 2004; Rao, 2004; Forgia and Nagpal, 2012).

India has been witnessing a plethora of central and state government-funded health insurance schemes (GFHIs) since the early 2000s. These GFHIs are largely pro-poor in nature. The state of Karnataka was a pioneer in launching a pro-poor GFHI called Yeshasvini Cooperative Farmers Health Care Insurance in 2003. In 2007, Andhra Pradesh launched the Rajiv Aarogyasri scheme for families possessing below poverty line (BPL) cards. The government of India's Ministry of Labour and Employment implemented a nationally representative health insurance scheme called Rashtriya Swasthya Bima Yojana (RSBY) on April 1, 2008. The scheme initially was designed to target the BPL households. Later on, it was extended to other defined categories of unorganised workers like building and construction workers, street vendors, Mahatma Gandhi National Rural Employment Guarantee Act (MGNREGA) workers (those who worked for more than 15 days), beedi workers, domestic workers, railway porters, sanitation workers, rickshaw drivers/pullers, mine workers, rag pickers, auto/taxi drivers, and weavers and textile workers. Many states implemented RSBY, though some states launched either their own version of the scheme with different names and/ or upgraded versions of RSBY (Hooda, 2020).

Most GFHIs are meant for poor families and, to some extent, informal sector workers. The coverage and coverage limits vary considerably, though. The annual coverage was Rs. 30,000 per family under nationally representative scheme RSBY. Himachal Pradesh launched RSBY Plus in 2010, with a coverage amount of Rs. 175,000 per family. Among other states, limits were fixed at Rs. 150,000 in Delhi under Apka Swasthya Bima Yojana 2011–2012, Rs. 2,00,000 under Yeshasvini Cooperative Farmers Healthcare Scheme 2003 of Karnataka, Rs. 1,50,000 per family per year plus buffer of Rs. 50,000 per year under Rajiv Aarogyasri Community Health Insurance Scheme 2007 of Andhra Pradesh, and Rs. 1,00,000 over four years per family under Chief Minister Kalaignar's Insurance Scheme of Tamil Nadu 2009. Chief Minister's Comprehensive Health Insurance Scheme of Tamil Nadu provides coverage up to Rs. 1 lakh and in critical cases up to Rs. 2 lakhs. Kerala's Comprehensive Health Insurance Scheme (CHIS) offers Rs. 30,000; however, since 2011, an additional amount of Rs. 70,000 is made available per family under CHIS Plus. It was Rs. 150,000 per family per year plus Rs. 50,000 per year buffer under Vajpayee Arogyashri Scheme 2009 of Karnataka. Maharashtra launched its flagship health insurance scheme called Rajiv Gandhi Jeevandayee Arogya Yojana (RGJAY) in July 2012 with coverage amount Rs. 1,50,000 per family per year, the scheme later renamed as Mahatma Jyotiba Phule Jan Arogya Yojana (MJPJAY) in April 2017. The Gujarat launched Mukhyamantri Amrutum Yojana in September 2012 with a coverage amount Rs. 3,00,000 per family per annum on family floater basis. The state of Rajasthan went ahead of all the states by setting the coverage limit Rs. 3,00,000 over and above the RSBY limit under Bhamashah Swasthya Bima Yojana 2015 making it Rs. 3,30,000 per annum per family.

In the 2018 budget, the government of India replaced the earlier nationally representative scheme RSBY with the National Health Protection Scheme under the ambit of Ayushman Bharat (renamed as Pradhan Mantri Jan Aarogya Yojana [PMJAY] at the time of its launch in September 2018). The coverage limit under PMJAY has been raised to Rs. 5,00,000 per annum per family, which is around 17 times higher than the earlier national health insurance scheme RSBY. Along with the coverage limit, the numbers of targeted families that are to be covered under different central-level and state-level schemes have also increased over time. For instance, the nationally representative scheme RSBY aimed to cover 7.0 crore BPL families comprising 35 crore persons and a defined categories of unorganised sector workers by 2017. The PMJAY set the higher target and identified 10.74 crore poor and vulnerable families (40% of India's population) using deprivation and occupational criteria. The benefits of this scheme also extended to families that were covered under earlier nationally representative government funded health insurance (GFHI) scheme RSBY.

Thus, the insurance-based system in India can be classified as employer-mandated social health insurance (SHI), commercial/voluntary health insurance (VHI), community-based health insurance, and target oriented government-funded health insurance (GFHI). In terms of coverage, the Insurance Regulatory and Development Authority report 2018–2019 reflects that the general and health insurance companies issued around 2.07 crore health insurance policies covering a total of 47.20 crore persons. Of the total, three-fourths of the persons are covered under government-sponsored health insurance schemes and the remaining one-fourth are by covered by group and individual policies (IRDA, 2019). The report suggests that coverage of persons under different health insurance schemes has been increasing over time. The number of people covered under government-sponsored schemes (including RSBY, CHGS and ESIS) has increased almost double, to around 3571 lakhs in 2018–2019 from 1891 lakhs in 2010–2011 (IRDA, 2019).

As regards to the population coverage, under RSBY, around 41.33 million families (a family of five members) were covered as of March 2016 – roughly 206 million persons. This is less than the target of 70 million families that were to be covered by the end of the Twelfth Five-Year Plan 2012–2017 (Hooda, 2020). The RSBY was operational only in 99 districts in the first year of its launch, 2009–2010; by October 2013, the scheme became operational in 27 states covering 447 districts. However, many states scaled down the scheme thereafter. Only 15 states continued with the scheme, covering 272 districts, as of March 2017. This is because, by the time, most of the states started implementing their own schemes. Now PMJAY is promised to 10.74 crore poor and vulnerable families – around 40% of India's population – and it is expected that all state schemes will come under its umbrella.

Different insurance schemes independently facilitate healthcare treatment for different sets of the population, though the level of care differs. They also vary considerably in terms of nature and coverage. The SHI generally serve the better-off, as they are exclusively meant for civil servants and workers working in the formal/organised sector. These schemes comprehensively cover inpatient as well as outpatient treatment expenses. The GFHIs, on the other hand, are explicitly a pro-poor financing strategy and are limited only for hospitalisation and inpatient care; outpatient care is not covered. However, they are mostly cashless. The amount of coverage under SHI for hospitalisation is unlimited, while GFHIs have limited coverage with a wide variation across state-level schemes.

One important feature of the currently promoted insurance-based system is that the resource-pooling mechanism is rather different from the funding nature of insurance-based models in other countries. The insurance-based system in India is almost entirely funded from public (tax) sources. This is simply because the contributions from employers in India are expected to be almost negligible because of the informal nature of the economy (around 93% of work-force in India is employed in the informal sector, which leaves little or no room to receive employer contributions) and the majority of informal workers have low paying capacity for insurance. Thus, the currently promoted insurance-based system in India is generally called government-funded health insurance (GFHIs) scheme or system, and this can have several implications ranging from financial, political, health-seeking behaviour and on cost, which are discussed in the following sections.

Financial implications of changing healthcare financing

Along with the coverage and coverage amounts, the treatments and procedures under GFHIs expanded over time. The PMJAY sets to cover pre-existing conditions on 1393 identified procedures, including – but not limited to – drugs, supplies, diagnostic services, physician's fees, room charges, surgeon charges, overtime and intensive care unit (ICU) charges, etc. This can certainly affect the rate of premiums paid by the government to the insurance companies. At the time of the launch of the earlier RSBY scheme, the average premium was less than Rs. 300 per family; the amount of premium paid by the government to insurance company increased to Rs. 600–800 per family in its later phases of implementation. The premium under Rajasthan's BSBY, which provides cover up to Rs. 3,30,000 per family, was around Rs. 600 in 2015, which increased to Rs. 1200 per family within a few years of implementation of this scheme (Hooda, 2020).

Despite the fact that the coverages and coverage amounts were the same in these two schemes, the average amount of premium paid increased over time. Such trends cost more for the government, as government has to allocate more tax resource to finance GFHI systems. Thus, insurance-based systems are likely to consume a significant proportion of total budget allocated for the healthcare sector. For instance, budgetary allocation by the central government for RSBY increased to Rs. 1002 crore in 2012–2013 from Rs. 103 crore in 2008–2009, which was further raised to Rs. 2000 crore in 2018–2019 budget. The budget for the recently launched national representative scheme PMJAY was raised to Rs. 6400 crore in 2019–2020. The state-level schemes have made substantial contribution ranges from Rs. 953 crore in Tamil Nadu, Maharashtra (Rs. 868 crore), Andhra Pradesh (Rs. 620 crore), Telangana (Rs. 437 crore), Karnataka (Rs. 285 crore), Kerala (Rs. 154 crore), Gujarat (Rs. 118 crore), to Odisha (Rs. 100 crore) (Hooda, 2020). The overall contribution of government health insurance is accounted at 12% (Rs. 5064 crore), the share of private insurance was 51% (Rs. 22,013 crore) and SHI was 37% (Rs. 15,889 crore) in 2015–2016 (NHA, 2018).

Health-seeking behaviour and insurance

It is important to understand how far health insurance is influencing health-seeking behaviour in terms of treatments received, the frequency of healthcare service received, and inpatient and outpatient care-seeking behaviour. We have observed that insurance beneficiaries generally have a tendency to sidetrack primary care in order to receive benefits of insurance which are meant only for medical care. For instance, uninsured persons have a high reporting rate for short-term morbidity as compared to the RSBY card holders. However, the rate of reporting for hospitalisation for major morbidity among RSBY card holders was higher than that of the uninsured. This may be because most of the short-term morbidities are not covered under RSBY. On the other hand, non-RSBY persons do not want to take the risk of occurring major morbidity, and report immediately to the hospital. The case is opposite for insurance holders (Figure 8.1). This is a clear case of sidetracking primary care. The reporting situation for short-term morbidity is worse in case of people residing in remote, less developed villages. In general, the card holders have a sense of security once they report for hospitalisation for major morbidities that they will receive free care, but not in case of short-term morbidities that are generally not covered under insurance packages. In the process, card holders sidetrack primary care and compromise on the health front.

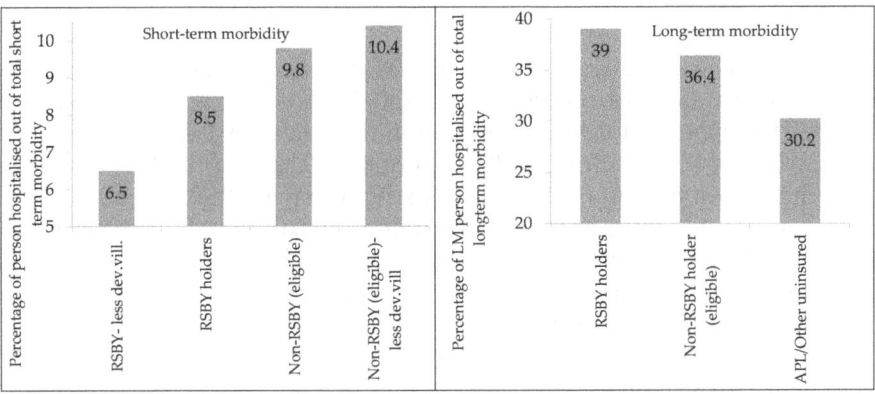

Figure 8.1 Sidetracking primary care: compromising health
Source: IHDS (2012)

The strengthening of primary care facilities in the country could easily address the problem of sidetracking of primary care and reduce the excessive burden on hospitals, as well. Examples also suggest that investment in primary care is not just important for promoting access to healthcare; it is a key strategy for achieving UHC and reducing healthcare costs by reducing the need for more expensive hospitalisation or tertiary care (Kruk et al., 2010; Starfield et al., 2005; Franks and Fiscella, 1998). The government of India started investing in primary care after the launch of the National Rural Health Mission in 2005, but expenditure has remained less than the required level of providing primary care in the country as reported in Chapter 2.

Over- or underutilisation of insurance cards is another problem of the insurance-based model. For instance, RSBY was implemented in the month of April through an insurance company model wherein the company has to enrol and renew the RSBY beneficiaries every year. In most states, the scheme

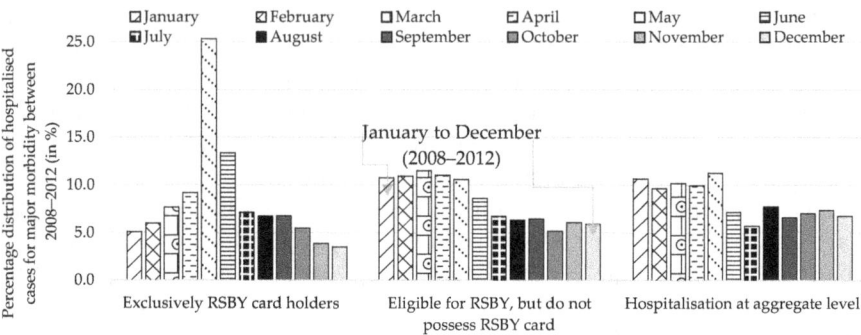

Figure 8.2 Inconsistency and overutilisation of medical care
Source: IHDS (2012)

was implemented between March and May. One can see that around the expiry date of the card, reporting for hospitalisation among card holders was high. The reporting for hospitalisation in the month of January is less than 5%, while in May it is over 25% (Figure 8.2). The abnormal reporting for hospitalisation only in the case of households having RSBY cards is a serious concern. Such reporting for hospitalisation for households that do not possess RSBY cards but are eligible have a similar hospitalisation patterns at aggregate level. One must not negate the case of corruption in reporting; it might have come either from the patient side and/or from the hospital side, but the fact is that reporting for hospitalisation reaches to enormously high level among card holders.

The insurance-based system influences the preference of accessing private facilities for medical care, while it is low for public facilities. That is, insurance is an instrument of promoting private healthcare in the country. For instance, Andhra Pradesh promoted an insurance-based model whereby more services are purchased from the private sector. A large percentage of households (around 62.4%) found to avail treatment from a private facility than the public in Andhra Pradesh (Figure 8.3). However, states like Himachal Pradesh and Mizoram have adopted various strategies to improve their public healthcare systems and spent large amounts (in per capita terms) of public funds on public healthcare systems. In these states, around 81–85% of households avail of care from public facilities and not private facilities. States like Tamil Nadu and Rajasthan adopted the mixed-model strategy. They have strengthened their public system as well as provided free access to medicine and pro-poor insurance schemes. This strategy has resulted in high access of public facilities and private facilities in these states, as well. The preference for public facilities in these two states, however, was reported to be lower than Himachal Pradesh and Mizoram, which have strengthened their public systems, indicating that there is no substitute for service delivery other than

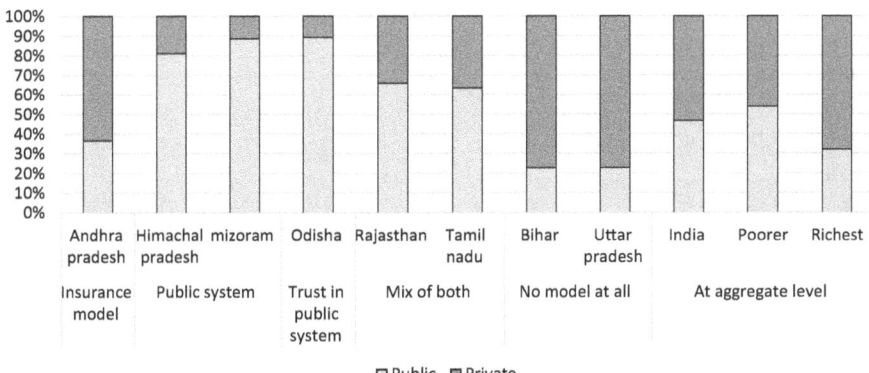

Figure 8.3 Choice of facility: percentage of households receiving treatment, by type of intervention strategy

Note: Share of service received from other source not reported

Source: NFHS (2016)

strengthening the public healthcare system. On the other hand, per capita public spending on health in Bihar and Uttar Pradesh is very low; people in these states are compelled/bound to use private facilities (Figure 8.3).

With the insurance penetration, frequency of visits for medical care increase. The frequency of service use was found to be 1.36 among insured relative to that of uninsured (1.24). Along with the frequency of service use, duration of stay of insured persons (6.68 days) was also found to be higher than that for the uninsured (5.82 days). The duration of stay was found to be even longer in private hospitals (7.0 days), maybe to increase unnecessary medical bills (Hooda, 2019). The duration of stay of the uninsured was 6.26 days in a private hospital as compared to 5.74 days in a public hospital. The duration of stay of those insured under GFHI/RSBY was recorded to be seven days in a private hospital as compared to 6.67 days in a public hospital. The duration of stay might have influenced the medical bill of the patient; however, this is beyond the scope of this chapter.

Healthcare access: the case of unequal opportunity to use insurance

The physical availability of health services is important for accessing healthcare. The low availability of facilities at one's doorstep puts serious limitations on access to healthcare. As reported in Chapter 7, there is a high concentration of empanelled hospitals across India's states, while it is lacking in many of the poor and remote area districts. This may have serious implications for access, as well as cost. In areas with high availability of

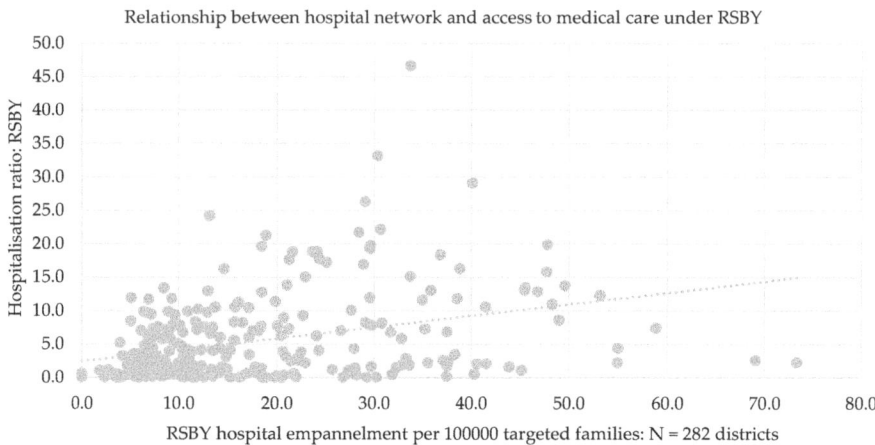

Figure 8.4 Hospital network and access to medical care under RSBY

Source: Government of India, https://www.rsby.gov.in

services, people will have more options to access healthcare and they have to travel less. In order to assess to what extent availability and concentration of hospital care impacts access to healthcare, results are reported using RSBY data from 282 districts and early experience of PMJAY scheme. RSBY data shows that access to hospital care (measured in terms of hospitalisation ratio) increases with the availability of empanelled hospitals in the districts (Figure 8.4). A further quantification of plotted dots in Figure 8.4, by classifying the districts in quintile using number of hospital per lakh targeted families, suggests that hospitalisation ratio was almost 9.3 times lower in districts where the number of healthcare providers (per targeted person) was low. The hospitalisation ratio was 1.27% in first-quintile-districts, while it is recorded 11.83% in fifth-quintile districts. The average size of empanelment of hospitals under RSBY in these districts was 3.39 and 50.99 hospitals per 100,000 targeted families, respectively.

It has already been reported in Chapter 7 that a high concentration of empanelled hospital in urban metropolitan areas, with facilities missing in the most remote rural areas, results in unequal access to healthcare. The GFHIs-based system so far has not been able to encourage and redirect private investment towards critical gap filling to meet the service demands of deficient areas.

The analysis from NSS 72nd Round on tourism (GOI, 2017a) shows that in the last 365, days nearly 4,87,92,883 people made overnight trips from their residences to seek healthcare and medical care (Hooda, 2020). Of these, over two-fifths had to travel outside either the district or state they reside in. In a majority of the states, a considerable number of patients had to

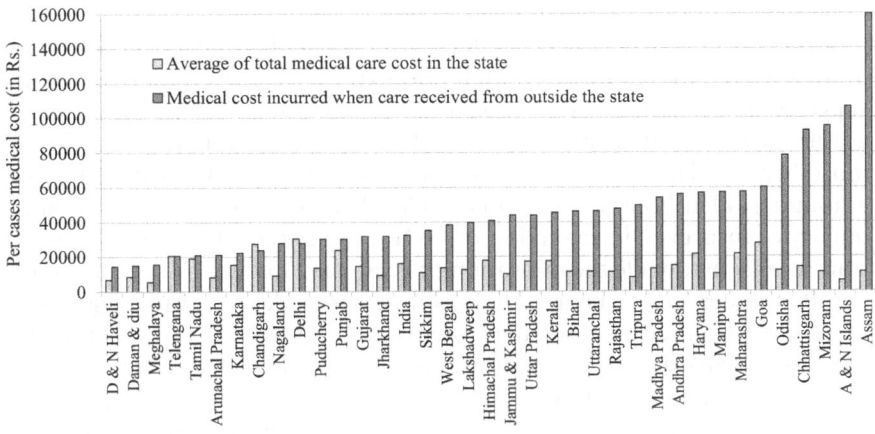

Figure 8.5 Medical care cost by location of service received
Source: GOI (2014)

travel outside to seek medical/hospitalisation care. This resulted in high costs. For instance, medical costs were around Rs. 22,403 and Rs. 15,938 when patients received service from outside the state and outside the district of the state, respectively, as against the Rs. 9766 when care is received from the district where they reside. Thus, moving out from state costs two times more. In some of the states, cost of care outside the state is 4–5 times higher as compared to the cost of care within the district. Mumbai, Delhi NCR, Chennai, Bangalore, Jaipur and some other metro cities, including Kolkata and Surat, have been centres of attraction for a large number of patients from neighbouring states. This is because of the high concentration of medical facilities in these cities. The estimates from health round data of NSS also reveals that cost of medical care increases manifold when care is received outside from a patient's own state. The cost of medical care outside the state was found to be almost 2–8 times higher than the average cost incurred in the home state. There is a considerable variation across states (Figure 8.5). The cost of care in Assam is 14 times higher when care received outside from the states.

Effectiveness of insurance-based systems

Experiences on the effectiveness of insurance-based systems in low- and middle-income countries are diverse and inconsistent (Erlangga et al., 2019). This study reported that out of the total 68 review studies, health insurance schemes in low- and middle-income countries are found to improve access to healthcare as measured by increased utilisation of healthcare facilities (32 of 40 studies), favourable effect on financial protection (26 of 46 studies) and moderate impact of health insurance in improving the health of the insured (nine of 12 studies). Several other remaining studies did not find significant impact of insurance on outcome indicators.

Several studies have been conducted to assess the impact of GFHIs on desired UHC targets in the Indian context, as well. An extensive review suggests that health service utilisation increased with the introduction of government-funded health insurance schemes (n = 7), along with a decline in mortality (n = 1), and a few have reported the decline in OOP expenditures among enrolled households, while 70% of the review studies showed no impact of insurance in reduction of OOP expenditure (Prinja et al., 2017). This reveals that while the utilisation of healthcare did improve among those enrolled under such schemes, there is no clear evidence yet to suggest that these have resulted in lowering down the OOP expenditure or financial risk due to healthcare payment. There is ample evidence which suggests that the existing public-funded health insurance schemes have largely been unsuccessful in reducing unit cost and OOP burden from households, and in protecting people falling below the poverty line (Bandyopadhyay and Sen, 2018; Ghosh and Gupta, 2017; Hooda, 2017; Karan et al., 2017; Sen and Gupta, 2017; Sood et al., 2014). While highlighting the relative importance of public provisioning systems over insurance-based systems, Hooda (2017) reported that public systems which deliver primary, secondary and tertiary care significantly help in reducing the overall OOP healthcare payments and catastrophic burden. Households are less likely to fall below the poverty line in districts where provision of the three-tier structure in the public healthcare system is high as compared to the districts where no or few facilities exist. However, insurance has the reverse effect.

The insurance-based system has attracted several criticisms historically, as this sector is highly characterised by intrinsic market failure with high degree of uncertainty associated to moral hazard and adverse selection (Arrow, 1963). Due to supplier-induced demand and information asymmetry between the principal and the agent, the patients, providers and insurers indulge in maximising their individual gains. In the healthcare market, insured patients have the incentive to indulge in excess demand; the providers, on the other hand, have a much bigger advantage over the patients, given the mystification of healthcare and the associated treatments. It may lead to increasing the level of inappropriate care, unwanted visits, unnecessary treatments, excessive laboratory tests or overcharging (GOI, 2011). Thus, the role of insurers in providing better health service access is highly questionable.

International experiences have shown difficulty in regulating the insurance-based system to keep costs down and ensure quality. It also does not mitigate inequitable access to health service in a fundamentally private healthcare–dominated delivery market. The US model of healthcare financing mechanism always cited has adopted an insurance-based financing model to deliver medical care. Robert H. Frank (2018) highlighted that the per capita health expenditures in the United States are more than twice the average of those in almost 35 advanced countries that make up the OECD. The high spending in the United States is largely due to the adoption of a market-oriented insurance-based financing model which has generated glaring inefficiencies, as well as high healthcare costs. The average cost of coronary bypass surgery is more than three times higher in the United States than in France, and a day in an American hospital costs 12 times as much as one in The Netherlands. The United States has more people in healthcare working as insurance administrators than as doctors which manifests in costs, and the United States still has not been able to regulate the market and control costs and prices (Frank, 2018).

Despite having huge financial implications, regulatory difficulties and ineffectiveness of the system, different political dispensations – as well as successive central governments and constitute states of India – have been experiencing sharp competition, especially in launching a scheme with enhanced insurance coverage and coverage limits. The sum assured amount gets enhanced over time from Rs. 30,000 to Rs. 5 lakh from nationally representative schemes RSBY to PMJAY. One predominant argument behind raising the coverage amount is that if the benefit packages and coverage amounts are less than adequate, several high-cost illnesses might leave families or individuals at risk of impoverishment. The merit in this argument whether high coverage amount had better achieve UHC targets has not been substantiated empirically.

We looked into this issue. Table 8.1 looks at the healthcare utilisation, an important indicator to assess the impact of GFHIs on access to healthcare, across rural-urban and socio-economic stratum households. The hospitalisation rate per 1,00,000 population found to be almost 26% higher among persons covered under GFHIs (around 6251 patients) as compared to persons not covered (4618 patients) under any insurance protection scheme. The poorest GFHI holders receive around 30.8% higher hospitalisation care than their poorest uninsured counterparts. The inured SC/STs, rural and urban residents, and the different employment category workers like the self-employed in agriculture and in non-agriculture, the regular wage workers, and the causal labour in agriculture and in non-agriculture, have access to high hospitalisation care as compared to the their uninsured counterparts. That is, the hospitalisation rates across poor-rich, rural-urban, STs-others, and the self-employed in agriculture-others are higher among those insured under GFHIs as compared to those who are not covered under any insurance protection measure.

The rate of hospitalisation in both low and high insurance coverage amount states is higher among the insured than the uninsured. The hospitalisation rate of insured persons living in high coverage amount states was found to be significantly higher, around 7089 patients, than the insured persons in states with low amounts of coverage, around 4993 patients per 100,000 population (Table 8.1). However, the hospitalisation rate in high insurance coverage states cannot directly attribute to the insurance coverage amount, because the hospitalisation rate of the

Table 8.1 Average rate of hospitalisation by level of insurance cover under GFHIs

	Low insurance coverage amount states			High insurance coverage amount states			At aggregate level – all states		
	Insured in GFHI	Uninsured	% diff.	Insured in GFHI	Uninsured	% diff.	Insured in GFHI	Uninsured	% diff.
Q1	5069	3426	32.4	6242	4987	20.1	5501	3805	30.8
Q2	3705	3560	3.9	6118	4941	19.2	4934	3945	20.0
Q3	4422	4084	7.6	5762	5408	6.1	5319	4561	14.3
Q4	6594	3968	39.8	6993	6764	3.3	6904	5012	27.4
Q5	7541	4956	34.3	11727	8070	31.2	10381	5990	42.3
Rural	4755	3860	18.8	6719	6205	7.6	5879	4477	23.9
Urban	6077	4281	29.6	8097	5801	28.4	7473	4965	33.6
STs	4040	3350	17.1	4738	4596	3.0	4293	3708	13.6
SCs	5831	4172	28.4	7762	6307	18.7	6950	4727	32.0
OBCs	4532	3723	17.9	7241	6224	14.0	6355	4599	27.6
Others	6357	4353	31.5	7069	5978	15.4	6793	4862	28.4
Self-emp. agricultural	4649	3869	16.8	6419	5790	9.8	5666	4434	21.7
Self-emp. non-agricultural	5485	4019	26.7	6923	5894	14.9	6400	4682	26.8
Regular wage/salary	4092	4302	-5.1	7773	6579	15.4	6655	5217	21.6
Casual labour, agricultural	4723	3611	23.5	7319	5449	25.6	6313	4262	32.5
Casual labour, non-agricultural	5108	3788	25.9	8007	5802	27.5	6590	4197	36.3
Others	7929	5052	36.3	7994	9117	-14.0	7965	6364	20.1
Total	**4993**	**3958**	**20.7**	**7089**	**6039**	**14.8**	**6251**	**4618**	**26.1**

Source: GOI (2014)

uninsured is also high in these states. The hospitalisation rate among the insured is significantly higher than that of uninsured in states with both low and high coverage amounts. The difference in hospitalisation rates is observed to be low (14.8%) in states with high coverage amounts. The rate is observed to be high (22%) in states with low coverage amounts. This indicates greater access to care in low coverage amount states than in high coverage amount states.

The package component is important to understand the impact of insurance, as under the GFHIs, a package of assured sums is provided. The insured persons are mostly treated under the package component. We have provided the analysis for first two income quintiles, as they are more likely to be covered under the insurance as mandated (Table 8.2). The analysis shows that the mean spending of insured patient (in GFHI/ RSBY) is significantly higher than uninsured at aggregate level and also in low insurance coverage amount states as well as in high insurance coverage amount states. The average medical spending on direct components is also noticed to be higher among the insured than the uninsured in low insurance coverage amount states as well as in high insurance coverage amount states. The indirect spending of the insured, however, is noticed to be lower than uninsured in both low and high insurance coverage amount states groups.

The prime objective of GFHIs is to provide free care. The households/ persons must not incur costs from their pocket, and the high amount of coverage must address this issue very effectively. The results from NSS 75th round data (2019) at aggregate level show that mean medical care spending among GFHIs holders (Rs. 24,170) found to be 8% higher than for uninsured patients (Rs. 22,353). When one looks at the mean medical OOP spending by insurance coverage amount, it gives an interesting result. No doubt, the mean medical spending in low and middle coverage limit states is higher among insured than the uninsured, with the difference in mean medical care spending between GFHIs holders and uninsured noticed to be very marginal. In the case of coverage amount of 2 lakh or higher, the mean spending of insured patients (Rs. 30,927) was around 45% greater than uninsured patients (Rs. 21,259) when care was received from private facility (Figure 8.6).

The public sector delivers services and care at low cost. The hospitalisation cost was noticed to be very low when an uninsured person received care from a public facility. The difference in hospitalisation cost for major morbidity among RSBY and non-RSBY holders was high on receiving service at a public hospital, while there is not much difference in cost when receiving service at a private facility (Figure 8.7), indicating that the private sector, rather than providing free care, promotes inflation and equalises the cost of care among insured and uninsured. The cost of care in the private sector is much high as compared to public sector.

244 *New financing and policy paradigms*

Table 8.2 Average medical care spending by insurance coverage amount under GFHIs

	For poorest (Q1)				For near poor (Q2)			
	Low insurance coverage amount states group		High insurance coverage amount states group		Low insurance coverage amount states group		High insurance coverage amount states group	
	GFHI/ RSBY	Uninsured	GFHI/ RSBY	Uninsured	GFHI/ RSBY	Uninsured	GFHI/ RSBY	Uninsured
Package components	8501	8365	22763	5807	13004	9278	19008	13165
Doctor fees	1151	1935	4495	3664	2330	2654	4013	4076
Medicines	2146	2958	3209	4336	2843	3364	4146	3807
Diagnostic tests	990	1349	1655	1624	1308	1400	2689	1599
Bed charges	751	1581	2090	2157	1353	1685	2758	2155
Other medical expenses	668	1175	1249	1257	1015	1548	1634	1267
Transportation for patients	536	553	420	448	559	561	503	521
Other non-medical expenses	918	950	1069	1056	1128	1073	1477	1103
Total medical expenditures, direct	6354	6095	9473	6034	8282	2031	12710	22395
Total expenditures, including indirect	6594	7970	8129	10513	8579	9769	11871	12484

Source: GOI (2014)

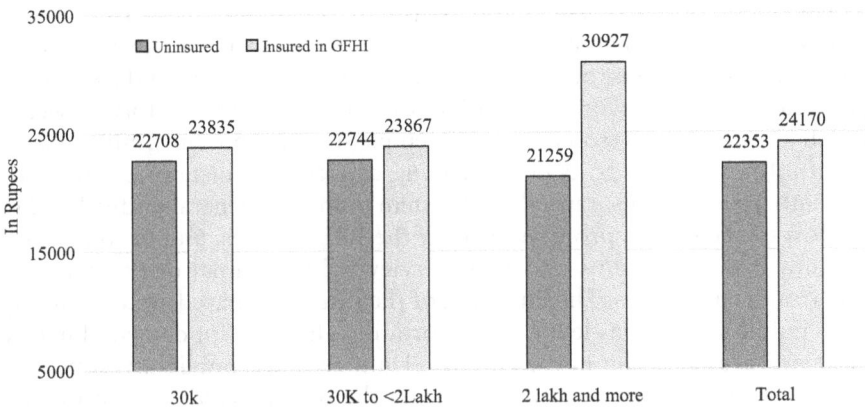

Figure 8.6 Comparing mean medical care spending in private facilities (per case)

Note and source: Estimated using unit-level records of 75th Health Round of NSS (GOI, 2019); reporting for 40% MPCE (monthly per capita consumption expenditure) households

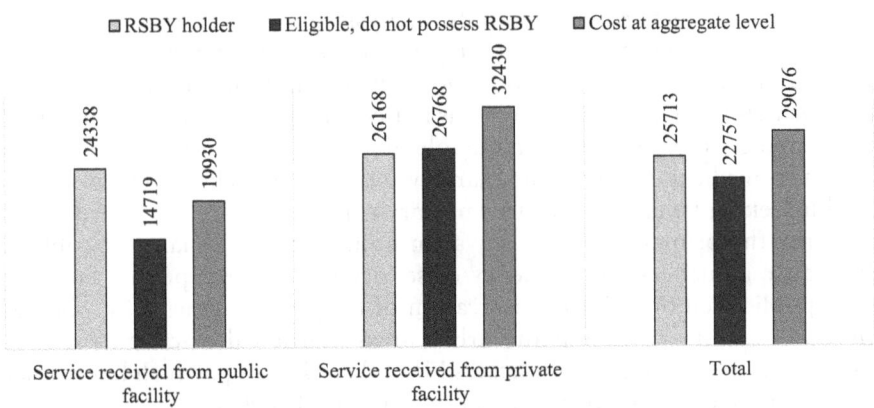

Figure 8.7 Per case net out-of-pocket spending on hospitalisation for major morbidity by insurance status and type of facility (in rupees)

Source: IHDS (2012)

Conclusion

Amongst the different risk-pooling mechanisms, it has increasingly been accepted internationally that health insurance coverage could enhance welfare of the society by providing an important safety net to low-income families by reducing the financial risk during health emergencies (Kasirajan, 2012), improve access to care and secure better health outcomes (Kenney et al., 2014) – but the resource-pooling mechanism in India is rather different from the funding nature of insurance-based models in other countries. The recently promoted insurance-based system in India is almost entirely funded from public (tax) sources. This is simply because the contribution from employers in India is expected to be almost negligible because of informal nature of the economy (around 93% of the workforce in India is employed in the informal sector, which leave little or no room to receive employer contributions), and a majority of informal workers have low paying capacity for insurance. Thus, the currently promoted insurance-based system in India is generally called GFHI.

Most of the GFHIs promise to cover the BPL families, and in some cases the informal community, under its purview with minimal or no contribution from beneficiaries. The financing of the insurance-based system entirely from public sources has led to an important shift in the fundamental nature of healthcare financing in the country. Until recently, public investment in healthcare was mostly used for financing the public health system for service provisioning; now, out of the total health budget, some (tax) funds will be diverted to finance the insurance-based system. That is, the currently promoted insurance-based system will also get financed in the same way as the public health sector. The difference lies in the fact that the provisioning would now be shifted almost entirely to the private sector.

About the effectiveness of GFHIs, analysis shows that access (in terms of utilisation) to hospital care among the insured is higher than that of the uninsured. The rate of utilisation among the insured rural-urban, rich-poor and formal-informal worker divides is noticed to be higher than among their uninsured counterparts, though the role of insurance in promoting equity in access to medical care remained largely insignificant. The GFHI promotes health-seeking behaviour towards tertiary care and tendency towards sidetracking the primary care. This system induces a moral hazard problem. Insurance influences the frequency of service use towards private facilities over public facilities. The concentration of hospitals in cities with populations of at least five million and urban areas of a few districts puts serious limitations on making services accessible at their doorstep, which has further resulted in unequal opportunity to use insurance benefits.

The prime objective of GFHIs is to provide financial protection against medical costs; that is, providing free medical care to the beneficiaries of the schemes. Unfortunately, after the implementation of pro-poor insurance schemes, per person monthly OOP of the poorest quintile households increased to a level of what the richest quintile spends on hospitalisation. The medical care spending of the insured recorded as higher than that of the uninsured. The increase in coverage amounts under different GFHIs have not made any significant difference in lowering the medical costs from the households or improved access.

Robust and comprehensive healthcare provisioning in the public system, however, significantly brings down the medical care costs and reduces overall health payment burdens from households. The estimates around the relative importance of tax-funded insurance and tax-funded public provisioning show that high provisioning of public facilities (namely sub-centres, primary health centres, community health centres, sub-divisional hospitals, civil/district hospitals and health personals which provide primary, secondary and tertiary care) in a district or area significantly brings down the overall health payment burden on individual pockets (Hooda, 2017). The public system is even more effective in bringing down the OOP burden when there is no insurance. After the rolling out of the insurance scheme, the health payment burden on households has only increased. High public provisioning also reduces the catastrophic health payment burden. The unit cost of hospitalisation of uninsured persons for major morbidities can be lowered in the public system, but not in the private setting. Rather than reducing the unit costs, insurance has increased the unit costs when services are received both at public and private facilities. Currently, India's healthcare system suffers from a fund crunch and an under-staffing problem, even though it has performed well in terms of ensuring high institutional child delivery and other maternal and child healthcare in the recent past, as reflected in pervious chapters.

Provider networks are essential for getting access to services through insurance, and also to check high cost of care. The National Health Policy (GOI, 2017b) floated the idea of strategic purchasing of health services promoted through a government-funded health insurance scheme. The intention of promoting strategic purchasing is to ensure access to affordable and quality secondary and tertiary care services from private providers in healthcare services deficit areas. It has been pointed out that strategic purchasing would play a stewardship role in directing private investment towards those areas and services for which currently there are no or few providers. The information available on private hospitals and facilities indicates the concentration of hospitals in urban metropolitan areas. Past experience shows that insurance so far does little to encourage and redirect private investment towards critical gap filling. This has wide implications for access to hospital care in vast areas where there are no or few providers. With the strengthening of the insurance-based model for financing care which provides paying capacity to the population, the medical industry may bust. However, one cannot negate the probability of high growth of large corporate hospitals in a few metro cities which may further generate monopoly in the country's medical market, as has happened in the United States, where a concentration of 5–7 big corporate hospitals caters to more than three-fourths of the medical care demand and has an inflationary impact on the medical sector.

References

Ahuja. 2004. *Health Insurance for the Poor in India*. ICRIER, WP No, 123. https://icrier.org/pdf/wp123.pdf

Arrow, K. J. 1963, December. Uncertainty and the Welfare Economics of Medical Care. *The American Economic Review*, Vol. 53, No. 5. www.elsevier.com/books/uncertainty-in-economics/diamond/978-0-12-214850-7

Bandyopadhyay, S., and Sen, K. 2018. Challenges of Rasthryia Swasthya Bima Yojana (RSBY) in West Bengal, India: An Exploratory Study. *The International Journal of Health Planning and Management*, Vol. 33, No. 2.

Barnes, A. J., Karpman, M., Long, S., Hanoch, Y., and Rice, T. 2017. More Intelligent Designs: Comparing the Effectiveness of Choice Architectures Used in Us Health Insurance Marketplaces. *Organizational Behavior and Human Decision Processes*, Vol. 163, pp. 142–164. https://doi.org/10.1016/j.obhdp.2019.02.002

Erlangga, D., Suhrcke, M., Bloor, K., and Ali, S. 2019. The Impact of Public Health Insurance on Health Care Utilisation, Financial Protection and Health Status in Low- and Middle-income Countries: A Systematic Review. *PLoS ONE*, Vol. 14, No. 8, p. e0219731. https://doi.org/10.1371/journal.pone.0219731

Forgia, G. M., and Nagpal, S. 2012. *Government-Sponsored Health Insurance in India: Are You Covered?* The World Bank, Washington, DC.

Frank, Robert H. 2018. Back to the Health Policy Drawing Board. *The New York Times*, March 16. https://www.nytimes.com/2018/03/16/business/back-to-the-health-policy-drawing-board.html; also see https://www.nytimes.com/2017/03/24/upshot/health-insurance-medicare-obamacare-american-health-care-act.html?rref=collection%2Fsectioncollection%2Fupshot&action=click&contentCollection=upshot&mtrref=undefined and https://www.fdlreporter.com/story/opinion/readers/2018/04/06/letter-u-s-has-failed-providing-healthcare-citizens/479404002/

Franks, P., and Fiscella, K. 1998. Primary Care Physicians and Specialists as Personal Physicians: Health Care Expenditures and Mortality Experience. *The Journal of Family Practice*, Vol. 47, No. 2, pp. 105–109.

Ghosh, S., and Gupta, N. D. 2017. Targeting and Effects of Rashtriya Swasthya Bima Yojana on Access to Care and Financial Protection. *Economic and Political Weekly*, Vol. 52, No. 4, pp. 61–70.

Government of India. 2011. *A Critical Assessment of the Existing Health Insurance Models in India*. Public Health Foundation of India Report submitted to Planning Commission of India, Government of India. http://planningcommission.nic.in/reports/sereport/ser/ser_heal1305.pdf

Government of India. 2014. *Social Consumption: Health – Unit Level Records*, National Sample Survey, 71st Round, Ministry of Statistics and Programme Implementation, Government of India.

Government of India. 2017a. *India – Domestic Tourism Expenditure*, NSS 72nd Round, Schedule 21.1, July 2014 – June 2015, Ministry of Statistics and Programme Implementation, Government of India.

Government of India. 2017b. *National Health Policy 2017*. Ministry of Health and Family Welfare, Government of India. https://mohfw.gov.in/sites/default/files/9147562941489753121.pdf

Government of India. 2018. *National Health Accounts (NHA, 2018) – Estimates for India 2015–16, National Health Systems Resource Centre (NHSRC)*. Ministry of Health and Family Welfare, Government of India. http://nhsrcindia.org/sites/default/files/NHA%20Estimates%20Report%20-%20November%202018.pdf

Government of India. 2019. *Social Consumption in India: Health – Unit Level Records*, National Sample Survey, 75th Round, Ministry of Statistics and Programme Implementation, Government of India.

Government of India. undated. *RSBY Webportal*. www.rsby.gov.in

Hooda, S. K. 2017, April 16–22. Health Payments and Household Well-being: How Effective Are Health Policy Interventions? *Economic and Political Weekly*, Vol. 52, No. 16, pp. 54–65.

Hooda, S. K. 2019. *Promoting Access to Healthcare in India: Role of Health Insurance and Hospital Network*. ISID Working Paper No. 215.

Hooda, S. K. 2020. Penetration and Coverage of Government-funded Health Insurance Schemes in India. *Clinical Epidemiology and Global Health*, No. 8, pp. 1017–1033.

IHDS-India Human Development Survey. 2012. *Unit Level Record of India Human Development Survey 2012*. NCAER. https://ihds.umd.edu/

IRDA. 2019. *Annual Report 2018–19*, Insurance Regulatory and Development Authority of India, Hyderabad, India.

Karan, A., Yip, W., and Mahal, A. 2017. Extending Health Insurance to the Poor in India: An Impact Evaluation of Rashtriya Swasthya Bima Yojana on Out of Pocket Spending for Healthcare. *Social Science and Medicine*, Vol. 181, pp. 83–92.

Kasirajan, G. 2012. Health Insurance – An Empirical Study of Consumer Behavior in Tuticorin District. *Indian Streams Research Journal*, Vol. 2, No. 3, pp. 1–4.

Kenney, G. M., Anderson, N., Long, S. K., et al. 2014. *Taking Stock: Health Insurance Coverage for Parents under the ACA in 2014. 9 September*. Urban Institute Health Policy Center. http://datatools.urban.org/features/hrmstest/102214/briefs/Health-Insurance-Coverage-for-Parents-under-the-ACA-in-2014.

Kruk, M. E., et al. 2010. The Contribution of Primary Care to Health and Health Systems in Low-and Middle-income Countries: A Critical Review of Major Primary Care Initiatives. *Social Science & Medicine*, Vol. 70, No. 6, pp. 904–911.

NFHS. 2016. *National Family Health Survey (NFHS-4) 2015–16*. International Institute for Population Sciences (IIPS), Mumbai, India and International Classification of Functioning, Disability and Health (ICF).

NHA. 2018. *National Health Accounts: Estimates for India 2015-16*. National Health Accounts Technical Secretariat (NHATS), National Health Systems Resource Centre (NHSRC), Ministry of Health and Family Welfare (MoHFW), Government of India, New Delhi.

NSS. 2019. Social Consumption: Health-Unit Level Records, National Sample Survey (NSS), 75th Round 2017-18, Ministry of Statistics and Programme Implementation. Government of India, New Delhi.

Prinja, S., et al. 2017. Impact of Publicly Financed Health Insurance Schemes on Healthcare Utilisation and Financial Risk Protection in India: A Systematic Review. *PLoS ONE*, Vol. 12, No. 2.

Rao, S. 2004. Health Insurance: Concepts, Issues and Challenges. *Economic & Political Weekly*, Vol. 39, No. 34, pp. 3835–3844.

Sen, K., and Gupta, S. 2017. Masking Poverty and Entitlement: RSBY in Selected Districts of West Bengal. *Social Change*, Vol. 47, No. 3, pp. 339–358.

Sood, N., et al. 2014. Government Health Insurance for People Below Poverty Line in India: Quasi-experimental Evaluation of Insurance and Health Outcomes. *British Medical Journal*, Vol. 349.

Starfield, B., Shi, L., and Macinko, J. 2005. Contribution of Primary Care to Health Systems and Health. *Milbank Quarterly*, Vol. 83, No. 3, pp. 457–502.

WHO. 2013. *World Health Report 2013: Research for Universal Health Coverage*. World Health Organisation, Luxembourg. https://www.who.int/publications/i/item/9789240690837

Index

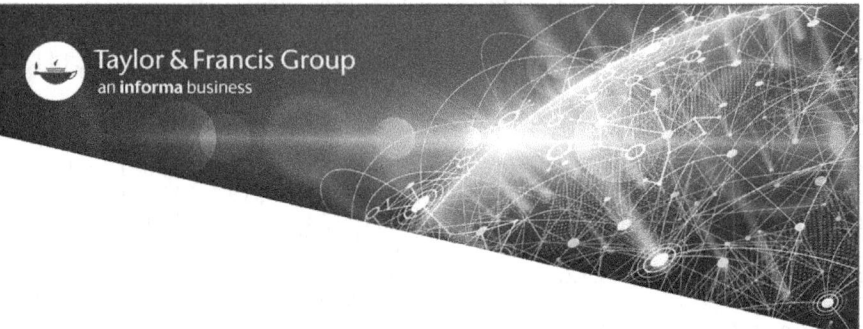
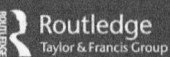
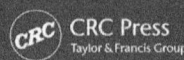